Praise for Ocean Robbins and
31-DAY FOOD REVOLUTION

"I've been watching the work that Ocean Robbins and his father, John, have been doing with Food Revolution Network for many years now, and I'm proud of what they've accomplished. The more people who hear this message and move toward diets marked by compassion and respect for life and the earth, the better off our world will be. The book that you hold in your hands is lighting the way for the future of your health and that of the planet."
—Paul McCartney

"With his passionate, playful, and persuasive style, Food Revolution leader and inspiration to millions, Ocean Robbins, shows you how to make healthy eating simple and irresistible."
—Kris Carr, *New York Times* bestselling author

"Ocean's genius four-step plan will help you build a better relationship with your food, your loved ones, and your community. Let him show you how to discover and practice everlasting habits that lead to a healthy and vibrant future. Your body will thank you for the rest of your life."
—Vani Hari, *New York Times* bestselling
author of *The Food Babe Way*

"Ocean Robbins advocates tirelessly for dietary practices that foster the health of people, protect the health of the planet, and respect the well-being of all other creatures. This compilation of his gentle, wise, and well-informed counsel is a wonderful asset for anyone wanting to eat well, be well, and do good."
—David Katz, MD, founding director, Yale-Griffin Prevention
Research Center; and immediate past-president,
American College of Lifestyle Medicine

"Ocean Robbins will show you how to put an end to procrastination and start getting the results you want. His straightforward, no-nonsense approach provides a brilliant pathway to a healthier life. And his book is a pleasure to read, too!"

—JJ Virgin, *New York Times* bestselling author and host of *The JJ Virgin Lifestyle Show*

"More than ever before, food is a hot topic in terms of our health, our politics, and even our spirituality. Ocean Robbins continues a family tradition of uplifting both our intellectual and moral understanding of the importance of our food choices, and how to make changes in our eating that better both ourselves and our world."

—Marianne Williamson, #1 *New York Times* bestselling author

"Ocean's new book has a depth, spirit, and breadth of information that makes it a must-read for anyone looking to up their game with the power of strong food. 31-DAY FOOD REVOLUTION shows how easy and delicious it can be for you to step into greater health for you and for your planet."

—Rip Esselstyn, firefighter, triathlete, and *New York Times* bestselling author of *The Engine 2 Diet*

"I learned so much that was new to me! This impeccably researched book made me realize that the food choices I make on a daily basis are BY FAR my biggest leverage point in making the world a better place. Ocean Robbins is probably the wisest, most brilliant, most visionary thinker I know."

—Susan Peirce Thompson, PhD, *New York Times* bestselling author of *Bright Line Eating* and founder, Institute for Sustainable Weight Loss

"31-DAY FOOD REVOLUTION provides a simple road map to a better future for you and for the planet. Combining the latest in nutritional science with practical implementation breakthroughs, Robbins will show you how easy it can be to lose weight, banish fatigue and brain fog, prevent diseases like heart disease, type 2 diabetes, and dementia, and contribute to a healthier world for you and all future generations."
—John Mackey, cofounder and co-CEO, Whole Foods Market, and author of *The Whole Foods Diet*

"Ocean Robbins is able to inform and influence people in a way that grips their interest and also touches their soul. His insight, warmth, and care for humanity are compelling and support the important scientific facts presented that are crucial for our world."
—Joel Fuhrman, MD, *New York Times* bestselling author and president, Nutritional Research Foundation

"In this accessible and timely book, Ocean Robbins provides the knowledge and guidance to help each of us become a creator of a new food future. One that protects our health and that of our families, revitalizes our farm communities, stops the suffering of countless animals, and affirms that healthy food will lead to a healthy planet. Get this critical road map for yourself, and share it with everyone you know. It opens a path to freedom from the toxic industrial food model—and a grounded hope that will empower you for life."
—Andrew Kimbrell, executive director, Center for Food Safety

"Ocean Robbins understands that we are smart, capable, and powerful beings who want what's best for our families and our planet. In 31-DAY FOOD REVOLUTION, he combines the light-giving, life-giving elements of food with a secret-telling and shadow-revealing exposé of the industry. When we know the truth, we can make informed choices and take action. Ocean is a wise being and we need him now. Lucky us that he has shared that wisdom in 31- DAY FOOD REVOLUTION."
—Geneen Roth, #1 *New York Times* bestselling author of *Women Food and God* and *When Food is Love*

31-DAY
FOOD
REVOLUTION

31-DAY FOOD REVOLUTION

Heal Your Body, Feel Great and Transform Your World

OCEAN ROBBINS

FOREWORD BY JOEL FUHRMAN, MD

Published in the United States by:
Grand Central Publishing, Hachette Book Group, 1290 Avenue of the Americas,
New York, NY 10104; grandcentrallifeandstyle.com

Published in the United Kingdom by:
Hay House UK Ltd, Astley House, 33 Notting Hill Gate, London W11 3JQ
Tel: +44 (0)20 3675 2450; Fax: +44 (0)20 3675 2451; www.hayhouse.co.uk

Published in Australia by:
Hay House Australia Ltd, 18/36 Ralph St, Alexandria NSW 2015
Tel: (61) 2 9669 4299; Fax: (61) 2 9669 4144; www.hayhouse.com.au

Published in India by:
Hay House Publishers India, Muskaan Complex, Plot No.3, B-2,
Vasant Kunj, New Delhi 110 070
Tel: (91) 11 4176 1620; Fax: (91) 11 4176 1630; www.hayhouse.co.in

A catalogue record for this book is available from the British Library.

Tradepaper ISBN: 978-1-78817-200-4
Ebook ISBN: 978-1-78817-238-7

Printed and bound by CPI Group (UK) Ltd, Croydon CR0 4YY

This book is dedicated to a world with healthy, ethical, and sustainable food for everyone who eats.

Author's Note

Trees for the Future

For every new copy of *31-Day Food Revolution* sold, Ocean Robbins is making a donation to Trees for the Future, enabling the organization to plant another organic fruit or nut tree in a low-income community.

Contents

Foreword

When I found out that Ocean Robbins was writing a book, I was thrilled, because his is a voice that is deeply needed in our times. You can trust what Ocean says. He's a renowned food movement leader who has devoted his life to being useful to others and to our fragile, troubled world.

We are faced with a food crisis whose tentacles penetrate deep into all aspects of society. This not only affects our own health; it also may intensify the damages for future generations. The decisions we make today may in fact dictate the survival of humans over the next hundred years. It is imperative that all of us be aware of the accumulating evidence and take action.

Many people know that heart disease, stroke, dementia, and cancer are predominantly the results of poor dietary choices. But most people are still unaware of the link between processed foods and lowered intelligence[1] and mental illness.[2] They also may not realize that highly processed food supplies the majority of calories in the modern industrialized diet, fueling food addictions and emotional overeating that can make it difficult to stop self-destructive eating habits. You may be shocked to learn that fast-food addiction and the consumption of junk food increase the risk of drug addiction and even crime.[3] Poor dietary habits also induce changes to our DNA that, when passed on to our children, increase the risk of autism, learning disabilities, birth defects, and even childhood cancers.[4] It is imperative to become informed with this knowledge so that you can protect yourself and your loved ones from needless tragedy.

Calorie-dense processed foods increase your risk of cancer, regardless of your body weight. Several cancers are considered weight-related—meaning that extra fat on the body increases their risk. These include colorectal, pancreatic, endometrial, ovarian, liver, kidney, gallbladder, and postmenopausal breast cancers.[5] But recently, researchers studying obesity-related cancers made an unexpected finding: an increase in risk of these cancers among women who were not overweight but consumed nutritionally barren, high-calorie foods.[6] Even if you're not obese, junk food is still damaging to your health. This was confirmed in a 15-year study of more than 92,000 postmenopausal women in the Women's Health Initiative.

Even moderate consumption of fast food or commercial baked goods doubles the risk of developing depression,[7] and just one serving of french fries per week has been demonstrated to increase risk of breast cancer by 27 percent.[8] In the long run, highly processed "Frankenfoods" can be lethal. Fast food today is like the asbestos of 20 years ago: a widely used silent killer.

Following a diet that is high in nutrients yet moderately low in calories is the secret to a long life free of medical suffering. This is the origin of my health equation $H = N/C$ (Health = Nutrients/Calories). A high ratio of micronutrients to calories forms the basis of a healthful diet.

What magnifies the risks associated with consuming unhealthy foods is medical care—and the widespread belief that taking drugs for high blood pressure, high cholesterol, and high blood sugars is the best way to address our dietary foolishness. Not only is medical care the third leading cause of death in the United States,[9] but medications make it seem as if people are safe because they have lower numbers on certain measurements and tests. These results allow people to rationalize (and continue) self-destructive eating behavior. Even worse, these unearned "positive" results also weaken motivation to change eating habits and thus to improve health. If we never had any medications at all, perhaps health professionals would be relentless and effective at inducing lifesaving dietary modification in their patients. Nutritional excellence is at least 100 times more effective than drugs for most chronic medical conditions, and it is the only way to achieve dramatic protection from heart disease, strokes, dementia, and even cancer.

When you follow the path laid out in this book and eat a diet with a high level and rich diversity of micronutrients and phytochemicals, you don't just age more slowly, you also boost your body's ability to protect against chronic illness. You'll add more health to your body, and more vibrancy to your life.

Ocean Robbins' *31-Day Food Revolution* will help you accomplish these goals. His knowledge, judgment, motivational skills, and compassion are all on display in a terrific book that can move you into a better life and help you to create a better world.

Ocean will show you how you can leverage the power of foods to heal your gut, lose excess weight, and dramatically lower your risk of disease. In this book you'll find heartwarming stories, solid science, and grounded inspiration to help you understand the true impact of your choices and to put these critical insights into action for your health and well-being.

We need a Food Revolution. I hope you will be part of it, for yourself, for our children, and for all of us.

Joel Fuhrman, MD
President, Nutritional Research Foundation
Author of Fast Food Genocide *and*
six other New York Times *bestsellers*

INTRODUCTION

Let's call it like it is. We live in a toxic food culture.

It's led us to epidemic rates of obesity, heart disease, cancer, type 2 diabetes, and Alzheimer's. Things have gotten so bad that most people think it's normal to have at least a few extra pounds around the middle, to depend on an ever-growing supply of prescription medications, and to lose a little more memory and mobility with every passing year.

This may be typical, but it sure as heck doesn't have to be normal.

Eating food is mandatory, but suffering from brain fog, living with ever-declining health, and feeling like crap are not. The fact is that right now, hundreds of millions of people are hurting from diseases that never, ever needed to happen in the first place.

Dangerous changes have been made to our food supply in just the last 25 years that impact how your food is grown and processed—and how safe it is to eat. The status quo is driving small farmers out of business, forcing animals to live in deplorable conditions, and producing food that's making us sick.

The medical industry and the processed food industry are earning trillions of dollars in a system that's devastating lives and threatening the very future of life on our planet.

It's my mission to help put an end to this madness, by sharing the truth about food and helping eaters put it into action. This is why I founded the 500,000+ member Food Revolution Network. And it's why I wrote the book you now hold in your hands.

In some ways, I might seem like a pretty unlikely food revolution-ary. After all, in 1953 my grandfather, Irvine Robbins, joined with his brother-in-law, Burt Baskin, to found the 31 flavors ice cream company—Baskin-Robbins.

In case anyone on the planet missed the memo, we're now pretty clear that ice cream is not a health food. But back in the 1950s, as my grandpa was pumping out delicious flavors by the dozen, not much was known about the connection between food and health. Up until then, most people seemed content with three flavors: vanilla, chocolate, and strawberry. My grandfather was a consummate entrepreneur, and he set his heart on offering consumers many more options—31, to be exact—one for each day of the month.

My dad, John, grew up with an ice-cream-cone-shaped swimming pool. Sometimes he even ate ice cream for breakfast. He was groomed from early childhood to one day run the family company. My dad's youthful innovations included Jamoca Almond Fudge (one of the company's most iconic flavors to this day) and the rollout to all the stores of the famous pink spoons that enabled customers to enjoy free samples.

But in 1967, my grandpa's brother-in-law and business partner, Burt Baskin, became very ill. His doctors informed him that he was dying of heart disease. I never knew my great-uncle Burt because he passed on a short time later, six years before I was born. But I do know that he was one of the greatest entrepreneurs in American history. He had tremendous wealth, a business he enjoyed, and a family he loved. He ate a lot of ice cream. And in the end, he lost his health and his life at the age of 54.

Grandpa Irv was faced with a choice: He could sell the company for a large sum of money, or he could keep the company in the family and take on my dad, then about to turn 20, as his business partner.

Grandpa Irv chose to invite his son aboard. But my dad declined his father's invitation, walking away from Baskin-Robbins and from any access to or dependence on the family wealth. For him, it was a choice for integrity, and it's a choice I've always respected.

My dad had seen ice cream bring smiles to a lot of people. But he also knew that unhealthy foods could fuel devastating consequences, and he didn't want to spend his life selling a product that might contribute to more people suffering and dying before their time. So he left a path that was practically paved with gold—and ice cream—to follow his own "rocky road."

My dad had suffered from polio as a child and grew up frequently fatigued and ill. In the 1960s, he fell in love with my mom in Berkeley and the two of them set out on a healthy living path. They stopped eating processed foods. They gave up ice cream. And they based their diet on vegetables and whole, natural foods.

As my dad's health and energy returned, he and my mom moved to a remote little island off the coast of British Columbia, Canada, where they built a one-room log cabin, grew most of their own food, practiced yoga and meditation for several hours a day, and named their kid Ocean.

They say that they almost named me Kale. I'm glad they took the more conservative route on this one.

In any case, we did eat a lot of kale—along with cabbage, carrots, onions, broccoli, turnips, Swiss chard, and many other vegetables that my parents grew, plus brown rice, sprouts, buckwheat, and beans. For a treat, once in a blue moon, we'd have a few drops of organic blackstrap molasses. I think we went through about a bottle a year.

Though my childhood diet was spartan and my family lived on very little money, I grew up feeling rich in health. I became an accomplished distance runner, completing my first marathon at the age of 10.

My dad went on to study the impact of food choices and to share what he was learning. His landmark bestsellers, including *Diet for a New America*, inspired millions of people and helped to galvanize the modern health food movement. The media was tickled by the notion of a would-be ice cream heir becoming a healthy-eating spokesperson and called him the "rebel without a cone," and "the prophet of non-profit."

Tens of thousands of people wrote my dad letters, often by hand, sharing how his work had changed—sometimes even saved—their lives. One of the lives his work impacted, as fate would have it, was that of my own Grandpa Irv.

Now my grandpa had been pretty mad when my dad walked away from the ice cream company. He and my dad went years without speaking. But then something remarkable happened.

In 1989 Grandpa Irv, then in his early seventies, was suffering from diabetes, heart disease, and weight problems. He'd always eaten the modern diet, with a double scoop of ice cream on top. His cardiologist told him that he didn't have long to live—unless he changed his diet. And then the good doctor handed him a copy of my dad's book, *Diet for a New America*. If my grandpa's cardiologist knew that the book was written by his patient's maverick son, he didn't let on. He simply gave Grandpa Irv the book and recommended following its advice. And Grandpa Irv didn't bother to tell his doctor that he knew the author.

Remarkably enough, my grandpa started eating fewer processed foods and less meat. He gave up sugar and, amazingly, he even gave up ice cream. He started eating a lot more veggies, fruits, and whole foods.

And he got results.

Before long, Grandpa Irv lost 30 pounds. He ditched all of his diabetes and blood-pressure medications. He was enjoying more energy than he'd had in decades. He bragged that his golf game had improved by seven strokes. He took morning walks with his dog, and soon he was traversing several miles each day. Despite the grim prognosis, he ended up living 19 more healthy years.

One morning, while we were visiting my grandparents at their home in Rancho Mirage, California, my grandpa went out for his usual walk. My dad and I were training for a marathon, and Grandpa Irv cheered for us as we cruised by. I'll always remember that morning as a vivid illustration of the power of food choices to fuel a healthy life—in every generation.

At the age of 16, inspired by my family's experiences and the legacy of leadership modeled by the two generations before me, I founded a nonprofit organization called Youth for Environmental Sanity (YES!). Our goal was to mobilize young people to say yes to choices that support healthy lives and a healthy planet.

Over the next 20 years I raised money, built an international organization, and led workshops and training programs for hundreds of thousands of grassroots activists from more than 65 nations.

As I traveled the globe, I had the privilege of being invited into the hearts and homes of people from many walks of life. I dined on hummus with Bedouins in the Middle Eastern desert; on quinoa with indigenous leaders in Peru; on black rice with villagers in Thailand; on potatoes and sweet corn with white farmers in Indiana; and on collards and black-eyed peas with African Americans in rural Alabama.

Everywhere I went, I was connecting and collaborating with leaders and change-makers. And everywhere, food was a force that brought us together. I met people all over the planet who were up to something good, often in extremely challenging circumstances. Their stories have humbled and shaped me, and they've galvanized my deep commitment to healthy food for all.

One of the things that most bothers me about the natural foods phenomenon is how elitist it can be. Most people are struggling just to survive. They don't have time or money to worry about which brand of MCT oil is best to add to their coffee, or which type of heirloom tomato contains the most lycopene. If they can get enough calories to feed their kids, then that's a freaking miracle.

Perhaps you can relate.

The thing is, it doesn't have to be this way. There's nothing about processing Mother Nature's bounty in a factory, stripping it of its fiber, vitamins, and minerals, wrapping it in a bunch of plastic, shipping it thousands of miles, and spending millions of dollars advertising it on television that inherently makes it cheaper than real, local, natural food. But we have governments and food policies that effectively subsidize the mass production of junk food, which artificially drives down its price.

In the developed world, there's a huge correlation not just between poverty and hunger, but also between poverty and obesity. As counterintuitive as it may seem, the less money you have, the more likely you are to struggle with your weight. Step into any big-city 7-Eleven and you'll see how many people feel dependent on products like Doritos and Coke. The brutal reality is that poverty typically makes it difficult to feed your family at all—and harder still to provide real, healthy food. Statistically, the poorer you are, the more likely you are to die of diet-fueled diseases like cancer, heart disease, Alzheimer's, and type 2 diabetes.

The people who can least afford to get sick are also the most likely to live and die with chronic illness. That's not the way I want it to be.

I don't think there's anything elitist about choosing real food, or about supporting family farmers who treat their land, animals, and workers right. What's elitist is a perverse system of subsidies (more on this in chapter 30) that makes crops grown with poisons and processed into junk food the cheapest to buy, in effect condemning the poor to diets that are nutritional disasters.

Working with people who are struggling, often against enormous odds, to live and to raise their families in a good way has inspired me, and it's also lit a fire in me. Food is more than a path to health. It's also a way to build a healthy world. It's personal. It's political. And it links us to people, policies, and practices around the globe.

I've learned so much from people for whom hunger and malnutrition aren't statistics on a UNICEF chart—they're a daily reality. Some of these people have lived through wars or have lost family to senseless violence, and are to this day grateful if they have anything to put in their bellies. These same people have built local, resilient economies that work to alleviate poverty and support health, from the ground up.

I've been blessed to learn from Tashka Yawanawá, chief of the Yawanawá tribe in the Brazilian Amazon rain forest, who shared with me the devastating impact that global meat consumption has on his people's home, as cattle ranchers burn the forest so Europeans and North Americans can buy cheap burgers at fast-food restaurants. I joined Tashka to raise money so the Yawanawá could buy airplanes to monitor their forest home for signs of illegal mining and cattle ranching—thus helping to save the tropical rain forests.

I've had the privilege of joining with community organizers in Detroit, Michigan, where the median home price in 2017 was $30,000 and where there are thousands of vacant lots and far too many financially destitute people. In 2009, the unemployment rate was as high as 28 percent.[1] A Yale University study found that in 2010 more than half of Detroit residents lived in areas with severely limited access to healthy food, and this made them "more likely to suffer or die prematurely from a diet-related disease."[2] And yet in the midst of this intense poverty—in spite of, or perhaps in some ways because of, the terrible food and health challenges Detroit faced—community leaders began to plant seeds of hope. By 2015, Detroit had become a world leader in the community garden movement, with more than 1,400 urban farms and gardens that now bring nourishment to food deserts and are helping to repair the city's ruptured fabric.[3]

As I neared the age of 40, I came to a crossroads. As much as I loved the work I was doing to support and empower grassroots organizers, I felt called to a bigger vision. The global food system is still churning out products laced with chemicals, pesticides, hormones, antibiotics, and other substances that don't belong in the human body. All over the world, Alzheimer's is crippling our elders, while attention-deficit/hyperactivity disorder (ADHD), diabetes, and obesity are devastating our kids. It's our children, our elderly, and our poor who are paying the heaviest price for a brutally toxic food system.

In many countries, including the United States, life expectancy is actually decreasing. Animals are still living in abject misery on factory farms. And industrialized agriculture is fueling desertification, drought, climate destabilization, and deforestation that seriously threaten the ability of coming generations to feed themselves.

In 2012, I decided I could make the greatest impact by joining my dad (and now colleague) in launching an online education and advocacy organization called Food Revolution Network. Since then I've had the privilege of working closely with some of the top food experts on the planet. (Some of them have contributed recipes for this book.)

Perhaps most importantly, I've had the opportunity to work with, learn from, and support a community of more than a million people from over 180 nations who have participated in our online Food Revolution Summits.

Time and time again, I hear from people who are fed up with toxic food, sick of feeling sick, and disillusioned with the status quo. What frustrates so many people is that they don't really know if there are solutions—and if there are, how to apply them to create lasting change.

Does this sound familiar? Chances are you know there's a lot of unhealthy food in the world, and you try to stay away from it. But in a junk-food–fueled society, it can feel as if you're being constantly pulled in the wrong direction. Family, habit, social pressure, price, confusion, and stress conspire to make healthy eating more difficult than it should be.

I wrote this book because I want to change all that for you. And I want to ask for your partnership in going a step further.

If you want healthy food not just for yourself but also for your loved ones and for your world, then I have a challenge, and an offer.

My challenge is this. Starting today, and for at least the next 31 days, I invite you to consider yourself a participant in the Food Revolution and to join me in taking a stand for healthy, ethical, sustainable food for everyone (including you!).

And my offer is simple. With this book, I'll show how it can be easier, more joyful, and more delicious than you imagined. I'll show how you can eat to prevent (and maybe even reverse) cancer, type 2 diabetes, heart disease, dementia, obesity, and other chronic ailments. I'll show how you can bring friends and loved ones together to create the support you need to thrive, and so the people you care about will benefit from what you're discovering. And I'll show how you can participate, in a meaningful way, in contributing to a world that we can be proud to pass on to our grandkids.

I'm interested in solutions that actually work, in the real world. I lost interest long ago in ivory tower theories that work only for the privileged few. Too many lives are at stake.

I'm a husband who knows what it's like to try to put good food on the table while my spouse and I are both working 60 hours a week. And despite the wealth of my grandparents, I didn't grow up rich.

I'm also a father of special-needs twins who, for reasons modern medicine can't explain, were born exceedingly prematurely. Today they're doing surprisingly well, but I don't know if they will ever live independently, and they require significant ongoing support. Even more than most teenagers, they hate being told what to do (and what to eat!). If these solutions can work for me and for our family, then they might work for you and yours, too.

HOW TO USE THIS BOOK

Here's how this is going to work. For the next 31 days, I invite you to join me in the Food Revolution.

In Part One, I'll help you **Detoxify** your life and set yourself up with the systems and the environment you need to succeed. We all know that health is priceless. Just ask anyone who doesn't have it. That's why the first order of business is your own wellness. I'll walk you through creating the conditions to leverage food as the true foundation for a healthy life.

In Part Two, **Nourish**, we'll dispel confusion and get you affordably and deliciously enjoying the foods that your brain, heart, cells, and muscles need to thrive. You'll find out how to enjoy warm breakfast porridges, creamy smoothies, hearty sandwiches, comforting casseroles, spicy stir-fries and curries, and other fabulous foods as good for your taste buds as they are for your health.

In Part Three, **Gather**, I'll help you navigate social and family dynamics, building a community and network of support that will sustain you in the journey. You may have some loved ones who are eager to share this adventure with you, and others could be fiercely resistant. If your family is anything like mine, you might even have a few members who are prone to acting like jerks on occasion. You can't control what anyone else does. But I'll help you to enroll loved ones, find allies, and navigate social relationships.

And in Part Four, **Transform**, you'll discover how you can make real, lasting change on the planet. (Spoiler alert: It can be *surprisingly easy*, because you're a lot more powerful than you know!)

The Food Revolution program works well when you spend a week honing each of these parts. But you can go at any pace and use this book in any way that helps you to apply what you're learning. If you like, you can read the entire book and then incorporate all four phases at once over the course of the following month.

I hope you can implement this revolution for at least 31 consecutive days. If you do, you'll see tremendous results—and I hope you'll never go back. But if you need to push "pause" while relatives visit or you're on vacation, or if you get distracted, it's okay to come back and pick up where you left off. Whether you take 31 days, or three days, or three years isn't the point.

What matters is that you're here, and that you're moving forward.

Every single chapter includes action steps with three options. Choose the ones that make the most sense for you. If some of the actions don't appeal to you, that's okay. I'll still celebrate every step you take. Doing five of the actions can make a very real difference. Ten will be game changing. Do them all, and your world will never be the same again.

The key is that you take action. That's how you get results. The truth is, cancer, like any other lifestyle-linked disease, doesn't care how much you know. But it does care, a lot, about what you eat and how you live. Cancer and heart disease and diabetes and obesity all want you to eat foods that undermine your joy and your vitality. I want something far better for you.

So what do you say? For the next 31 days, will you join me in this healing Food Revolution?

Shall we get started?

PART ONE

DETOXIFY

People often ask me what is the best way to detoxify. Am I a fan of infrared saunas, or of chelation to remove heavy metals? What about intermittent fasting, coffee enemas, cleansing programs, Epsom salt baths, or megadoses of vitamin C?

Some of these ideas can have value. But if you want to detoxify, the first thing to do is to stop bringing toxins into your body in the first place. And the place to start is with the food on your plate.

In the developed world, we now have the dubious distinction of having the most addictive and obesogenic (obesity-causing) food in the history of humanity. The sheer number of chemical food additives in use today is staggering, and the galling reality is that many of them have been declared safe only by the companies making them, without any testing or oversight from governmental agencies.

The food industry often tells us that there are "good for you" foods and "fun for you" foods, and the key is a healthy balance. But it's amazing how often these "fun for you" foods turn out to fuel suffering, disease, and addiction.

I've had my own journey with craving foods that weren't in my own or my family's best interests.

When my twin sons, River and Bodhi, were nine, I had conflicts with Bodhi (the elder twin by six minutes)—over potato chips. I'll be honest: I was the reason we had the chips in the first place. Potato chips are one of my weaknesses. Something about the salty, crunchy flavor really does it for me. The only ones around the house were organic Kettle chips—but they were, after all, still deep-fried potato slices.

Bodhi, too, enjoyed potato chips. But knowing that fried foods are loaded with free radicals and that most chips are nearly devoid of vitamins and minerals, I felt a responsibility to limit his consumption of them.

Whenever Bodhi found a bag of potato chips, I'd invite him to take five chips, and he'd take ten or twenty. I'd say that was enough, and he'd erupt into a tantrum or grab the bag, run to his room, lock the door, and eat the whole thing.

No matter how hard I tried to hide my stash, Bodhi always seemed to find it. He'd snoop through desk drawers, cupboards, the laundry closet... one day he even found them hidden under my bed. He wore an especially satisfied grin after plundering the loot that day.

And when we went shopping, Bodhi would demand that we start on aisle 4 so he could grab a bag of you-know-what to munch as we moved through the store. If I said no, all shopping cooperation went out the window. More than once, I faced scornful looks from annoyed shoppers as my son sat screaming on the floor.

I asked Bodhi's mom (my beloved of 24 years and counting, Phoenix) for advice. She suggested—sensibly enough—that I stop buying potato chips. If no chips were around, Bodhi would eventually stop looking for them. And of course he'd stop eating them.

It sounded simple. So simple that I could scarcely believe I hadn't thought of it myself. But then it hit me: I had to stop eating potato chips, too.

So that was it. Parental love forced me to change my ways. I stopped buying chips. Once Bodhi realized that his house-wide searching was fruitless, he stopped looking. Within a few weeks, he no longer even asked to visit aisle 4.

Okay, I admit it. I still enjoy potato chips once in a while when I'm traveling or at other people's houses. But they don't come home with me anymore.

When your eating environment is filled with things that you know aren't in your best interests, it can feel like you're constantly swimming upstream. My goal in this Detoxify phase is to help you clear the space and create your home environment so you can minimize stress and set yourself up for success.

In the next few chapters, you'll learn what the science really says about food and health, and what are the overall dietary patterns that have been proven to uplift millions of people. You'll learn how to listen to your own body wisdom so you can eat in ways that make sense for your utterly unique life. I'll share how you can break bad habits and set up your home and your life to make healthy eating as simple and automatic as brushing your teeth. And I'll show you some of the hidden dangers that are likely lurking in your kitchen right now (I bet some of them will surprise you!)—and how you can affordably add safer nontoxic alternatives.

If you share a kitchen with other people who aren't on this journey with you, that can add complications. But you can still choose to define your environment in the best possible way. (We'll look more closely at how you can navigate social dynamics, and be a positive influence on loved ones, in Part Three.)

Now, let's get going with clearing out toxins and making space for the life that you deserve!

Take the Quiz: How Toxic Is Your Food Environment?

Which of these items are currently in your kitchen?

Packaged and fried chips (such as corn chips or potato chips)
  0. A lot.   **1.** At least a package.   **2.** None.

Meat, eggs, or dairy products not from wild or pasture-raised animals
  0. A lot.   **1.** A little.   **2.** None.

Products with added sugars or sweeteners (whether from agave, honey, beetroots, cane, corn, coconut, maple trees, or factory products like high-fructose corn syrup, aspartame, or sucralose)
  0. At least ten.   **1.** Between one and nine.   **2.** None.

A source of purified/filtered water free from chlorine and other contaminants that doesn't depend on plastic bottles
  0. No.   **1.** Yes, but I don't entirely trust it.   **2.** Yes.

Teflon or other "nonstick" cookware whose surface is not specifically ceramic, enamel, stainless steel, or cast iron
  0. Yes.   **1.** Not sure.   **2.** No.

Organically grown foods
  0. None.   **1.** Some.   **2.** Everything.

Plastic containers for storing food
  0. A lot.   **1.** A few.   **2.** None.

Your score will be between 0 and 14. The higher the better! Go to 31day foodrevolution.com/quiz1 if you want to take the quiz online, compare your results with others, and share in the 31-Day Food Revolution with cohorts.

Regardless of your score, I guarantee one thing: The Food Revolution isn't about getting to some destination of perfection and setting up camp. It's about starting where you are and taking steps in a positive direction. And it's about helping other people and our world to move forward with you.

CHAPTER 1

The Food Revolution Diet Plan

Eric Adams is a former New York state senator who now serves as president of Brooklyn Borough. In 2017, Eric was startled by a diagnosis of type 2 diabetes. He was suffering from tingly hands and feet, and doctors told him he'd need to be on medications for the rest of his life and that he faced a high probability of blindness and amputation.

Rather than be defined by this fate, Eric did further research and came across the book *How Not to Die* by Dr. Michael Greger. He followed its advice, replacing the processed-food- and meat-filled diet he'd known his entire life with a whole-foods, plant-based diet centered around vegetables, beans, whole grains, and fruit.

Within three weeks, Eric's extremities stopped tingling, and a few months later, his blood glucose levels had normalized and his diabetes had been effectively cured. No amputations. No blindness. No more of the medications he'd been told he would be on for the rest of his life.

Now Eric's using his political office to help others obtain the same benefits. Thanks to his leadership, all events at Brooklyn Borough Hall must offer plant-based meal options. And he's organizing for a ruling that would require Brooklyn hospitals to have a well-educated department focused on promoting plant-based options and a mandate that doctors inform patients about the role of nutrition when treating lifestyle-fueled illnesses.

Many people know that food's important, but are confused about what, exactly, they should be eating.

We have access, today, to more information about diet and disease than any population that's ever lived. We can review the findings of tens of thousands of studies published in peer-reviewed medical journals from any laptop or smartphone. Thousands of nutrition and diet books are published every year, while billions of websites tell you what to eat and what to avoid.

Unfortunately, many of them are wrong.

I've seen different so-called experts delivering wildly conflicting dogma—with some telling people to avoid legumes and açai berries, while others say to eat all calories in two hours of the day; to never go more than three waking hours without eating; to eat nothing blended; to eat everything blended; to go raw; to go 100 percent cooked; to avoid oils; or to make sure that 90 percent of calories are from fat. We've got different folks telling us to eat lots of meat, to go vegan, or to eat nothing but fruit before noon.

When I hear all the conflicting information, I'm reminded of the old saying: "A man with one watch knows what time it is. A man with two watches is never quite sure."

In a sea of confusion, all too often the status quo prevails. When you don't have a clear path forward, you're more inclined to take the path of least resistance. In a toxic food culture, we know where that leads.

The truth is, most serious food and health researchers aren't clueless about the basic care and feeding of humans. Modern medical science is quite clear about the dietary patterns that can, in the vast majority of cases, help prevent or even reverse many of the chronic ailments of our times.

THE OPTIMAL DIET FOR HUMANS
(MOST OF THE TIME!)

In his study of what he terms the "Blue Zones," National Geographic Fellow and explorer Dan Buettner identifies the five regions where people enjoy not only the longest life spans but also the most abundant health spans. His studies focus on Sardinia, Italy; Loma Linda, California; Nicoya Peninsula, Costa Rica; Ikaria, Greece; and the islands of Okinawa, Japan.

Dan describes asking a 102-year-old Okinawan woman what it feels like to hold her great-great-great-granddaughter. She tells him that "it feels like leaping into heaven."

Most of us fear growing old. But in the Blue Zones, many people look forward to it. Perhaps we all would if we had role models like Dr. Ellsworth Wareham, a surgeon from Loma Linda, who still enjoyed his practice in the operating room at age 95—conducting open-heart surgery on 20 patients every month. (Dr. Wareham retired in 2009, but he is still living happily, as of this writing, at the age of 103.)

Remarkably, despite spanning the globe, all of the Blue Zone regions have a number of things in common. Residents have strong social and family ties, low rates of smoking, a plant-rich and predominantly (though not often exclusively) vegetarian diet, and enjoyment of consistent and moderate physical activity.

Inspired to explore the overarching principles that lead to positive outcomes, Yale-Griffin Prevention Research Center founding director David Katz, MD, assembled a global coalition of experts called the True Health Initiative. As a member of this initiative myself, I'm joined by more than 450 of the world's leading doctors, scientists, researchers, clinicians, and health advocates. Our goal is to clarify and communicate an emerging consensus that there is a way of eating and living that massively promotes longevity, vitality, and overall health.

Our overarching conclusion, which is reflected in the findings from all the Blue Zones, is summarized in Michael Pollan's famous seven words: **"Eat food. Not too much. Mostly plants."**

By "**eat food**," we mean "eat real food," not the ultraprocessed food-like substances that make up most of the calories in the modern diet in the industrialized world. On this point, there's little controversy. We find vast agreement among very nearly every scientist and research organization in the world, calling for us to eat fresh whole foods that are grown and produced sustainably and that are minimally processed, if they are processed at all.

The good news is that real foods don't tend to stimulate addiction, because they provide more nutrition than calories. This means that when you eat them, it's easier to feel full and deeply satisfied while eating "**not too much**."

And what about eating "**mostly plants**"? We now know that plant foods, and in particular fresh vegetables and fruits, are the most concentrated sources of many of the nutrients the human body needs in order to thrive. Fruits and vegetables provide antioxidants, phytochemicals, phytosterols, fiber, enzymes, prebiotics, probiotics, essential fats and proteins, vitamins, and minerals.

Flavonoids, with their tremendous nutritive value, are the pigments that give plants their colors—like the deep blue of blueberries, the purple in grapes, the orange in pumpkins, the green in leafy greens, and the red of tomatoes. In general, the darker orange the carrot, or the darker green the leaf, the more nutritious and flavorful it will be. You may have noticed that as vegetables age, they become pale. This reflects a decline in nutrition and flavor.

Researcher Alec Baxt once ran a fascinating experiment. He tested a variety of carrots for their nutrient density. He distributed representative samples to volunteers and had them rate the carrots on flavor. The ones that people said tasted the most "carrot-y," bursting with the most flavor, were also the ones that offered the highest nutrient value.

When you cook with fresh fruits and vegetables, the flavors speak with a distinct elegance and boldness. The taste of a midsummer heirloom tomato, perhaps lightly seasoned with sea salt, is incomparably more delicious than a beefsteak tomato that was picked green and then trucked thousands of miles. The same goes for eating an orchard-fresh apple—it has a crisp, snappy sweetness that conveys a refreshing sparkle.

The good news is that, as you'll see in chapter 28, when you eat **"mostly plants**," you walk on the earth with a lighter footprint, which means you help save forests, water, topsoil, animals, and our climate from suffering and destruction.

What about meat, fish, eggs, and dairy? Thoughtful researchers generally agree that most people would benefit from eating more plants and fewer animals. Whether the optimal level of animal products in the human diet (from a health perspective) is zero, or 5 percent or 10 percent of calories, is a subject of debate—probably because the answer isn't the same for everyone. But the average American gets 34 percent of calories from meat, dairy, and eggs, while less than 6 percent of calories come from vegetables and less than 3 percent come from fruits.[1]

For almost all of us, the optimal direction seems clear: mostly plants.

BUT WHERE DO YOU GET YOUR PROTEIN?

Anyone who adopts a plant-based diet or even considers going vegetarian is likely to hear this question with alarming frequency. But it's actually not quite the problem it's been made out to be.

Protein is an essential nutrient for the building, maintenance, and repair of almost all the tissues in your body. The question is, how much is enough—or too much?

In the United States, the official recommended daily allowance is 0.36 grams of protein for every pound of body weight. (To meet this target, at 160 pounds, you'd need about 58 grams of protein per day.) If you're an athlete trying to build muscle, or you're pregnant or lactating, or if you're under physical stress, the recommendation is to get at least 0.45 grams of protein daily per pound of body weight (which means, at 160 pounds, you'd need about 72 grams of protein daily).

New research is finding that protein needs for seniors are somewhat higher because as we get older, we don't tend to absorb protein as efficiently. Carol Greenwood, PhD, a specialist in geriatric nutrition at the University of Toronto, suggests that people over the age of 70 should get at least 1 daily gram of protein per kilogram of body weight.[2] This means that a senior who weighs 160 pounds should be getting at least 73 grams of protein per day. At 200 pounds, we might need 90 grams per day.

But protein deficiency is shockingly rare. Most American adults eat about 100 grams of protein per day, or nearly twice the amount that's recommended for most people.[3] Most Europeans get far more than they need, too.[4] And although meat and other animal products are usually high in protein, the reality is that many vegetarian food sources contain abundant protein. For example, the percentage of calories coming from protein in tempeh, tofu, or green lentils is actually higher than in bacon or in cow's milk.

Here's a chart, developed by *New York Times* bestselling author and healthy living advocate Kris Carr, that can help you assess your protein needs and see where your protein might come from on a plant-based diet.

Your Protein Needs

1. Find your "P" value.
   Kids ages 4 to 13 = 0.43
   Adolescents ages 14 to 18 = 0.39
   Adults ages 19 to 64 (moderately active) = 0.36
   Seniors ages 65+ = 0.44 to 0.52
2. To calculate your needs, multiply your lean body weight (in pounds) by your "P" value to find out how many grams are recommended for you each day. (If you are significantly overweight, you may adjust the formula down to base it on what you might consider to be a healthy body weight.)
3. Take a look at these plant-based food sources, and see how they stack up with your protein needs. Remember that you don't have to get all your protein from one source. Virtually everything you eat adds to your daily protein total. Many drops fill a bucket!
   Tempeh (4 ounces): 20 grams
   Lentils—cooked (1 cup): 18 grams
   Beans—cooked (1 cup): 14.5 grams
   Hemp seeds (3 tablespoons): 10 grams
   Quinoa—cooked (1 cup): 9 grams
   Tofu—extra firm (3 ounces): 9 grams
   Almonds—raw (¼ cup): 8 grams
   Sunflower seeds—raw (¼ cup): 7 grams
   Porridge—cooked (1 cup): 6 grams
   Chia seeds (2 tablespoons): 6 grams
   Broccoli—chopped (1 cup): 3 grams

Based on the available research, these recommendations are intended for general health, disease prevention, and longevity. But for specific contexts, such as power athletes and weightlifters, there is also research showing that higher protein intakes may be advisable in some instances.

If you want to boost your protein levels, you might consider using shelled hemp seeds or flax or chia powder, so you get all the benefits of the whole food. If you're considering a more refined protein supplement, be forewarned: In 2018, when the Clean Label Project tested the most popular protein powders on the market, researchers found that virtually all of the 134 products tested contained detectable levels of at least one heavy metal and 55 percent tested positive for BPA.[5] The plant-based and organic protein powders were no better, and in many cases fared the worst. But the good news is that so long as you eat a varied diet based around whole foods, and get enough total calories, chances are you have no need for protein supplements anyway.

For the hundreds of millions of people on the planet who don't have enough food to eat, protein deficiency can be a serious and even life-threatening problem. It can also become a concern for "junk food vegans" who eat no animal products but a lot of processed food. Remember, there's no protein in sugar or bottled oils, and very little in fries or chips.

But in the industrialized world, where starvation is relatively rare, inadequate protein consumption is remarkably rare. If you eat 2,400 calories in a day, and 15 percent of your calories are coming from protein, you'll be eating 90 grams of protein.

And as surprising as it may sound, we're beginning to understand that many people may be suffering from getting too *much* protein.

When the International Scholarly Research Network published a meta-analysis of 31 studies on protein intake and disease, it concluded that overconsumption of protein was associated with higher rates of cancer, osteoporosis, renal disease, disorders of liver function, and coronary artery disease.[6]

Valter Longo, PhD, director of the Longevity Institute at the University of Southern California, led a 2014 study that tracked 6,381 adults over the age of 50 for nearly 20 years. The study found that between the ages of 50 and 65, participants who ate a high-protein diet (defined as 20 percent or more of calories coming from protein) were four times more likely to die of cancer than those who consumed a low-protein diet (with less than 10 percent of calories coming from protein).[7] The increase in cancer risk associated with a high-protein diet during these years was on par with smoking 20 cigarettes per day.

Once over the age of 65, however, cancer mortality data leveled off, indicating that for people over age 65, there is no meaningful cancer-fighting benefit to a low-protein diet. At each age, however, those participants who ate a high-protein diet had a five times greater risk of mortality from diabetes. Overall, the study found that people with a high-protein diet were 74 percent more likely to die of any cause within the 20-year study period than their low-protein counterparts.

What if we've had it all backward? Is it really possible that most of us are actually getting too much? Dr. Longo thinks so. Summarizing the findings, he concludes that the study provided "convincing evidence that a high-protein diet—particularly if the proteins are derived from animals—is nearly as bad as smoking for your health."

But what about food combining? Do plant-based eaters, especially, need to worry about getting the right mix of amino acids? Well, here's how it works: What we call *protein* is actually made up of 21 amino acids. Your body can make 12 of them, but there are 9 that are called the "essential" amino acids because you need to get them directly from your food. As long as you're eating a variety of whole, natural foods, and getting enough total calories and enough overall protein, your need for all 9 essential amino acids should be easily met.

THE PLAN I RECOMMEND

I've developed four core principles that I call the Food Revolution Diet Plan. Unlike a lot of diets you hear about, these principles are flexible. They're more about pointing in a direction than insisting on a set destination.

I have way too much respect for biochemical individuality, and for the diversity of life experiences and contexts, to try to tell anyone exactly what they should or shouldn't eat. But there are some overarching principles that are beneficial for just about everyone.

The Four Principles of the Food Revolution Diet Plan Are:

1. **Eat fewer processed foods.** Our bodies weren't designed for sugar, white flour, bottled oils, or chemicals.

2. **Eat fewer animal products.** Modern meat and dairy products—especially from factory farms—are leading drivers of heart disease, cancer, diabetes, and obesity, as well as culprits in widespread environmental destruction.

3. **Eat more whole plant foods.** Fruits, vegetables, and other whole plant foods give you an abundance of the vitamins, minerals, antioxidants, flavonoids, and other phytonutrients your brain, lungs, heart, immune system, and cells need to thrive.

4. **Source consciously.** When you buy more organic, non-GMO, humane, local, and fair-trade foods, you're taking a stand for your health and for your planet, as well as supporting farmers who do the right thing.

Let's make one thing totally clear: I'm not asking you to sign a purity pact or to be subjected to regular inspections by the food police. If you want to pig out on pizza occasionally, or go out for ice cream now and then, I'll still love you. (And I hope that you'll still love you, too!) It's not what you do on occasion that matters most. In the long run, it's the choices you make day in and day out, and the habits you forge and sustain, that chart the course of your destiny.

RHONDA'S STORY

In 2014, Rhonda Hogan of Tempe, Arizona, was diagnosed with stage 3 chronic kidney disease and a bone marrow cancer in her abdomen. She was a mother and grandmother. Her family depended on her. And now, she feared for her life.

I first met Rhonda a short time later, when she enrolled in a healthy eating course that we were leading through Food Revolution Network. I was struck by her passion for life. She didn't want to die, and she was willing to make big changes.

Rhonda adopted the principles of the Food Revolution Diet Plan. Her new diet not only saved time and money—it also may have saved her life. Today Rhonda is cancer-free and her kidney disease has gone in reverse. Instead of wondering if she'll be alive next year, she's eagerly looking forward to dancing at her grandchildren's weddings.

The overarching principles of healthy eating are pretty clear, but every human being is different. In the next chapter, we'll look at why it's critically important to understand your uniqueness and to listen to your body's signals and wisdom to establish the habits that are right for you.

ACTION:

Option 1: Go meat-free for a day.

Option 2: Give up all animal products (meat, dairy, and eggs) for a week, and eat more vegetables.

Option 3: Eat nothing this week that comes from a package listing more than seven ingredients.

You'll find a fabulous five-day meal plan at the end of the delicious recipes in the back. If you want a 31-day meal plan, with suggestions for breakfast, lunch, dinner, and snacks, you're in luck! Download a plan from 31dayfood revolution.com/mealplan. It's one of many online resources that I created to help you get the most out of our journey together. You can join our virtual community of friends, readers, and fellow food revolutionaries to share struggles, tips, recipes, and breakthroughs.

CHAPTER 2

Know What's Right for You

There are many kinds of diversity. From ethnicity to religion, and from cuisine to political perspective, no

> Always remember that you are absolutely unique. Just like everyone else.
> —*Margaret Mead*

two of us are exactly alike. Sometimes even within families we find huge differences, and how we interact across these spans is crucial in shaping a family's culture.

I know a bit about this from personal experience. My wife, Phoenix, and I are parents of adorable, love-filled identical twins. River and Bodhi were born in 2001, nine weeks prematurely. They've grown to be beautiful, generous young men. And they're autistic.

They have extraordinary memories and display forms of intelligence that are unique. And they have to work much harder than their neurotypical peers to manage many of the life tasks and functions that most of us might consider basic.

Why are they autistic? I wish I knew! Autism diagnosis rates have risen exponentially in the last generation. While some people blame vaccinations, GMOs, environmental contamination, religious proclivities, or poor diet, any serious scientist knows that we don't have causal certainty. And most likely there's more than one factor at play.

I'm pretty clear that our kids' autism wasn't a result of vaccines, GMOs, or direct pesticide exposure. They've been raised in an exceptionally nontoxic environment, and were given no vaccines prior to their unique neurology revealing itself. And I believe that genetics are involved.

In 2011, the California Autism Twins Study reported finding that when one identical twin develops autism, the chances of the other twin developing it as well are 70 percent.[1] A large-scale study involving more than 300,000 children found that those whose fathers had IQs of 111 and above had a 31 percent higher chance of being autistic.[2] And another study found a significant and distinct genetic commonality between child prodigies and autistic children.[3]

Autism is, among other things, a form of neurological diversity. I believe that autistic people's brains work differently from the norm, and that the very factors that can make them brilliant in some domains can also make them uniquely vulnerable to the spread of chemicals, pesticides, and other pollutants that increasingly contaminate our world.

No matter how hard we try to minimize our children's exposure to environmental toxins, there are many factors beyond our control.

For example, the egg that later became River and Bodhi was formed when their mother, my beloved Phoenix, was in the womb of her mother, Diane, in 1975. At that time, River and Bodhi's grandma Diane was living in Michigan—which had just two years earlier been the site of the most catastrophic agricultural disaster in U.S. history.[4] Ten to twenty bags of the highly toxic and potent flame retardants polybrominated biphenyls (PBBs) were accidentally added to cattle feed, leading to PBB exposure for 90 percent of state residents and eventually to the forced destruction of tens of thousands of cattle. There's little doubt Diane was exposed—and studies suggest that exposure to PBBs can persist for a lifetime and may impact future generations. Grandma Diane was also at the time eating fish from Lake Michigan. We now know that this fish was seriously contaminated with PCBs (another damaging chemical), and that consumption of it in the 1970s has been clearly linked to brain damage as well as to birth defects in the next generation.[5] And it doesn't stop there. According to groundbreaking research from biologist Michael Skinner, toxic exposure is showing up two and even three generations downstream.[6]

We don't know, and we may never know, what could have led to River and Bodhi's premature birth or autism.

But I do know this: Being River and Bodhi's dad has humbled me, and taught me much about who I am and about what really matters. Life brings each of us more than our share of hardships and challenges. I believe that how we respond to those challenges is part of what defines us as human beings.

OUR AUTISM BREAKTHROUGH

As River and Bodhi were growing up, we tried what seemed like gazillions of dietary and therapeutic approaches. But still, at the age of 10, our kids were not potty-trained. They had frequent violent outbursts and enjoyed almost no positive social interactions with peers.

Then we discovered an approach to autism called The Son-Rise Program. Instead of focusing on modifying behavior, Son-Rise focuses on building relationships. It's based on the notion that autistic people lack the ability to filter sensory input and are overwhelmed with hyperstimulation. They retreat from contact and resort to familiar and repetitive behaviors to find safety.

With the Son-Rise approach, instead of trying to drag them into our world, we learned to join theirs. As we made contact on their terms, we befriended them, and then in time, we could show them the doorway out, into our world.

For example, River and I never shared meaningful eye contact during his first 10 years. Sometimes his eyes would drift past mine, but I never had the experience of dropping into sustained connection. It was one of the things that I missed the most.

But that was about to change.

At the age of 11, River went through a phase of being passionate about, of all things, Barbie dolls. He loved to play with them, to change their clothes, and mostly, to chew on their feet. One day River was chewing on a Barbie's foot while staring into space.

I worried about what toxins in the plastic might be leaching into River's body. I also began to fear that my son could never have a dating life if he insisted on chewing on Barbie feet. I was tempted to pull it out of his mouth.

But instead, I tried the Son-Rise approach. I picked up another Barbie and chewed on her foot. I went from seeing River's behavior as pathological to seeing it as playful, and I joined him in it.

To my amazement, River came out of his chewing trance enough to look at me and grin. I could almost hear him thinking, "Oh my God! There is intelligent life on this planet after all!"

After a minute or so that felt like a beautiful eternity, River gestured for me to come closer. He was inviting me to chew the other foot of his Barbie. I found myself three inches from River's face, beaming into his eyes—chewing on a Barbie foot.

It was one of the happiest moments of my life.

WHAT THIS MEANS

River has grown up a lot. He now knows how to use the toilet (most of the time, anyway). He has a growing number of friends of all ages. He demonstrates profound caring and compassion for others. And he hasn't chewed on any Barbie dolls in years. He and his brother still struggle, but to me they are living miracles.

Now, nearly every time we hang out, River and I have some moment in which we look into each other's eyes and smile. And invariably, some part of my heart melts.

So what does this have to do with the Food Revolution? Quite a lot.

You see, your brain isn't the only thing about you that's unique. Your hormones, cardiovascular system, neurology, digestion, and even your psychological and emotional state all have an effect on how you respond to food and everything else you encounter.

When we fall prey to the illusion that we have anyone (including ourselves!) figured out, and when we try to make people conform to our beliefs about the right way to eat or to behave, we run the risk of ceasing to pay attention, and not listening.

River taught me about the importance of meeting him where he is, and being willing to learn new things in unexpected ways rather than expecting him to conform to my existing worldview.

The same principle is true with your diet. When you approach your body and dietary path with open-minded curiosity, you create the conditions out of which real learning is possible. And from that learning, you can grow, over time, into some degree of wisdom.

YOU'RE MORE UNIQUE THAN YOU IMAGINE

Does a grandparent need the same food as a child? Does a sedentary office worker require the same diet as an athlete?

The answer is unequivocally no. When a dietary doctrine or one-size-fits-all approach becomes part of our identity, we deny our individuality.

In 2015, a comprehensive study published in the journal *Cell* found that people metabolize the same foods in very different ways.[7] To measure how food was digested, researchers recruited 800 people and measured their responses to 46,898 meals. During the study, participants were asked to log every bite, sip, exercise session, bowel movement, and sleep session on a phone app. Their blood sugar levels were measured every five minutes by a device attached to their bodies, and they turned in stool samples for gut bacteria analysis. They also gave blood samples, and everyone ate the same meals for breakfast.

As they analyzed a mountain of data, the researchers were struck to discover how differently the participants responded. Sushi caused one man's blood sugar to spike higher than ice cream did. For another participant, eating a seemingly healthy food—tomatoes—spiked her blood sugar. Some glucose levels would spike after consuming fresh fruit but not a glass of beer. For others, the exact opposite was the case.

Some people thrive with a hearty, protein-packed breakfast, while others feel best eating more lightly, with just fruit or a smoothie in the morning. And what's best for your body might change over time.

THE DIFFERENCE BETWEEN CRAVING AND HUNGER

Sometimes I crave a slice of bread or a nibble of my favorite vegan "cheeze." Now that I don't eat potato chips anymore (at least, not at home), these have become my go-to indulgences. My cravings usually emerge if I stay up late—past the time that my body may have wanted to go to sleep. When I override my body's natural signals, I notice that I'm drawn to oral stimulation that will provide comfort and sensation.

But I also know that late-night eaters are more likely to be drawn to the foods that are least healthy, and that eating before bed can be bad for digestion and metabolism and can increase the chance of weight gain. I allow myself a slice or two of bread or "cheeze" from time to time at night, but I try not to let it become a habit.

Many people confuse emotionally sourced craving, or physiological addiction, with genuine hunger. Physical hunger signals usually come from your stomach, with growls or hollow feelings, or from your brain, with fogginess, lack of concentration, headache, or fatigue. Emotionally driven cravings, on the other hand, may take the form of obsession with specific things—and more often than not, they aren't things that are good for you.

It helps to look for root cause. Many cravings arise in response to stress. Stress-reduction techniques could include taking a hot bath, going for a walk, practicing relaxation exercises or yoga, or cuddling with a loved one. Sometimes when you think you're hungry, you might really just be thirsty. Drinking water can help. If the urge persists, try eating something healthy, like whole fruit (I love slices of apple, peach, pear, or orange) or vegetable sticks. (It can be fun to munch on carrots, destringed celery, or slices of cucumber or jicama.)

Heather Fleming of San Diego, California, likes to look at what's underneath her craving—and often she finds something deeper at work. One Easter holiday, she was craving a doughnut. She inquired more deeply, without judgment, asking herself what she was really craving. A childhood memory emerged of having a doughnut with her parents and grandparents after church. She realized it was actually a feeling of connection with her family that she was longing for. Heather grabbed a cup of tea and called her mom, and amazingly, the doughnut craving disappeared.

Food cravings can be triggered by emotional, psychological, and physical factors. Some people are biochemically addicted to foods, and for them, no amount of willpower or psychological prowess will lead to lasting freedom. But there are tools that have been proven to work (more on them in chapter 5).

HOW TO TELL IF YOUR BODY NEEDS SOMETHING MORE

There are some nutrients that most of us, even if we're eating a wholesome diet, should pay attention to—specifically vitamins B_{12}, D_3, and K_2, as well as zinc and the omega-3 fatty acids. If you're unsure how your levels are holding up, you can ask your health care provider to prescribe blood tests for the important nutrients.

Some people do better with small amounts of consciously sourced wild fish and/or other animal products, while others feel healthiest maintaining a boundary that avoids all meat and dairy. As we'll discuss later, many people thrive optimally with some whole grains and legumes. But not everyone.

Some people accustomed to eating sweets or refined foods might find that small amounts provide a sense of psychological relaxation and ease. But for others, anything sweet can stimulate cravings that lead to an addictive cycle of dependency. The point is that a diverse, whole-foods diet is ultimately best for just about all of us, but there's always room for finessing.

If you're already eating a whole-foods, plant-centered diet and still have symptoms such as inflammation or digestive problems, you may want to try an elimination diet, a process used to identify specific problem-causing foods by eliminating all suspected foods and then reintroducing them one at a time. Many elimination diets involve steering clear of the commonly allergenic foods, including nuts, corn, soy, dairy, citrus fruits, nightshade vegetables (tomatoes, potatoes, peppers, and aubergine), gluten (which comes with wheat, rye, and barley), pork, eggs, and seafood, for two to three weeks. For digestive problems, some elimination diets also omit legumes. If symptoms disappear, you can try adding food items or categories back on a methodical basis and seeing if the symptoms return.

The placebo effect is well known for its medical potency. When you have a bias toward thinking that a certain food may be bad for you, then any time you eat it, you risk experiencing symptoms of indigestion, brain fog, or other ailments that could be caused more by your expectations than by your body's native response. One way to establish a bit of objectivity is with a journal. Record everything you eat, how much you sleep and exercise, how you're feeling, and how much energy you have, and review your results over time to observe any trends.

What I learned from my son River is that when we judge or pathologize what we don't understand, we lose traction in our relationship to it. So if you experience symptoms or challenges that don't make sense, my suggestion is to greet them with curiosity and, as much as possible, with kindness.

When you bring caring attention to what you eat, to your body, and to your health, it's a precious blessing. You'll almost certainly learn new things that shape the wisdom of your choices.

Just like everyone else alive, you deserve total and unconditional love.

ACTION:

Option 1: *Write down one thing that's unique about you, and one thing you appreciate about it—some gift, resource, or contribution that this part of you makes possible.*

Option 2: *Start a food journal. Write down what you eat and anything else you want to track. See what you discover.*

Option 3: *Go on an elimination diet and steer clear of all nuts, corn, soy, dairy, citrus fruits, nightshade vegetables, wheat and other foods containing gluten (rye and barley), pork, eggs, and seafood for two weeks. See if any surprising symptoms or challenges disappear. If they do, slowly and methodically add food groups back in, introducing another group of foods every three days. Monitor closely with a journal to see if any symptoms return. If they do, back that food group out of your diet again until the symptoms disappear, and then try adding another class of foods every three days. It can take up to six weeks, but this process can help you identify the culprits.*

CHAPTER 3

Foods to Eat and Foods to Avoid

Dorothy Prabhu grew up in India. Shortly after she met and married her husband, Mark, they moved to the United States and began eating a variation of the modern industrialized diet. Dorothy developed a series of problems, including sinusitis, uterine fibroids, and chronic fatigue. She struggled to get out of bed in the morning. Dorothy's doctors prescribed drugs, some with major side effects. They never told her that diet might be a factor in her suffering.

Instinctively, Dorothy felt that something better must be possible. She began to learn about nutrition, and she adopted a whole-foods, plant-strong diet. Today her fibroids are gone, and she has more physical and mental energy than ever. But her husband, Mark, did not follow her lead. In 2016, following his sustained bout with diabetes, she lost him to renal disease. They had been together 36 years.

Dorothy's deeper research revealed that both type 2 diabetes and renal disease can be reversed with a healthy diet. As far as she's concerned, it was the modern industrialized diet that took her husband's life. Now she lives with a devastating hole in her life, and she's still paying off his medical bills. But she's also passionate to learn all she can. Dorothy doesn't want anyone else to suffer. She's been one of the editors of this book and a growing force in the Food Revolution community.

We hope you'll join us.

While the status quo is so ubiquitous that most people think chronic suffering is normal, the truth is, it doesn't have to be. The modern industrialized diet and the nightmares it fuels are a relatively recent invention.

And we're only now beginning to understand the immense impact that stems from this way of eating.

In 2013, an international collaborative of scientists led by the Institute for Health Metrics and Evaluation at the University of Washington completed the largest study of risk factors for death and disabilities ever conducted in human history.[1] Their study analyzed impacts of 291 diseases, conditions, and injuries, as well as 67 different possible risk factors (such as diet, exercise, and economic status) over the course of 20 years.

Their resulting report, *Global Burden of Disease*, concluded that unhealthy diet is the biggest contributor to tens of millions of deaths worldwide, and to more than 678,282 deaths annually in the United States.[2] This means that more Americans are dying from diet-fueled disease *each year* than died in World War I, World War II, the Korean War, the Vietnam War, the war in Afghanistan, and both Iraq wars *combined*. This time the enemy is our own food choices.

Pat Spensley, MD, is a family practice doctor in Newberg, Oregon. Like most doctors, he learned very little in medical school about nutrition. In 2013, faced with severe asthma and obesity, Dr. Spensley participated in a Food Revolution Summit that my dad and I hosted. After changing to a whole-foods, plant-rich diet, Dr. Spensley lost 50 pounds, and his health and energy levels improved dramatically. Now instead of only prescribing drugs and surgeries, he talks to his patients about how diet can help prevent osteoporosis, cancer, hypertension, obesity, and heart disease.

I look forward to the day when we have more doctors like Pat Spensley, who get the education they need to make healthy eating a foundation of their medical practice.

It's up to you to decide what makes sense given your priorities, values, and health goals. But to start you out with some guidance on the Food Revolution Diet Plan, I put together a chart suggesting foods to eat abundantly, foods to eat moderately (if at all), and foods to minimize or eliminate.

HOW TO USE THIS CHART

These guidelines are based on extensive data and medical research, but they're not universal rules. While more than 400 foods are listed, the chart is by necessity very general. How a food is produced and processed, what pesticides it may or may not have been grown with, how an animal was treated, and many other factors can lead to very different results. As in all things, listen to your body and, where applicable, to your health professional, and use your own best judgment.

If you're susceptible to the pull of addictive foods, draw sharp, firm lines with your choices of what to eliminate. Think of how most alcoholics can't have "just one drink." Likewise, if you're suffering from a serious medical condition, you may want to be strict and even, perhaps, a bit dogmatic. For example, someone with celiac disease or serious gluten sensitivity should avoid all forms of wheat and other gluten-containing grains. But for many other people, wheat, barley, and rye in their healthiest forms can be part of a good diet—that's why they're in the "Eat Moderately" category.

I know people who eat modest amounts of grass-fed beef and report positive benefits. But the medical research is also pretty consistent that for the vast majority, red meat is associated with higher rates of heart disease, cancer, dementia, and other ailments. So for the sake of simplicity, I've placed all forms of beef in the "Minimize or Eliminate" category.

See if you can find items from the "Eat Moderately" or the "Minimize or Eliminate" groups that are part of your diet now but that you might be ready to give up.

VEGETABLES	Eat Abundantly	Eat Moderately	Minimize or Eliminate
	Artichokes		
	Arugula/Rocket		
	Asparagus		
	Beet greens		
	Blackberries		
	Bok choy		
	Broccoli		
	Brussels sprouts		
	Cabbage		
	Carrots		
	Cauliflower		
	Celery		
	Chard		
	Chicory		
	Chinese cabbage		

VEGETABLES	Eat Abundantly	Eat Moderately	Minimize or Eliminate
	Aubergine		
	Chives		
	Collard greens		
	Cucumbers		
	Dandelion greens		
			French fries
	Green beans		
	Jicama		
	Kale		
	Kohlrabi		
	Leafy green vegetables		
	Leeks		
	Lettuce, leaf or romaine	Lettuce, iceberg	
	Mushrooms		
	Mustard greens		
	Okra		
	Onions		
	Parsley		
	Parsnips		
	Peppers		
		Potatoes, white or red (with skin)	
	Pumpkin		
	Radishes		
	Rutabagas/swede		
	Seaweed		
	Spinach		
	Spring onions		
	Summer squash, all varieties		
	Sweet potatoes		
	Tomatoes		
	Tomato paste		
	Tomato sauce		
	Turnips		
	Turnip greens		
	Vegetables, frozen	Vegetables, canned	
	Water chestnuts		
	Watercress		
	Winter squash, all varieties		
	Yams		

FRUITS	Eat Abundantly	Eat Moderately	Minimize or Eliminate
	Apples	Apple juice (unfiltered)	Apple juice (filtered)
	Apricots		
	Avocados		
	Bananas		
	Black currants		
	Blackberries		
	Blueberries		
	Cantaloupe		
	Cherries		
	Cranberries		
		Dates	
	Elderberries		
	Figs, fresh	Figs, dried	
	Fruit, fresh or frozen	Fruit, canned or dried (no sugar added)	Fruit, canned in syrup or dried (sugar added)
	Gooseberries		
	Grapefruit		
	Grapes		
	Guavas		
		Honeydew melon	
	Kiwifruit		
	Lemons		
	Limes		
	Mangoes		
	Nectarines		
	Oranges	Orange juice, fresh squeezed	Orange juice, from concentrate
	Papayas		
	Peaches		
	Pears		
	Persimmons		
	Pineapples	Pineapple juice	
	Plums		
	Pomegranates		
	Quinces		
		Raisins	
	Raspberries		
	Rhubarb		
	Sapote		
	Star fruit		
	Strawberries		
	Tangerines		
	Watermelon		

GRAINS	Eat Abundantly	Eat Moderately	Minimize or Eliminate
		Barley	
			Biscuits
		Bran	
			Bread, fried
		Breads and bread products, whole grain	Breads and bread products, white
	Buckwheat		
		Bulgur	
			Cakes
		Cereals, whole grain (sugar-free)	Cereals, refined grain
			Cookies
	Corn*		
		Corn flour*	
	Cornmeal*		
		Couscous	
			Croissants
			Doughnuts
			Farina
		Flour, 100% whole wheat	Flour, white
	Kamut		
	Millet		
		Noodles, udon	Noodles, fried
	Oats: whole, steel cut, or slow-cooking	Oats: quick-cooking or instant	
		Orzo, whole grain	
	Pasta, legume	Pasta, brown rice or whole wheat	Pasta, semolina/white
			Pastries
	Polenta*		
	Quinoa		
		Rice, all varieties	Rice, fried
		Rice cakes	
		Rye	
			Semolina
		Sorghum	
	Spelt		
	Teff		
		Tortillas, corn* or whole wheat	Tortillas, white
		Wheat	

LEGUMES	Eat Abundantly	Eat Moderately	Minimize or Eliminate
	Beans, all varieties	Beans, refried	
	Beans, sprouted		
	Chickpeas		
	Dal		
	Edamame*		
	Lentils, all varieties		
	Miso		
	Peas		
			Soy cheeze*
			Soy mayonnaise*
			Soy protein*
			Soy sour cream*
		Soy yogurt*	
	Tempeh*		
			Textured soy protein*
	Tofu*	Tofu, baked (as typically seasoned in packages with salt and sweeteners)*	Tofu, fried
NUTS & SEEDS	**Eat Abundantly**	**Eat Moderately**	**Minimize or Eliminate**
	Almond butter, raw	Almond butter, roasted	
	Almonds, raw	Almonds, roasted	
	Beech nuts		
	Brazil nuts		
	Cashews, raw	Cashews, roasted	
	Chestnuts		
	Chia seeds		
	Coconut		
	Filberts		
	Flaxseed		
	Hazelnuts		
	Hemp seeds		
	Hickory nuts		
	Macadamia nuts		
	Peanut butter*		
	Peanuts, raw**	Peanuts, roasted**	
	Pecans		
	Pine nuts		
	Pistachio nuts, raw	Pistachio nuts, roasted	
		Poppy seeds	

NUTS & SEEDS	Eat Abundantly	Eat Moderately	Minimize or Eliminate
	Pumpkin seeds		
	Sesame seeds		
		Soy nuts, lightly roasted**	Soy nuts, dark roasted**
	Sunflower seeds		
	Tahini, raw	Tahini, roasted	
	Walnuts		

FATS/OILS	Eat Abundantly	Eat Moderately	Minimize or Eliminate
		Canola oil, organic*	
		Coconut oil, organic*	
			Corn oil*
			Cottonseed oil*
	Flax oil, fresh, unheated		
		Hemp oil	
			Lard
	MCT oil, unheated, from coconuts		
		Olive oil, extra virgin	
	Omega-3 oils, from algae or fish		
			Palm kernel oil
			Palm oil
			Partially hydrogenated oils, all*
			Peanut oil (groundnut oil)
			Safflower oil
			Sesame oil
			Soybean oil
			Sunflower oil

SWEETENERS	Eat Abundantly	Eat Moderately	Minimize or Eliminate
			Agave
		Barley malt	
			Brown rice syrup
		Coconut sugar	
			Corn sweetener*
			Corn syrup, high-fructose*
		Dates	
			Erythritol
		Figs (dried)	
		Honey, raw	Honey, pasteurized

SWEETENERS	Eat Abundantly	Eat Moderately	Minimize or Eliminate
	Jam/preserves, 100% fruit	Jam/preserves, sweetened	
		Maple syrup	
		Molasses	
			No-calorie sweeteners (Splenda, saccharin, NutraSweet, aspartame*, etc.)
			Sorbitol
		Stevia	
		Sugar: brown, turbinado, evaporated cane juice	Sugar: white
		Xylitol	

BEVERAGES	Drink Abundantly	Drink Moderately	Minimize or Eliminate
			Beer
			Cocktails and alcoholic mixed drinks
	Coconut water		
	Coffee, cold brewed, unsweetened	Coffee, hot brewed, unsweetened	Coffee, flavored or sweetened
		Coffee, decaffeinated	
		Fruit juices	
	Grape juice, red		
			Hard alcohol
			Hard cider
		Kombucha	
			Sake
		Sodas: natural, sugar-free	Sodas: colas, regular
	Sparkling water		
	Tea, unsweetened: black, green, herbal, oolong, white, yerba maté	Tea, sweetened	
	Water		
		Wine, red	Wine, white

HERBS, SPICES, & CONDIMENTS	Eat Abundantly	Eat Moderately	Minimize or Eliminate
		Arrowroot	
			Barbecue sauce
		Bragg Liquid Aminos*	
	Broth: vegetable		Broth: beef or chicken

HERBS, SPICES, & CONDIMENTS	Eat Abundantly	Eat Moderately	Minimize or Eliminate
	Fresh & dried herbs/spices: allspice, basil, bay leaves, caraway seed, cardamom, cayenne pepper, celery leaf, celery seed, ground chilis, cinnamon, clove, coriander, cumin, curry, dill, fennel, fenugreek, galangal, garam masala, garlic, ginger, herbs de Provence, kaffir lime leaves, lemongrass, lemon pepper, marjoram, mint, mustard powder, nutmeg, oregano, paprika, parsley, pepper, rosemary, saffron, sage, tarragon, thyme, turmeric		
			Ketchup
			Mayonnaise
	Miso		
		Mustard, prepared	
	Nutritional yeast		
	Pickles, unsweetened		
		Pickle relish	
	Salsa/picante sauce		
		Salt	
	Sauerkraut		
			Soy sauce, commercial*
		Tamari/soy sauce, traditional*	
	Vanilla extract		
	Vinegar: apple cider, red wine, balsamic	Vinegar: grain*, rice wine	
SNACKS	Eat Abundantly	Eat Moderately	Minimize or Eliminate
	Almonds, raw	Almonds, roasted and seasoned	
	Bars: raw fruit and nut (Lärabar, Rawbite, Nakd Nudie, etc.)	Bars: nutrition/health/ protein (Clif, Kind, etc.)	Bars: granola (Chewy, Nature Valley, Quaker, etc.)
			Candy
	Cashews, raw	Cashews, roasted	
			Cheese dip
	Chips: kale		Chips: corn, potato, rice

SNACKS	Eat Abundantly	Eat Moderately	Minimize or Eliminate
		Chocolate, dark	Chocolate, milk
		Crackers: rice or whole-grain flour	Crackers, refined flour
		Fruit, dried	
	Guacamole		
		Gum, xylitol-sweetened	Gum, conventionally sweetened
	Hummus		
	Pistachios		
	Trail Mix		

* Soy, corn, cottonseed, sugar beets, and canola are frequently grown with genetic modification. I recommend going with organic or certified non-GMO for foods made from these crops. I'll discuss why I recommend avoiding GMOs in chapter 25.

** Technically a legume, but often considered an "honorary nut" on account of a nutlike flavor and nutritional profile.

A Word About Animal Products

Industrial meat and dairy production has become a nightmare to the planet, directly using up enormous amounts of fresh water, causing massive water pollution, and producing more greenhouse gases than all the cars, trucks, airplanes, ships, and railroads combined.[3] Its products are relatively cheap, but that low cost is achieved through the systematic abuse of animals and workers as well as the externalization of environmental impact. And consumption of industrial meat and dairy products is strongly linked to higher rates of heart disease, type 2 diabetes, Alzheimer's disease, obesity, some forms of cancer, and most of the other chronic diseases pervasive today.[4] For these and other reasons, many people eschew animal products and base their diets completely, or nearly completely, on plants. However, some people report feeling better and having more energy if they include some animal products in their diets. If you are or might be one of those people, and if you don't have an ethical stand against killing animals for food, I've created this chart to show you how I think various animal products stack up, strictly from a health perspective. I'll discuss this controversial topic in more depth in chapter 29.

FISH & SEAFOOD***	Eat Abundantly	Eat Moderately	Minimize or Eliminate
	Anchovies		
			Bass: sea, striped
		Catfish	

FISH & SEAFOOD***	Eat Abundantly	Eat Moderately	Minimize or Eliminate
			Caviar
			Cod
		Crab	
		Crawfish	
			Eel
		Flounder	
			Grouper
			Haddock
			Halibut
	Herring		
			Lobster
			Mackerel
			Mahi mahi
			Mollusks
			Monkfish
		Mullet	
		Mussels	
			Octopus
		Oysters	
			Pollock
		Prawns	
	Salmon, wild	Salmon, farmed	
	Sardines		
		Scallops	
			Shark
		Shrimp	
			Snapper
		Sole: Dover, petrale	
			Squid
			Sturgeon
			Swordfish
		Tilapia	
			Tilefish
		Trout: rainbow, steelhead	
			Tuna: albacore, ahi, bluefin, yellow
		Whitefish	

*** Fish can be farmed or wild. There are many methods of farming—most of which are high in toxins. If the fish is wild, then it will be heavily impacted by the level of pollution in the water in which it swam. Mercury and other toxins tend to accumulate up the food chain, and many fish are at the top of very long food chains. This chart takes general toxicity levels into account, as well as environmental concerns, concentrations of omega-3 fatty acids, and overall nutritional profile. But it's highly imprecise because there are so many variables. There are also substantial ethical and environmental factors to consider with fish. For a directory of sustainable seafood, visit fishwatch.gov.

EGGS, DAIRY, & DAIRY SUBSTITUTES	Eat Abundantly	Eat Moderately	Minimize or Eliminate
		Butter, pasture-raised cow	
			Buttermilk
		Buttery spreads: Earth Balance, Nutiva coconut oil (buttery flavor)	Buttery spreads: margarine, Smart Balance
	Cheese: cultured nut		Cheese: dairy, soy
		Coconut milk	
			Coffee creamer
			Cottage cheese
		Cream cheese: nut	Cream cheese: dairy
		Eggs, pasture-raised	Eggs, conventional
			Ghee
			Ice cream
			Margarine
	Milk, unsweetened: almond, hemp, oat, or soy*	Milk, sweetened: almond, hemp, oat, pea protein, rice, or soy*	Milk: cow, goat
			Sour cream
			Whipping cream
	Yogurt, unsweetened: almond or coconut	Yogurt: sweetened soy*; unsweetened cow	Yogurt, sweetened: almond, coconut, cow

MEATS & MEAT SUBSTITUTES	Eat Abundantly	Eat Moderately	Minimize or Eliminate
			Bacon
			Beef
		Bison, grass-fed	Bison, conventional
			Canned meats
		Caribou, wild	
			Chicken
			Cured/salted meats
			Dried meats
			Duck
			Ham
			Hot dogs: meat or soy
			Lamb
			Luncheon meats
			Mutton (sheep)
			Pork

MEATS & MEAT SUBSTITUTES	Eat Abundantly	Eat Moderately	Minimize or Eliminate
			Quail
			Rabbit
			Sausage (meat-based and veggie-based)
			Smoked meats
			Spam
	Tempeh, organic*		
	Tofu, organic*		
			Turkey
			Veal
		Veggie burgers	
		Venison (deer, elk)	

* I recommend going with organic or certified non-GMO soy. I'll discuss why in chapter 25.

For a downloadable version of this chart, visit 31dayfoodrevolution.com/chart.

CHAPTER 4

Vote with Your Dollars

I love grocery shopping. There's something fun about roaming the aisles and looking for good foods and great deals. Perhaps it harkens to our ancient history as hunter-gatherers, or for me to my childhood foraging for wild berries on a small Canadian island. Or maybe I just like food.

As a natural-foods advocate, I find it exciting to see the steady expansion in the range of available natural and organic foods. When I was a kid, the only natural-foods store in our town had a tiny (and very expensive) produce section. The only whole-grain breads tasted an awful lot like cardboard. And to be honest, most natural-foods stores were pretty dingy.

My, how things have changed.

In the last few decades, natural and organic foods have become big business. Annual revenues in the United States alone have nearly tripled since 2001, and they now exceed $69 billion.[1] Sales of organic foods in Europe have also been on the rise, exceeding €27 billion in 2015.[2] Healthy food isn't just for hippies anymore, and the corporate food industry is getting in on the action.

But not everything is cheery in Organic Land. Some natural-foods lovers are uncomfortable with the fact that most of their treasured brands have been bought by corporate behemoths.

Clorox bought Burt's Bees. General Mills claimed Cascadian Farm and Muir Glen. Coca-Cola bought Odwalla and Honest Tea. Even Kellogg's got into the buy-up bonanza by purchasing popular brands like Kashi and Gardenburger. In the United States, 80 percent of organic brands are now reportedly owned by megacorporations.[3]

And in 2017, in the most significant purchase in natural-foods industry history, Amazon bought Whole Foods Market for a reported $13.7 billion.[4]

Natural foods are going mainstream, but the mainstream is also entering, and changing, natural foods. Standards are shifting, and increasing numbers of natural brands now incorporate practices and ingredients that might have been unthinkable a few short years ago.[5]

Does this mean there's no longer a difference between, for example, Walmart and Whole Foods? Hardly.

Whole Foods Market states that it considers certain ingredients to be "unacceptable in food." In 2014 Ben Blatt of *Slate* conducted a study to determine how many of the grocery products on a Walmart shelf are banned from Whole Foods. He concluded that Whole Foods banned roughly 54 percent of Walmart's fare.[6] From Minute Maid lemonade to Doritos to Wonder Bread, there were numerous items that Walmart sold and Whole Foods didn't.

Whole Foods may or may not change policies, but as of this writing the company provides a list of 78 items deemed "unacceptable ingredients for foods."[7] This includes everything from high-fructose corn syrup to MSG to chemicals most humans find impossible to pronounce, such as dimethylpolysiloxane.

Does this mean that everything sold at a Whole Foods Market is good for you? Not even close. Recently, I went to the Whole Foods in Santa Cruz, California. In their bakery, they offered dozens of freshly baked breads. How many of the breads made in-house by "Whole" Foods Market contained 100 percent *whole* grains?

None.

But I did find six varieties of freshly made vegan "natural" doughnuts, some gluten-free. These were basically deep-fried sugar and refined flour with added flavoring. They might not include any of the 78 ingredients that the chain has banned, but that hardly makes them a health food.

So if you shop at a store, whether it's Walmart or Whole Foods Market, there's no way around the fact that you need to pay attention—you can't take your health or your safety for granted.

ALTERNATIVE SOLUTIONS ARE ON THE RISE

Shopping at big-box grocery stores isn't the only option. In spite of, or perhaps in part because of, the corporate takeover of the natural and organics industries, new alternatives are springing up. And some of them can be fun!

Some people are growing gardens. (More on that in chapter 28.) And more and more people are choosing farmer's markets, community-supported agriculture, and online retailers.

Farmer's Markets

Between 1994 and 2014, the number of farmer's markets in the United States quadrupled.[8] These markets provide consumers with fresh produce, much of it organically grown and often picked on the day of sale. By eliminating the distributors and the typical grocery store overhead, farmers earn a higher price while consumers may pay a lower one. And the food is definitely fresher.

In the most recently available nationwide survey of 1,400 farmer's market managers in the U.S., most reported steady expansion in sales, number of vendors, and number of customers.[9] In addition, almost three-quarters of farmer's markets now have at least one vendor accepting federal nutrition assistance as payment. Programs like the Supplemental Nutrition Assistance Program (SNAP—also referred to as "food stamps") can expand the customer base for farmers, give recipients access to healthy foods, and encourage the sale of locally sourced produce.

I love walking down the aisle of a farmer's market and meeting the actual people who grew the fruits and vegetables in front of me. I can ask questions about their growing practices, about how the weather is affecting their harvest, and about which variety of peach is the most flavorful this week. I enjoy the feeling of community that emerges as locals gather to support and be nourished by our farmers.

Community-Supported Agriculture

Community-supported agriculture (CSA) programs allow people to purchase seasonal produce directly from local farmers. Typically, a CSA-participating farm will offer a certain number of "shares" to the public and will then commit to grow food for participating members. Community members, in turn, agree to support the farm through financial contributions, typically paid on a steady and recurring basis. Membership dues help pay for seeds and plants, greenhouse expenses, equipment, labor, and other costs related to the workings of the farm. Members receive a weekly or biweekly share of the harvest. Essentially, the community members become shareholders in the farm—and the farm has a consistent source of revenue.

The concept of CSA began in Japan in the mid-1960s and 1970s, in response to consumer concern about the increasing use of pesticides in industrial farming. It began to spread around the world in the 1980s.

Since then, many farms and communities have tailored the model to their own needs. CSAs can operate on very different scales, with some serving just a dozen families and others providing food for more than a thousand households. In France alone in 2016, an estimated 400,000 people enjoyed food from CSA farms.[10]

Some CSAs offer home delivery options, some distribute shares at farmer's markets, and others require members to pick up their shares at the farm. Members at some farms choose what kinds of produce they want in their share each week, while other farms let the weekly harvest dictate what will be included.

Our family belongs to a CSA. Every week, we drop by to collect a box with our share of the week's harvest. We enjoy seeing how foods vary with the seasons. It's fun to get some varieties of lettuce in June, others in July, and still others in October.

Phoenix and I decided to make a family game out of using up each week's order before Wednesday rolled around for our next pickup. Succulent apricots would be gone within minutes. But then there was the time we opened our box to find, along with everything else, three pounds of... celeriac root.

If you're wondering what celeriac is, you're not alone. I like to think that I know a bit about different varieties of vegetables, but I'll be honest—I didn't know what it was. Our sons River and Bodhi researched it online and explained that celeriac is, in fact, the root of the celery plant. Websites describe it as "the ugly root," a "by-product of the celery industry," and even "pig feed."

At first, I was annoyed. I figured that our local farmers were harvesting their celery and trying to get rid of a root that nobody wanted. And worse yet, because of our family game, we had to figure out some way to eat it.

River and Bodhi saved the day. They Googled celeriac recipes, and before long I was peeling and chopping it up by the pound—so we could add it to soups, stir-fries, and salads.

The challenge of incorporating a new food brought creativity and a spirit of adventure to our family. And only later did I learn that celeriac is one of the healthiest foods around. It's been linked to benefits for digestion, heart health, bone health, and even your immune system.[11]

I love that our local CSA brought us a new experience and helped our family to bond around healthy food. I like that being part of a CSA keeps our family connected to the local environment and the seasons, reduces food transportation, supports local commerce, and provides farmers with financial security. And sometimes, with a bit of luck, it adds a splash of adventure.

You might even find that if you're exposed to a new food, you wind up making a new friend. Sarah Medlicott of Santa Cruz, California, learned of Freewheelin' Farm, a CSA that delivers produce to its members on bicycle. She signed up, and immediately discovered the joys of delicata squash. Having never been exposed to this delicious squash before, Sarah found multiple ways to prepare it—including roasting, baking, and blending into soup. Sarah soon became known as the delicata queen, bringing this roasted veggie to numerous social gatherings.

If you're in the United States, you can get information on CSA programs, and help finding one near you, by visiting localharvest.org/csa.

Shopping Online

More and more people are shopping for food online. It doesn't support local business, but it does provide compelling convenience. And while delivery trucks have a problematic environmental impact, this is balanced by the savings generated by customers not driving to the store and by retailers not needing to keep a brightly lit and climate-controlled storefront open for business.[12] Delivered foods come in boxes, and some people worry about the environmental impact of all the packaging. But retailers go through a massive quantity of boxes, too. It's just that consumers never see them.

While Amazon is pushing hard to dominate online grocery sales, it's facing stiff competition from Thrive Market, another company with a different set of goals. Amazon aims to be the "everything store." But Thrive Market was founded for a very different purpose: to make healthy food accessible and affordable for everyone.

Thrive Market uses a membership-based online model to sell more than 4,000 nonperishable natural, non-GMO, and organic foods for wholesale prices. By financing its core operations with membership fees, Thrive Market is able to pass heavily discounted food prices on to its members. And by providing screening for criteria such as organic, gluten-free, soy-free, raw, vegan, and Paleo, the store makes it relatively easy to see what you want without being tempted to buy anything that doesn't fit with your food priorities. Thus far it doesn't offer fresh fruits and vegetables, so Thrive Market isn't a "one-stop shop," but it does pair well with a CSA, farmer's market, or vegetable garden.

In keeping with its mission to democratize access to healthy food for low-income communities and people living in "food deserts," for every paid membership, Thrive Market gives a free membership to a person of low income through a program called Thrive Gives.

Sharon, a Thrive Gives member, is a single mother of three. She works full-time as a registered nurse. When he was an infant, her now 12-year-old son suffered a brain injury, and he's required special care ever since, making it hard for Sharon to support her family of four on her own. But Thrive Gives has made it possible for her to afford healthy organic food. This makes a tangible, positive difference for her peace of mind and her family's well-being.

So far, Thrive Market is available only in the United States. You can find out more and get a free trial membership at 31dayfoodrevolution.com/thrive.

ACTION:

Option 1: List all the places you shop for groceries. Rank them based on how much of your total budget you think you spend in each establishment. Decide whether your list feels congruent with your values and goals.

Option 2: Find at least one food outlet that you haven't used before (such as a natural-foods store, farmer's market, or online food source like Thrive Market) and buy something healthy from it.

Option 3: Join (or help start) a CSA membership program and initiate a regular flow of healthy foods into your life.

CHAPTER 5

Build Healthy Eating Habits

Not long ago, Josh LaJaunie of Thibodaux, Louisiana, was en route to a family vacation when he was told that, due to his size, the small plane he was on could only fly safely if he moved closer to the front. When he got home, Josh stepped on the scale and got an error message, because it couldn't measure above 400 pounds.

Knowing that obesity and heart disease ran in his family, Josh realized that his life was on a very dangerous path. He set about making major changes, trading in hamburgers for vegetables. Before long, Josh had released 230 pounds. And incredibly, he became an ultramarathon runner. In 2016, Josh competed in a one-hundred-mile race and landed on the cover of *Runner's World*. Today, Josh is a local celebrity in his Louisiana town and a passionate advocate for healthy habits.

But we all know it can take more than knowledge to change old habits. Have you ever gotten inspired about a new choice or decision—only to look back months later and realize you didn't follow through? Have you ever resolved to stop eating a certain food, or to work out regularly, or to stop snacking...but after a while, the force of old habits won out?

Habits develop when you stick with the same routine for a long time. And they can be powerful. Over millennia, a steady flow of water in the same place carved the mile-deep Grand Canyon.

THE FAILURE OF THE WEIGHT-LOSS INDUSTRY

There may be no domain in which habits are harder to break than those that impact weight loss. Hundreds of millions of people feel trapped by habits and addictions that seem to keep pulling them away from the right-sized body they desire.

Recently I was speaking at an event in San Francisco. Afterward, a woman named Jen came up to me. In her mid-fifties, she'd been eating what she thought was a healthy diet for 23 years. Yet she continued to struggle with weight problems. She'd tried dozens of diets, cleanses, supplements, and protocols but always wound up where she'd started—still overweight, with just as many cravings and a little less hope.

Jen's story is all too common.

More than half of Europeans, and more than two-thirds of Americans, are overweight or obese.[1] Right now more than 108 million Americans are on a diet.[2] Nevertheless, fewer than 1 percent of diets result in successful and sustained weight loss.[3]

Is there any other domain in which so many people try so hard and so often, yet experience so few positive results?

WHY WILLPOWER USUALLY ISN'T ENOUGH

For many years I believed, as many people still do, that weight problems stemmed from a lack of willpower. I thought that if people knew what to do and stuck with it, then their habits would change and their excess pounds would melt away for good.

But for people prone to food addiction, lasting weight loss takes a lot more than willpower or desire. Many problems can be solved by the application of intelligence, ambition, motivation, and perseverance. Often, though, that just isn't true for weight issues. Think about this: Every year a million diabetic people worldwide undergo a limb amputation surgery because they're unable to make the dietary changes that could reverse their condition.[4]

New York Times bestselling author Susan Peirce Thompson, PhD, a brain and cognitive scientist and adjunct associate professor at the University of Rochester, spent two decades studying the root causes of the obesity epidemic. She concluded that our most popular programs are fundamentally flawed because they depend in large part on sustained willpower. That approach will fail, she explains, because all of us have a very limited pool of willpower from which to draw. The average person makes many dozens of food-related choices per day. If you're relying on willpower to navigate all of them successfully, you're set up for failure.

It's when you're tired, on automatic pilot, or under a lot of stress that you're most susceptible to cravings and addictions. When it comes to breaking unhealthful habits, how you show up at the hardest times is what really matters. Because all it takes is a moment of slipping up, and you might slide right back to where you started.

IT'S HOW YOUR BRAIN IS WIRED

Jordan Gaines Lewis, PhD, explains how neuroscientists recognize that in order for us to survive as a species, things like caring for others, eating, and reproducing must be pleasurable to the brain so that these behaviors will be repeated.[5]

When you do something pleasurable, such as eating a piece of chocolate, your brain releases the neurotransmitter dopamine, particularly in areas called the nucleus accumbens and the prefrontal cortex. The prefrontal cortex is what governs many of your more sophisticated thoughts and decisions—such as determining whether or not to take another bite of that delicious chocolate. The release of dopamine anchors the pleasure-reward cycle into your brain, reminding you to repeat a positive behavior. Now your body will know that the chocolate tastes really good—and it will remember this important reality in the future.

The brain is extraordinarily skilled at convincing you that you need to do what it has been wired to think is in your best interests.

If you want to test how this works, imagine that I offer you $1,000 if you can hold your breath for two minutes. You'll likely start off feeling reasonably comfortable. Two minutes, after all, isn't terribly long. It's not likely to kill anyone. But if you manage to reach past one minute, you'll probably begin to be flooded with anxiety.

Your survival won't be threatened. Your body probably has more than enough oxygen stored for you to live another minute. But evolutionary wiring far beneath your conscious mind will have your brain sending signals of life-threatening urgency. Wait a little longer, and the intensity of those signals will rise exponentially.

The point is that eating is like breathing. You're hard-wired to need it. And sooner or later your brain will convince you to eat, one way or the other.

Most of us prefer sweet foods over bitter ones because, in the course of evolution, the human brain learned that sweet things provide a healthy source of rapid energy. When our ancestors scavenged for berries, sour meant "not yet ripe" and bitter often meant "poisonous." Sweet not only tasted pleasurable, but it also provided a burst of blood sugar that led our brains to activate the release of dopamine. And this remains true.

THE MODERN WORLD HAS CHANGED EVERYTHING

In the modern world, the challenge is that we've gone quite a way beyond ripe berries. The average American eats more than 77 pounds of added sugar per year.[6] And most people in developed countries aren't far behind, consuming more than 50 pounds of added sugar annually.

Our evolutionary history has left us utterly unprepared for the onslaught of brain-stimulating pleasure that the industrialized food industry provides.

Sugar addiction hijacks the brain's reward pathway in a manner very similar to the way that cocaine, heroin, and alcohol addiction function. But there's one critical difference. Most of us don't start on cocaine, heroin, or alcohol in infancy, whereas most of us feed our kids added sugar starting close to day one. Some mothers give their babies Coke in baby bottles. (Both Coca-Cola and Pepsi happily sell baby bottles with their corporate logos prominently displayed.) The addictive response is being wired into little ones before they can even talk.

Today, neuroscientists are discovering that for food addicts, it's not only sugar that's driving their struggles.[7] Flour, too, plays a critical role. The simple act of grinding grain causes an exponential increase in particle surface area. This means that flour—even whole wheat flour—can be digested very rapidly, changing to sugar almost immediately. A healthy insulin response will enable the body to adapt—but not before the brain has released dopamine and sent out the message, "Yes! This is great! Do it again!" (Flours higher in protein or fat and lower in carbohydrates, such as those made from legumes, almonds, or coconut, have a bit of the same problem, though it's much milder.)

Powerful addiction triggers are fortified by a society that celebrates birthdays and weddings with cake and rewards children with doughnuts and candy. From the beginning of our lives, we're conditioned to associate junk foods with pleasure, self-care, and celebration.

MY FIRST SUGAR STORY

When I was seven years old, my mom and dad started to drop me off for birthday parties at the houses of my fellow second-graders, and in the process, I was exposed to foods that I didn't normally eat.

One day, I decided to try a piece of the chocolate cake that my friends were eating, and I was stunned to discover how good it tasted.

I was a little nervous to tell my dad, because I didn't know what he would think. But I summoned the courage later that day, and with my voice shaking a little, I confessed what I'd eaten.

He said that he loved me no matter what I ate and would always thank me for telling him the truth. Emboldened, I took the plunge and added that the cake tasted pretty delicious.

My dad replied that he knew only too well how tasty sugar could be, considering that he'd grown up eating more ice cream than probably any kid who ever lived. He suggested I try an experiment. The next time I was at a party, I could observe how eating cake affected everyone's moods and see if it led to any change in behavior. Feeling a bit like an undercover investigator, I agreed.

The next time I went to a birthday party, everyone was having a great time. Then the cake came out, and all the kids enjoyed it.

But then I noticed something. Within about 10 minutes, a bunch of fighting erupted. Nathan and Jeremy had been playing Ping-Pong, and they didn't want to let anyone else have a turn, which made Susan and Penny start screaming at them. Quarrels erupted over how much cake everyone had gotten, and over who was responsible for breaking Seth's Chewbacca action figure. Some kids were crying, and pandemonium was breaking out.

I repeated this experiment several more times as different kids had their birthday parties, and each time I observed similar outcomes. The scientific explanation might have been that my classmates were experiencing a blood sugar spike that caused an insulin response, triggering mood instability. But as a seven-year-old, I summed it all up in five words: "Cake causes fighting and misery."

A BRIGHT LINE SOLUTION

In 2014, Dr. Susan Peirce Thompson founded Bright Line Eating. Since 2015, I've had the privilege of joining forces with her to share her message on a global scale. We've organized a series of eight-week online programs, called Boot Camps, which she's led and which have guided more than 7,000 people into releasing over 100,000 pounds.

Most remarkable of all, most of Susan's program participants experience sustained and continued weight loss after the Boot Camp. Thousands report not only continuing to lose weight but also getting off diabetes and blood pressure medications, lowering their LDL cholesterol and triglyceride levels, and feeling more energetic.

One of those people turns out to be Jen, who you may recall came up to thank me at my event in San Francisco. You see, Jen didn't just share her struggles. She also told me about a tremendous victory. Jen had heard from me about Susan's work and signed up for one of Susan's programs. In two years, Jen had released 50 pounds and overcome cravings she'd thought she could never shake. "I have my life back," she told me, "and I can't tell you how much that means to me."

What's the key curriculum that Susan promotes? At its core is the recognition that if you're highly susceptible to the addictive pull of unhealthy foods, you probably need to draw some "bright lines" with food, just as drug addicts must draw bright lines with their drug of choice—lines they commit to never crossing. The major lines that Susan encourages her addiction-prone clients to draw are:

1. No sugar
2. No flour
3. No snacking outside of official, planned meals
4. No seconds after ample firsts

For many people, especially those with an addictive relationship to unhealthy food, following bright lines doesn't feel like restriction, it feels like freedom. After Susan's eight-week Boot Camp, 97 percent of participants report that they have little to no food cravings anymore, 88 percent report that their peace and serenity with food has increased, and 86 percent report feeling confident that they will finally reach and maintain their goals.

> To find out more about Susan's work, or to take her online quiz to discover how susceptible you are to food addiction, go to 31dayfoodrevolution.com/foodquiz.

After years of cyclical dieting, self-sabotage, and steady weight gain, Angela D'Amico of Syracuse, New York, found herself weighing nearly 400 pounds—trapped in a body that made it difficult for her to breathe, move, or sleep. Overwhelmed, overworked, and overstressed, Angela faced that she had developed a life-threatening addiction to food. She resolved to move toward a clean diet, to give up sugar, and to never eat when she was angry, lonely, or tired.

It took discipline to establish new bright-line habits, but once they were in place, Angela found it got easier and easier to stick with them. Now, whenever cravings set in, the first thing Angela does is move her body. Exercise distracts her from the addictive pull and resets her brain in a positive direction. She's released more than 150 pounds so far, and while she has a ways to go, she's grateful to be on the right track.

Whatever habits you're trying to shift, bright lines and positive alternatives can help. Some people adopt different ones at home than when traveling. For example, I have a friend who's 100 percent vegan at home, but sometimes when he's at restaurants, he'll order fish. Another friend only spends her money on 100 percent organic and non-GMO foods. But if she's at a friend's house for dinner, she eats (almost) whatever is served.

Clarify the rules of the game you want to play, and then follow through and play it well.

Ginny Trierweiler of Denver, Colorado, was 65 pounds overweight when she decided to cut out all sugars, flours, and alcohol. She knew it was going to be a challenge, so she went to a hypnotherapist who, at her request, helped her to view sweet foods through a negative lens. Ginny essentially trained her brain to see those foods as toxic and disgusting.

It worked! Ginny's been sugar-, flour-, and alcohol-free for two years. She's lost 66 pounds and has dropped from a size 16–18 to a size 6, which she hasn't been since high school. She's gained tremendous vitality and confidence—and she's even dating again.

Not everyone is going to want to work with a hypnotherapist. But Ginny's story is a powerful illustration of the power of the brain to support (or hinder) sustainable habit change.

Pathways to Positive Habit Change

- Restructure your environment to remove temptation. This might mean getting rid of certain foods or activities in your home. Minimize your exposure to regressive influences.
- Make clear commitments, with unambiguous bright lines. These may get more tangible if you tell a friend or write them down. Could you give up flour and sugar for a whole day? How about a week? A month?
- Ask loved ones to support (or at least respect) your commitments. Find nonthreatening ways to share boundaries. For instance, you might say, "I'm choosing not to eat anything with sugar."
- Commit to staying with your plan for 31 days. Many neuroscientists believe that if you can stick with a new habit for a month, it will begin to take root in your life.
- Leave notes in conspicuous places or create calendar alerts for things you want to remember (or avoid) at certain times of the day.
- Spend time with people you want to emulate. When you surround yourself with positive role models, they'll pull you along your path.
- If you're obese or struggling with food addiction, you may want to participate in one of the programs offered by Dr. Susan Peirce Thompson. You'll find not only a proven road map you can follow, but also a potent community of peer support.

ACTION:

Option 1: Identify one "bad" habit you'd like to change. Apply what you've learned in this chapter to come up with a strategy for implementing the change.

Option 2: For 24 hours, avoid consuming any added sugar or flour products. Can you do it? (Note how you feel. Flu-like symptoms can sometimes be a sign of withdrawal from this hugely underestimated addiction.)

Option 3: Give up all sugar and flour for a set period of time. My time recommendation, if you really want results, is 31 days. (If you don't think you can do this, you might check out Susan's quiz at 31dayfoodrevolution.com/foodquiz to see if you're addicted to food.) At the end of your sugar-and-flour-free period, check in with your body. If you're craving sugar or flour products, chances are you need to stay with the practice longer. Or you might be someone who can add them in judiciously without getting sucked down the addiction rabbit hole.

CHAPTER 6

You Deserve a Toxin-Free Home

We all know that toxins lurk in many modern foods. But there are other insidious sources of toxins that may be entering your mouth every day. They can come from your pots, pans, food storage containers...and even your water.

NONSTICK DOESN'T MEAN NONTOXIC

Nonstick cookware has become popular because, well, it keeps foods from sticking—making it convenient to use and to clean. But did you know that when it's overheated, most of the nonstick cookware in widespread use emits toxic fumes?

Manufacturers' labels often warn consumers to avoid high heat when cooking with Teflon and other nonstick materials.[1] But tests commissioned by the Environmental Working Group show that in just two to five minutes on a typical stove, cookware coated with Teflon and other nonstick materials could exceed temperatures at which the coating breaks apart and consequently emits toxic particles and gases.[2]

Avian (bird) veterinarians have known for decades that many forms of nonstick cookware, including those that are Teflon-coated, can produce fumes that are dangerous to pet birds.[3] As early as 1986, a Chicago-area expert on "Teflon toxicosis" called the phenomenon a "leading cause of death among birds," estimating that hundreds of pet birds are killed by the fumes and particles emitted from Teflon-coated products each year.[4]

Have you ever heard of the "canary in the coal mine"? Birds can be more sensitive to dangerous gases than humans—but if something is lethal to birds, then it doesn't take a coal miner to guess that it probably isn't good for you or me, either.

Aluminum cookware can present problems, too. Studies show the metal can leach into foods, especially when you're cooking tomato products or other acidic foods.

So what are the alternatives?

If you're steaming or boiling food, you don't really need your pot to be nonstick coated. And for frying pans, there are a few options that seem substantially safer than Teflon and many of the other nonstick pans.

Some people like stainless steel, but my experience is that food tends to stick to it unless you use a lot of oil. Others love cast iron. If that's your thing, terrific. But cast iron is heavy and takes some maintenance. And while eating a certain amount of iron can be a good thing, many people with cast-iron pans get too much of it, which can become a problem.[5]

There are new types of nonstick pans coming out all the time. My current favorites are enamel-coated cast iron and ceramic-coated cookware. Both of these are highly effective in preventing food from sticking, without the toxins found in most nonstick pans.

WHAT ABOUT FOOD STORAGE CONTAINERS?

Storing leftovers is wonderful. Unfortunately, most modern kitchens are stocked with plastic food storage containers (and plastic water bottles) that leach bisphenol A (BPA).[6]

BPA is a known hormone disrupter and has been linked to obesity, diabetes, cardiovascular disease, asthma, cancer, infertility, low sperm count, liver problems, and ADHD.[7]

As news started coming out about the dangers of BPA, many manufacturers began phasing this nasty chemical out of their products. At first that seemed like a good thing. But then the National Institutes of Health funded research on BPA-free plastics.[8] They found that "almost all" commercially available plastics that were tested leached synthetic estrogens—even when the plastics weren't exposed to conditions known to unlock potentially harmful chemicals, such as the heat of a microwave oven, the steam of a dishwasher, or the sun's ultraviolet rays. According to this NIH-funded research, some BPA-free products released synthetic estrogens that were even more potent than BPA.

At this point, we don't have reliably safe forms of plastic to use for food storage. If you need to use plastic containers, I advise against storing highly acidic foods such as tomato products in them, and never expose them to direct sunlight, put them in the dishwasher, or add hot foods to them.

Our family used to love plastic food-storage containers, but my wife and I didn't want to expose any of us to synthetic estrogens. So one day we bit the bullet and threw out all but a few backup plastic containers. We ordered glass and stainless-steel ones, and I'm glad we did.

Today just might be your day to do that, too.

We do most of our food storage in glass containers that come with clear snap-on plastic lids. For traveling, I prefer airtight stainless-steel containers with snap-on lids that have a silicone seal (like the kind made by Onyx) because they're lighter and more break-proof than glass. But unless you're Superman and have X-ray vision, you can't see through these, which is why I prefer glass at home because it helps to keep the fridge organized when you can see your food.

BE WATER SAFE

Drinking plenty of clean water is one of the top things you and I can do to boost our health. But hundreds of millions of people don't have access to an adequate, safe supply.

For many people in developing countries, the biggest problem is that most of the water is contaminated with bacterial pathogens. Worldwide, contaminated water causes more than a million deaths each year, mostly from diarrheal diseases.[9]

Many cities and developed regions have water-treatment systems that rely heavily on chlorination. When chlorine was first introduced to the water supply, it brought a rapid reduction in the spread of disease and other waterborne ailments. Chlorination made it easier for cities and towns to purify drinking water, and it helped keep residents safe.

It's better to have chlorine in our public drinking water than to risk widespread bacterial contamination. But there's a dark side to mass chlorination.[10] According to research published in *Environmental Health Perspectives*, the by-products of chlorine are associated with an increased risk of bladder and rectal cancers.[11] A 2008 study based on an analysis of nearly 400,000 infants in Taiwan found that when pregnant women drank water that contained chlorine, there was an increase in the risk of them having children with heart problems, cleft palates, or major brain defects.[12] Still other studies have found a possible correlation between chlorinated water and increased rates of heart disease.[13]

I wish I could tell you that chlorine was the biggest water danger in the industrialized world. But it's not.

In 2015, Flint, Michigan, suddenly dominated the news with headlines describing the high levels of lead in the drinking water.[14] Lead can disrupt brain cells, lower IQ, and foster learning disabilities and behavioral problems in children.

Despite all the attention on Flint, it isn't the only area with a lead problem—not by a long shot. According to an investigation published in the *Washington Post* in 2016, "Lead taints water across the U.S., EPA records show."[15] The report went on to describe that an estimated 20 percent of the water systems in the United States have unsafe levels of lead. Among these water systems, 350 day care centers and schools failed lead tests a total of 470 times between 2012 and 2015. In New Jersey alone, 11 cities had even more dangerously high lead levels than Flint.

Is this problem limited to the United States? No. According to a 2014 story in the *Irish Times*, lead contamination levels up to 80 times the legal limit were detected in drinking water in Dublin.[16] And an estimated 40 percent of properties in the United Kingdom are connected to the water supply main by lead pipes that are leaching lead into municipal drinking water.[17]

Chlorine and lead aren't the only contaminants that we need to be concerned about. Recent tests have found that chromium-6, the cancer-causing chemical made famous in the movie *Erin Brockovich*, is contaminating the water supplies that more than 200 million Americans depend upon.[18] Despite these tests, lobbying from industry and utility companies has prevented strong regulations that would bring the chromium-6 levels down into safe zones.

As if chlorine, lead, and chromium-6 weren't serious enough, studies also show that our water supplies can contain a variety of other toxic chemicals, including drug residues such as antibiotics, antidepressants, hormones from birth control pills, and painkillers.[19]

Want to test your tap water to find out what's in it? You can call local water authorities to ask if they can recommend a trustworthy independent lab. Local labs may be able to advise you on what you should be testing for given the particular concerns in your area. Once you've done a thorough one-time test, you'll have a basis for deciding what (if anything) to test for on an ongoing basis.

BOTTLED WATER

One of the popular solutions is to purchase bottled water. Consumers worldwide are buying more than 20,000 bottles of water every second, at a cost of more than $170 billion per year.[20]

But bottled water isn't always as safe as we might like to think. In some cases, it's merely high-priced tap water encased in plastic. And it gets expensive. One person drinking eight glasses of bottled water per day might spend $400 to $1,600 on it each year.

What about the plastic bottles containing the water? Thousands of chemical additives (often including BPA) are used in the manufacture of plastics. When these plastics are heated, which can happen when they are washed in hot water or left in a hot car, they have been found to leach some of these chemicals.[21] Bottled water often travels many miles and through a range of climates, so the chance of it being heated at some point on its journey is very real.

Disposal of plastic bottles also poses a risk for the environment. Fewer than half of the bottles bought in 2016 were collected for recycling, and just 7 percent of those collected were made into new bottles.[22] Most plastic bottles ended up in landfills, incinerators, or, worse yet, the ocean.

WHAT'S THE WATER SOLUTION?

Creating a truly safe and clean water supply for billions of people is difficult. Even if water is clean at its source or is purified perfectly in a plant, during the time it flows through many miles of pipes and into a home, it can easily pick up contamination. For this reason, filtering water right in your home is usually the best way for you to protect yourself and your loved ones.

Establishing a reliable source of clean water is one of the best things you can do for your health. In our home, we use a reverse osmosis water filter system. But there are also strong arguments (and passionate advocates) for carbon, distilled, and many other water filtration options. To download a report with my review of the available options, visit 31day foodrevolution.com/wateroptions.

In our house we keep a supply of stainless steel water bottles on hand, so any time we're going out, we can bring along a bottle of water, tea, or some other drink. Personally, I love sparkling water—so much so that I bought a home carbonation system, and now I can make "bubbly water" for a few pennies per liter. Sparkling water with ice and a squeeze of lemon or a splash of red grape juice is one of my favorite drinks with dinner.

But what about the 700 million people in the world who don't have access to safe water or, frankly, any water at all? Instead of working or going to school, many women and girls must spend hours every day traveling on foot to fetch their family dirty water in barrels and drums.

Last year, Food Revolution Network raised more than $50,000 in support of Charity: Water, which helps to lift communities out of sickness and poverty by building wells, thus saving millions of lives and freeing up girls to go to school or make a living. And we intend to raise a lot more in the years to come. Find out more about this organization's inspiring story, and if you like, pitch in too, at 31dayfoodrevolution.com/charitywater.

ACTIONS (YOU CAN DO ALL OF THESE!):

Option 1: Get rid of Teflon or other conventional nonstick cookware in your kitchen. Replace it with cast-iron, enamel-coated cast-iron, or ceramic-coated cookware.

Option 2: Discard plastic water bottles and food storage containers, replacing them with glass or stainless steel. (Word to the wise: Get a good bottle brush to clean your bottles well!)

Option 3: Get a good water treatment system that fits your budget and enables your family to have a steady flow of delicious water you can trust. You can download my review of water filtration options at 31dayfoodrevolution.com/wateroptions.

CHAPTER 7

How to Make a Happy, Healthy Kitchen

From the earliest days I can remember, I've loved food. When I was 10, I went so far as to start a home bakery. I called it Ocean's Bakery and sold natural and organic baked goods. Every day after school, I'd make bran muffins, banana bread, carrot cake, whole wheat bread, or other goodies. Then I'd bag up my wares and head off with my little red wagon, selling door-to-door around the neighborhood. I had more than 100 customers and even landed on the front page of my local paper, the *Santa Cruz Sentinel*, under the headline "Boy Isn't Very Rich, But He's Got Dough."

As a man, and as the father of twin sons, I've always felt that food should not be the domain of only women. Men can cook and nurture, too. I believe that if there were more men and boys learning to cook, we'd have stronger and more cohesive families.

We live in a time when sexual harassment of women, normalized for far too long, is finally being exposed. Sometimes the process is messy, but in my view, the movement to end harassment and objectification is vitally important.

The gendering of kitchen life is another domain in which our society has some long overdue room for growth. I have male friends who act as if cooking is unmanly. But what's manly about not knowing how to prepare food? No matter what your gender identity is, knowing how to feed yourself and your family good food can be empowering. And in a toxic food culture, it can even be an essential skill for survival.

AND IT DOES TAKE TIME

One thing that's in short supply these days for everyone, of every gender and age, is time. Most people want more time to sleep and more time to play and share with loved ones. And a surprising number want more time to cook.

But it can be hard when you feel stressed just trying to address the bare essentials. Some days feel like a never-ending series of reactions to the demands of people and circumstances beyond your control.

It's amazing how often healthy eating can be one of the first casualties of a triage-filled life. When we're faced with too much to do and too little time to do it, we tend to fall back into old habits. Because we live in a food culture that's often toxic, for many of us our old habits around food can be downright dangerous.

Unless you happen to be rich, our industrialized food system doesn't make it especially easy to do the best thing for your health or your family. Most of our "fast foods" and "convenience foods" are junk foods.

Sure, there are expensive options for people who don't mind spending an arm and a leg for convenient nutrition. Some folks partake of things like the vegetable- and sprouted-seed crackers that my local natural-foods store sells for $11 per five-ounce package. (For the math whizzes, that comes to somewhere north of $34 a pound.) But assuming you're like most humans in the world and have a limited amount of money as well as time, it becomes important to bring affordable efficiency into your life. That way, no matter how busy you get, your health doesn't have to suffer.

Over the last 25 years, I've seen where people get stuck. And I've also seen some simple solutions that save time and money. Here are my favorites. Are you already applying them?

GO BIG

When you buy staple foods in bulk, you don't have to shop as often. The difference between shopping twice a week and shopping every day could save you hours otherwise spent driving, parking, and waiting in line to check out. (Buying in bulk generally requires a car, so if you don't have one, you may want to borrow one, rent a Zipcar, or take a Lyft, Uber, or taxi on shopping day.)

Prepare food in quantity, maybe on the weekend, so you have ready-to-heat meals in your fridge or freezer. Store individual servings in stainless steel or glass containers and you have lunch or a quick dinner ready to go! When you make a soup or casserole, making a larger amount doesn't increase clean-up time much. The bonus is that leftovers can keep you fed for days.

Ginny from Colorado prepares three or four days' worth of salads twice each week, and a week's worth of roasted vegetables every weekend. In her salads, she combines lettuce, carrots, celery, radishes, peppers, purple cabbage, cut tomatoes, cucumbers, beetroots, and a nut (usually pistachios). She roasts brussels sprouts, beetroots, carrots, parsnips, and butternut squash. She loves having a giant colorful salad for lunch every day and coming home to delicious roasted vegetables for dinner.

And now, a word on behalf of leftovers. Many of us think of them as second-rate. But delicious food stored properly in the fridge or freezer can be a way of "paying it forward" with an abundance of health. Think of it as a bit like putting money in a savings account. You're expressing thoughtfulness and foresight that you can draw on later, in the midst of a busy week.

PREPARE BREAKFAST AND LUNCH BEFORE BEDTIME

I don't know about you, but my mornings are hectic. Once I get out of bed, it's a race to get everyone fed and in motion, to jump in the shower and scramble to pull together food for the day, and then I'm off to work.

I'd be willing to bet you don't spend your mornings lounging around watching the drapes fade, either.

For most people, morning isn't a great time to spend hours in the kitchen. This is why Phoenix and I love to prepare food the night before.

In our home, dinner typically includes a big salad, steamed vegetables, and an entrée. Occasionally we'll add a dessert.

Cleaning up from dinner can be a perfect time to pack up lunch for the next day. Most of my lunches (and more than a few of my breakfasts!) consist of dinner leftovers.

I often eat at least a meal or two each day at my desk. I'm not recommending this as the optimal way to absorb nutrition. I'm just sharing that I live in the real world, and sometimes that works best for me. A healthy meal, often prepared the night before, nourishes me even when my attention is on all sorts of other things.

And that, ultimately, is the key. You want to be doing good things even when you aren't paying attention. Healthy habits make it easier and easier to do the right thing, day in and day out.

This might sound obvious or mundane. But sometimes we can get so enamored with newfangled things that we forget the basics. Packing a good meal isn't exactly on the cutting edge of dietary innovation. But in the end, it just might do more for your long-term health than an army of modern hospital surgeons, which you may never need if you treat your body right in the first place.

BE SHOPPING-LIST SMART

The simple act of making and sticking with a shopping list can save you significant money. How?

First of all, people who use shopping lists typically waste less food. And that's a big deal, because collectively, we waste more than you probably imagined. Every year, Americans throw away 70 billion pounds of food, worth more than $165 billion (with a *b*).[1] That adds up to an average of $2,200 per year for an average family of four. European habits are a little better, but Europeans still waste 22 million tons of food annually.[2]

People with shopping lists are also less likely to make impulse purchases. Have you ever gone to the store to get one thing but ended up buying a bunch of other stuff? Or added something to your basket while waiting to check out?

Most grocery retailers design their store layout methodically, with the goal of tempting customers into impulse buying. They place some of their top impulse-fueling products with the highest markups, such as candy, chips, and soda, in locations that everyone will pass.

If you don't fall prey to the tactic of impulse-provocative marketing, you'll avoid some of the least healthy foods while achieving financial benefit. Researchers from the University of Pennsylvania found that people who make it a habit to steer clear of impulse spending can wind up saving up to 23 percent on their grocery bills.[3] A family that spends $1,000 per month on food could save as much as $230 every month—simply by avoiding this shopping hazard.

Between not wasting money on impulse purchases and steering clear of food waste, a family can save hundreds of dollars every month. My favorite tool to support this goal is the mighty shopping list. Here are three very different ways to implement a shopping list system.

Smart Shopping List Version 1: Paper and Pen

This is absurdly simple—but it works. Secure a piece of paper to your fridge with magnets, buy a magnetic pad and put it up on your fridge, or keep a pad on a counter. Record needed items throughout the week, and take the list with you when you go shopping.

Smart Shopping List Version 2: The Master List with Checkboxes

Create a master list of all the things you typically buy, organized by different zones of the store, such as Produce, Freezer, Bulk, and so on, with a checkbox preceding each item in each category. Print copies and post one somewhere convenient. When you run out of something, simply check the appropriate box. Take your list to navigate the store, zone by zone.

You can download the version my family sometimes uses at 31day foodrevolution.com/shoppinglist and customize it for your preferences.

Smart Shopping List Version 3: The Menu Planner

There are many solid online menu-planning applications. For example, BigOven.com lets you search an index of more than 350,000 recipes by main ingredient, type of cuisine, special considerations, preparation method, season/occasion, and course/dish. All recipes come with ratings, user reviews, and nutrient information. The app lets you select and add reci-pes to a simple yet powerful meal-planning calendar, and then add needed ingredients, with quantities factored in, to your grocery list with one click. You can take the app to the store and let it guide you through different zones as you check off items. Or choose any app that you prefer. This technology boost can help you discover how easy and fun menu planning can be.

MAKE YOUR KITCHEN A HAPPY PLACE

Okay, let me ask you a question: How often do you cook?

Life happens, we get busy, and we wind up scrounging, snacking, eat-ing out, or dumping a can of prepared soup in a pot. How much time do you think you actually spend preparing food in your kitchen?

And how do you feel about that? With all your various priorities and values, does it seem like the right amount? Would you like it to be more? Or less?

The answers will be different for each of us. The more aware you are of how things are, and of how you'd like them to be, the more likely it is that you can create the life, and the lifestyle, that you desire.

Now I'm curious how you feel when you prepare food. Do you feel stressed and hassled, as if you're trying to do too many things at once? Or are you calm and happy? Right now, when you picture yourself prepar-ing food, what feelings and images come to mind?

And one final question: How would you *like* to feel while prepar-ing food? Do you want to feel confident that you're doing the right thing for your family? Do you want to be relaxed, clear, and on task? Do you want to feel spaciousness—that you have enough time to enjoy the experience?

These are some things Food Revolution members told me they do to add vibrancy and beauty to their kitchen lives:

- Patricia Stevens says: "I play Debbie Gibson's 'Only in My Dreams,'" and a kitchen dance party ensues.
- If dishes are dirty, Anjali Bhavanani will wash them so she has a clean space to start cooking. (Somehow, her kitchen never stays clean for long—but she still loves to start with a clean slate!)

- April Hansen likes to prepare meals with her family, so that the process can be a source of connection and bonding.
- Adele Mandagie starts off with a prayer. Some people light incense or turn on an aromatherapy diffuser or pour themselves a glass of sparkling water to start things off in a fun way.

Maybe some of these will work for you—and maybe they won't. My advice is that you make your kitchen the happiest place it can be. McDonald's might have tried to co-opt the term, but I think that real happy meals come from a healthy, fun kitchen.

Once you've got your home environment set up to support your healthy eating path, it's time to focus on enjoying delicious food. In Part Two, we'll look at how you can optimally nourish your body. I want you to have all the insight you need about what to eat—and what not to eat—to fight disease, lose weight, and thrive. I'm also going to dispel some damaging and widely held myths, so you can know what the science actually says about some of the most controversial, and important, food topics of our times.

ACTION:

Option 1: Before you go to bed tonight, make a delicious and healthy breakfast for tomorrow.

Option 2: Make a big pot or casserole of something healthy, and freeze some to "pay it forward."

Option 3: Upgrade your shopping list system to optimize how organized and efficient it is. A few minutes setting up a better system, or learning about a new app, could save you time and stress, not to mention money, every week for years or even decades to come.

PART TWO

NOURISH

I have an adopted aunt named Carol. I've treasured her for more than 25 years. As is often the case with family, we're united more by love than by diet. Aunt Carol's approach to eating is relatively typical of the modern industrialized world, and she's never been overly keen to hear from me on the topic.

In 2015, dear Aunt Carol came down with bladder cancer and wound up undergoing chemotherapy and life-altering surgeries. I'm glad to say that after a great deal of suffering, she made it through.

The irony is that not once, in all of Aunt Carol's medical treatments, did her oncologist mention diet or nutrition. He never asked about what she ate, or recommended any dietary protocols to help her through treatment or prevent recurrence of the cancer—despite the fact that we now know that the vast majority of cases of cancer are caused not by genetics but rather by a combination of diet, lifestyle, and environmental factors.

As I saw my aunt undergoing brutal medical treatments in desperate hope that they would save her, I felt sad that her doctors seemed to be ignoring the massive dietary underpinnings that fuel health and disease. I feared that the odds of my aunt facing a later recurrence remained disturbingly high.

I felt a flash of anger at her doctor. But then I realized something: Her doctor truly didn't know. A doctor who doesn't know about nutrition is a little like a firefighter who doesn't know about water. And yet most doctors are painfully ignorant about the relationship between food and health. And it's not really their fault. You might think medical schools would teach doctors about nutrition, but for the most part, they don't.

A study in the *Journal of Biomedical Education* in 2015 found that the average physician graduates medical school having received just 19 hours of nutritional education.[1] In the United States, only a quarter of all medical schools require even a single course in nutrition. And of the limited nutritional education that's offered, most focuses on the specific problems that can arise from deficiency of isolated nutrients. There is virtually no attention given to helping patients prevent disease or optimize health by eating healthy food.

The truth is, we have a health care system that often acts as if food doesn't matter. And of course, at the same time, we have a food system that often acts as if health doesn't matter.

I wrote this book because I don't want you, or the people you love, to be dependent on nutritional leadership from a medical system that's unprepared to provide it, or a food system that profits most from selling junk food. I want you to have the knowledge you need to take your health into your own hands—where it belongs.

There's an old saying that pain pushes and vision pulls. Some people are motivated by fear of suffering. If that's true for you, then fearing or experiencing aches and pains, fatigue, or illness could be a powerful motivating force. And some people are called forward by visions and dreams of what they want. You might be inspired about looking great in a pair of skinny jeans, or by wanting abundant energy to play with your grandkids. You might want to improve your running times or to have expanded mental clarity for the long haul.

When you replace sugar, refined flour, processed carbs, and factory-farmed animal products with real, wholesome food, you set your body up to fight cancer, dementia, and diabetes—and just as important, to replenish, recharge, and revitalize yourself.

One of the things I like about the Food Revolution is that it isn't just about saying no to the bad stuff. It's also about saying "Heck yeah!" to the good stuff. It's an opportunity to clear away toxins and to saturate your body and brain with life-giving, artery-opening, mind-clearing nutrients that can add not only years to your life but life to your years.

We hear a lot of talk about exotic "superfoods" like Himalayan goji berries, $300-a-pound ginseng, and Brazilian açai berries. No doubt these foods are potent, but how "super" is a food that only the wealthiest people can afford? The superfoods that interest me are the ones that do the most good for the most people. And what we're discovering is that there are vegetables, as well as berries, legumes, nuts, herbs, and spices, that make a world of difference. They provide antioxidants, flavonoids, and micronutrients that are stunningly powerful in fighting cancer, dementia, heart disease, and even wrinkles. These nutritional powerhouses can boost your immune system, improve your digestion, give you better energy, and contribute to a more satisfying sex life.

Healthy food is the foundation of a healthy life. So let's get building!

Take the Quiz: How Nutrient-Rich Is Your Diet?

How much of these items do you eat (or drink) in a typical week?

Green leafy vegetables
0. Fewer than four ½-cup servings.
1. Four to six servings.
2. At least seven servings.

Nuts and seeds
0. Fewer than three ¼-cup servings.
1. Three or four servings.
2. At least five servings.

Mushrooms
0. Fewer than two ¼-cup servings.
1. Two to four servings.
2. At least five servings.

Legumes (including beans, split peas, or lentils)
0. Fewer than two ½-cup servings.
1. Two to four ½-cup servings.
2. At least five servings.

Berries (fresh or frozen—including blueberries, strawberries, black-berries, raspberries, etc.)

0. Fewer than two ½-cup servings.

1. Two to four ¼-cup servings.

2. At least five servings.

Fermented foods (kimchi, raw sauerkraut, unsweetened yogurt, coconut kefir, natto, etc.)?

0. Less than three times.

1. At least three times.

2. At least five times.

Unsweetened green tea, white tea, black tea, hibiscus tea, and/or coffee

0. Less than three cups.

1. Three to six cups.

2. At least seven cups

Add up your points to get a score from 0 to 14. The higher, the better! To take your quiz online and then see how you compare to other quiz takers, join the 31-Day Food Revolution with cohorts by going online to 31dayfoodrevolution .com/quiz2.

CHAPTER 8

Eat to Beat Cancer

There's one sentence that's probably more feared than any other: "You have cancer."

Despite the billions of dollars spent in the war on cancer, despite the pink ribbons and races for the cure, cancer now takes the lives of more than 8 million people annually. And the devastating toll keeps rising.

What's causing so many people to get cancer? Is it just that we're living longer, and human cells malfunction with age? Are we prone to a genetic defect that causes cells to go rogue and threaten the organism that brought them into being? Do we simply lack some as-yet-uninvented drug that will protect or cure us? Or is cancer somehow being caused by the way we're living?

In 2008, researchers at the University of Texas MD Anderson Cancer Center set out to understand what was driving the global cancer epidemic. They conducted a meta-analysis of studies in peer-reviewed journals and then published their own summary report in *Pharmaceutical Research*.[1]

The researchers concluded that only 5 to 10 percent of all cancers have their roots in genetic defects. The other 90 to 95 percent are caused by a combination of diet, lifestyle, and environmental factors. They found, not surprisingly, that of all cancer deaths, 25 to 30 percent are caused by tobacco consumption. But there was another factor that the researchers determined was even more significant than smoking.

Diet.

In fact, the researchers reported, diet causes 30 to 35 percent of all cancer cases worldwide—totaling more than two million deaths per year. Based on their analysis of all available data, what cancer-prevention diet did these scientists recommend?

"Increased ingestion of fruits and vegetables...[and] minimal meat consumption."

DOES THIS MAKE SENSE?

Sometimes I wonder if we've got it all wrong. The United States' National Cancer Institute alone has spent more than $90 billion on cancer research.[2] Global spending on cancer medications exceeds $100 billion annually.[3] And yet more than two million people worldwide are dying from diet-fueled cancer every year, while fewer than half of all Americans even realize that a diet high in fruits and vegetables, and low in red meat and processed foods, can help prevent this horrible disease.[4]

Can you imagine what would happen if even a fraction of the tens of billions of dollars now being spent on drugs and surgeries were to be spent on educational campaigns, or on truly healthy food? Wouldn't we save more lives if we focused on preventing cancer from happening in the first place?

Why don't we?

Is it possible that part of the reason is that established interests are profiting from selling foods that are making us sick, and that as long as we're spending hundreds of billions of dollars on drugs and medical care, some folks are earning a lot of money? If there was as much money to be made off of broccoli as there is for chemo, do you think we'd see more broccoli eaten?

Mother Nature gives us a huge pharmacy of natural foods, herbs, and spices that are stunningly effective in promoting health. And the only side effects of feasting on nature's pantry turn out to be good ones.

But natural products, by definition, can't be patented—and drugs can. A study from the Tufts Center for the Study of Drug Development found that pharmaceutical companies spend an average of $2.6 billion for each new drug they bring to market.[5]

No one's about to spend that much proving that plants are safe and effective as medicines, because they can't be patented. Whoever financed the $2.6 billion would be out all that money, with no more ability to profit than your local farmer.

So natural products are at a fundamental disadvantage in the marketplace. And the vast majority of doctors and insurance companies are stuck prescribing and covering what's been proven—in a system that effectively mandates that only patentable drugs can become approved as medicines.

Unfortunately, when it comes to nutrition, sometimes it seems as if the medical establishment is intent on ignoring the basic facts.

In 2014, the American Association for Cancer Research convened more than 18,000 researchers, doctors, and other health professionals for the organization's annual meeting.[6] During the entire conference, there was almost no mention of the role that diet can play in reducing cancer risk. But there was an evening reception at which guests partook of a sumptuous buffet that included thick slabs of roast beef and a large variety of rich cheeses. Afterward came the cancer research association's grand celebration, renowned for its dessert buffet. As if harkening back to the days, just a generation ago, when doctors smoked at medical conferences, we now had a carcinogenic food binge served at a medical convention—at a time when we know that diet causes more fatal cancers than cigarettes.

Is it possible that we can make a change in our lifetimes?

I think so.

But in order to get there, we're going to have to uproot some established interests. And some of them sell their products in pretty pink buckets and other eye-catching packages.

LIKE KFC, FOR EXAMPLE

Starting in 2010, the largest grassroots breast cancer advocacy group in the world, a group called Susan G. Komen for the Cure, launched a partnership with the fast-food chain KFC in a U.S.-wide "Buckets for the Cure" campaign.

KFC took every chance it could drum up to trumpet the fact that it donated 50 cents to Komen for every pink bucket of chicken sold.[7]

For its part, Komen's group announced on its website that "KFC and Susan G. Komen for the Cure are teaming up . . . to . . . spread educational messaging via a major national campaign which will reach thousands of communities served by nearly 5,000 KFC restaurants."[8]

How often do you think this "educational messaging" provided information about the critical importance diet plays in maintaining a healthy weight and preventing cancer? How often do you think it referred to the many studies that, according to the National Cancer Institute's website, "have shown that an increased risk of developing colorectal, pancreatic, and breast cancer is associated with high intakes of well-done, fried, or barbecued meats"?[9]

If you guessed zero, you're exactly right.

Meanwhile, the American Institute for Cancer Research reports that *up to 70 percent of all cancers can be prevented with lifestyle changes.*[10] Their number one dietary recommendation is: "Choose predominantly plant-based diets rich in a variety of vegetables and fruits, legumes, and minimally processed starchy staple foods."

That doesn't sound like pink buckets of fried chicken to me.

THE TOP FOODS THAT DO FIGHT CANCER

As you might be able to tell, I'm more than a little passionate about food. It bothers me that so few people know the truth, despite the fact that it can save millions of lives. I don't want you to suffer needlessly.

So let's look at some of the top foods that are especially potent in helping to fight cancer.

The Magical Fungi

The ancient Egyptians believed that eating mushrooms brought long life. Now modern scientists are likewise discovering that mushrooms have some fascinating medicinal properties.

In 2004, researchers from the University of Western Australia in Perth conducted a study of 2,000 Chinese women, about half of whom had breast cancer.[11] The scientists reviewed the women's eating habits and factored out other variables that contribute to cancer, such as being overweight, lack of exercise, and smoking. They came to a startling conclusion about mushrooms.[12]

Women who consumed at least one-third of an ounce of fresh mushrooms per day (less than one typical-sized mushroom) were 64 percent less likely to develop breast cancer. Dried mushrooms had a slightly smaller protective effect, reducing the risk by around half. What was even more impressive is that women who combined eating mushrooms with regular consumption of green tea saw an even greater benefit—they reduced their breast cancer risk by an astounding 89 percent.

Why are mushrooms so powerful? They are thought to protect against breast and other hormone-related cancers because they inhibit an enzyme called aromatase, which produces estrogen.[13] Mushrooms also contain specialized lectins that recognize cancer cells and prevent these cells from growing and dividing. (Lectins, a type of carbohydrate-binding protein, have gotten a bad reputation in some circles, but some of them, such as the ones in mushrooms, can be beneficial.)

Which types of mushrooms are best? There are thousands of varieties, and our understanding of their properties is growing rapidly—but it is still in its infancy.[14]

All edible mushrooms we know of, including button, white, cremini, shiitake, oyster, portobello, maitake, turkey tail, and reishi mushrooms, contain bioactive compounds with the potential for potent anticancer activity. These mushroom phytochemicals have anticancer effects that show promise against stomach, colorectal, breast, and prostate cancers.[15]

But it's important to cook mushrooms and generally not to eat them raw. Mushrooms contain agaritine, a natural toxin that has been found to be carcinogenic. Agaritine is destroyed by heat, so as long as you cook mushrooms you don't have anything to worry about. (And of course, never eat wild mushrooms unless you're absolutely certain they're edible and not poisonous.)

Since I heard about the power of mushrooms, I've made it a habit to eat cooked ones almost every day. Searing or roasting them allows them to caramelize, which highlights their fantastic umami flavor and satisfying texture. You can enjoy mushrooms sautéed with greens, on top of a salad or pizza, on warm and creamy polenta, blended into a soup, grilled like a burger, or stirred into soba noodles with ginger and garlic.

Cruciferous Vegetables

Cruciferous vegetables have four-petal flowers that resemble a cross or "crucifer." Cabbage is the best known, but other cruciferous vegetables include broccoli, brussels sprouts, rocket, cauliflower, kale, mustard greens, turnips, and collards. When it comes to protecting you from cancer, cabbage and the other crucifers could be some of the most powerful nutritional superheroes on the planet.

Researchers have found that components in these veggies can protect you from free radicals that can damage your cells' DNA.[16] Cruciferous vegetables might also help you eliminate cancer-causing chemicals, and studies have linked increased consumption of cruciferous vegetables with a decrease in rates of breast, lung, colorectal, and prostate cancers.[17]

For chemistry fans, here's an explanation of how cruciferous veggies work their magic: They contain glucosinolates and an enzyme called myrosinase. When we blend, chop, or chew these vegetables, we break up the plant cells, allowing myrosinase to come into contact with glucosinolates, initiating a chemical reaction that produces isothiocyanates (ITCs). ITCs have been shown to detoxify and remove carcinogens and to stimulate a process called apoptosis in which cancer cells self-destruct.[18]

In case you don't have any great love for chemistry, here's the punch line: Cruciferous veggies are good for you and for your cells, too.

Cruciferous vegetables also provide vitamin C (known for protecting cells as an antioxidant and for supporting the immune system). And most are good sources of manganese, folate, potassium, dietary fiber, and carotenoids, such as beta-carotene, which promote cell communication and help control abnormal cells.

Enjoy cruciferous vegetables raw and shredded (try making a coleslaw—you'll find a delicious recipe on page 299), or try them steamed, baked, sautéed, in a wrap, or even broiled. Broccoli adds a beautiful emerald color when puréed into a rich soup. Sautéed collards are superb when tossed with pasta and caramelized onions. Cauliflower is delightful in creamy Indian curries served atop steaming-hot quinoa or fragrant basmati rice. Kale is wonderful wilted into a pot of hearty Italian minestrone. The possibilities are endless—and exquisite.

And Then There's Celery

Celery is mostly water, and it's rarely regarded as a nutritional powerhouse. But this crunchy food has been known for its health-giving properties since the ninth century, when it was used as a medicine.[19]

According to studies performed in China, eating just two medium-size stalks of celery two or three times per week could reduce your risk of lung cancer by an amazing 60 percent.[20] Other studies have found celery to be potentially effective at killing ovarian, pancreatic, prostate, breast, and liver cancer cells.[21]

What makes celery such a powerful anticancer food? Its crispy green stalks contain two anticancer compounds, apigenin and luteolin—both of which are bioactive flavonoids that work as antioxidants and neutralize free radicals in the body.

Apigenin is effective at causing apoptosis (cell suicide) in many types of cancer cells.[22] In a 2013 in vitro study, it was found to kill up to 86 percent of lung cancer cells.[23] Apigenin is also a powerful anti-inflammatory that rivals commercial anti-inflammatory drugs.[24]

As for luteolin, it may be able to short-circuit the replication cycle of cancer cells. In a study published in the *BMC Gastroenterology* journal, researchers discovered that luteolin blocked the signal pathways necessary for the growth of colorectal cancer cells.[25]

I'm not a fan of studies on lab animals, because, frankly, I think most of them are cruel. But once they've been conducted, I don't think there's any benefit to the poor mice, rats, or other critters who may have been through them if we ignore whatever was learned in the process. So you'll hear me mention lab studies a few times, not because I ethically condone them, but because I think we might find some value in the insights we can glean from them.

In one very sad laboratory study, mice were fed a strong mutagen to induce fibrosarcoma (a form of bone cancer).[26] When these mice were supplemented with luteolin in their diet, researchers noted a nearly 50 percent drop in tumor rates, and slower tumor progression as well.

Celery is naturally rich in vitamins A, C, and K, minerals folate and potassium, and more. It's been found to help with calming your nervous system, aiding digestion, reducing inflammation, and lowering blood pressure.[27] Because it's rich in fiber, celery can also help prevent constipation.

Chopped celery adds a juicy crunch to all kinds of salads, and you can cook it into soups, stew, and casseroles. It's a lovely addition to green juices and green smoothies, and it can be delicious with a dollop of hummus or another tasty dip. For a timeless treat, destring a stalk and smear peanut butter down the middle. Adding a few raisins creates a favorite childhood snack known as "ants on a log."

ACTION:

Option 1: Bring cooked mushrooms into your life! Make a recipe that features them.

Option 2: Find a delicious way to prepare a cruciferous vegetable (cabbage, broccoli, brussels sprouts, cauliflower, kale, mustard greens, turnips, or collards), using one of the following ideas for inspiration. **1) Stir-fry:** Thinly slice your cruciferous vegetable and stir-fry it in olive oil, along with an assortment of other favorite vegetables, onions, and garlic. Add soy sauce and any desired spices, and serve atop quinoa, rice, or another whole grain. **2) Salad:** Thinly slice your chosen vegetable, and toss with avocado, fresh lemon juice or apple cider vinegar, salt, and nutritional yeast— then top with roasted pumpkin seeds or sunflower seeds. **3) Buddha Bowl:** Roast or sauté the vegetable and pair with quinoa, chopped walnuts, shredded dark leafy greens, baked tofu, and a dab of tahini.

Option 3: Take the triple-health challenge. Make a meal that includes all three of these anticancer powerhouses: mushrooms, cruciferous vegetables, and celery. Enjoy it regularly!

CHAPTER 9

Heal Your Gut

Deep in your gut, 40 trillion chemists are hard at work helping you digest your meals, making essential nutrients you can't produce on your own, protecting you from disease, and even shaping which parts of your DNA manifest and which remain dormant.[1] These talented creatures are fungi, bacteria, and other single-celled organisms. And they are a bigger part of who you are than you have probably ever imagined!

While your body includes about 22,000 human genes, it also hosts as many as two trillion microbial genes that are technically not "you," but rather benevolent guests working in exquisite harmony with your body. Some of these microbes flourish on your skin, but the vast majority take up residence in your digestive tract.

Study of the microbiome—the community of microorganisms living inside your body—could well be the most compelling frontier of health science.

The digestive process breaks down food and beverage particles so that your body can absorb the nutrients it wants and excrete the rest. Trillions of organisms join in the effort. These microbes also play a critical role in shaping your appetite, allergies, metabolism, and neurological function. In fact, scientists have found that gut bacteria produce neurotransmitters such as serotonin, dopamine, and GABA, all of which play a key role in determining your mood.[2]

Studies suggest that your gut microbiota may factor into your risk of developing neuropsychiatric illnesses like schizophrenia, ADHD, obsessive-compulsive disorder, and chronic fatigue syndrome.[3]

In other words, the bacteria living in your gut have a huge impact on the way you feel.

WHICH ONE ARE YOU FEEDING?

There's an often-told story, reportedly from Cherokee folklore, about a Cherokee elder who is teaching his grandson about life. "A fight is going on inside me," he says to the boy. "It's a terrible fight between two wolves. One is evil—he is anger, envy, sorrow, regret, greed, arrogance, self-pity, guilt, resentment, lies, false pride, and ego. The other is good—he is joy, peace, love, hope, serenity, humility, kindness, empathy, generosity, truth, and compassion. The same fight is going on inside you—and inside every other person, too."

The grandson thinks for a minute and then asks, "Which wolf will win?"

The old Cherokee replies, "The one you feed."

When it comes to the bacteria in your gut, every time you eat, you are feeding somebody. Unfortunately, the modern industrialized diet is all too often feeding the bad guys and, just as important, starving the good.

To put it simply, "bad" bacteria tend to feed on sugar and unhealthy fats (yes, I'm talking about you, junk food!).[4] And the single most important nutrient that good bacteria need to thrive inside you is fiber. When they have plenty of fiber, they can do their job—and your digestion, mental function, and even your mood reap the benefits.

It's clear that fiber is critical to gut health. But less than 5 percent of Americans get the recommended 25 to 30 grams per day.[5] It's estimated that our Paleolithic ancestors got an average of up to 100 grams per day.[6] Compare that to the average Brit, who gets only 18 grams per day, and the average American, who gets even less—just 15.[7]

Most of us are literally starving the good bacteria that would, if we only gave them the chance, be digesting our food and making the brain-boosting chemicals we need to thrive.

THE INFLAMMATION CONNECTION

Inflammation is the defense response that focuses your immune system's attention toward fighting a perceived threat—such as bacteria, a virus, or a toxin. When part of your body becomes reddened, swollen, hot, or painful, this is inflammation in action.

So far so good. But when inflammation becomes chronic, your body's natural defenses get depleted and become unable to do their job properly because they are worn out. Constant alarms put the body in chronic stress, until its defenses are unable to function properly.

We've known for some time that chronic inflammation can result when your body is inundated with a barrage of threats—often stemming from food allergies, poor diet, toxins, or stress. But now, researchers are coming to believe that an often-critical piece of the inflammation puzzle actually lives in your gut bacteria.

How does this work?

From the esophagus all the way to the anus, your digestive tract contains a lining called the epithelium, which is only one cell thick. The portion that runs through your small intestine is exquisitely designed to absorb the nutrients your body needs to thrive, while keeping out whatever might be harmful or inadequately digested. But since it's only one cell thick, it's very vulnerable.

According to Lita Proctor of the Human Microbiome Project at the National Institutes of Health, the "bad bacteria" that are fed by sugar and unhealthy fats can emit chemicals that compromise your intestinal lining.[8]

When your gut lining is damaged, or "leaky," certain chemicals and proteins can cross the lining and activate an immune or inflammatory response in your body.

HOW GLYPHOSATE COULD BE ADDING FUEL TO THE FIRE

Nearly all the soy and corn grown in the United States today, and most of the soy and corn grown worldwide, was genetically engineered by Monsanto (now Bayer) to withstand the company's proprietary herbicide, Roundup. The primary active ingredient in Roundup is glyphosate.

There are many problems with glyphosate, including the fact that it's considered probably carcinogenic by the World Health Organization and by the state of California, which wants it to carry warning labels when sold.[9]

But there's another issue with glyphosate that's received shockingly little attention.

In 2012, the weed killer was patented by Monsanto as an antibiotic. Antibiotics kill microbes, such as bacteria.[10] Increasing numbers of scientists believe that this chemical, millions of tons of which have been applied directly to food crops destined for human consumption, may disrupt and kill beneficial bacteria in your gut, leading to impaired immune function and a cascade of other ill effects.[11]

Prior to being purchased by Bayer in 2016, Monsanto frequently told us that Roundup was nontoxic to humans. They paid many scientists to reiterate this claim,[12] and some pointed out that glyphosate killed weeds by interrupting a process called the shikimate pathway.[13] The shikimate pathway is the process by which plants take carbohydrates and change them into amino acids, which are the building blocks for protein. We humans don't have that pathway in our cells, so we were told that we had nothing to worry about. It was a pathway found only in plants and bacteria.

But this is where the company's story began to fall apart. Many of the 40 trillion microbial cells in your body are bacteria that do, in fact, depend on the shikimate pathway for the production of what are called aromatic amino acids (in case you're wondering, aromatic amino acids don't emit some special scent—I'm just telling you what they're called!).[14] The aromatic amino acids produced by bacteria in this way are phenylalanine, tyrosine, and tryptophan, and they are all essential to human health.

What's becoming increasingly apparent is that glyphosate, found at increasingly high levels in and on today's genetically engineered foods, is having a significant and potentially damaging impact on the human microbiome.

Of course, Monsanto was quick to tell us that this was all a bunch of hogwash.[15] But keep in mind, Monsanto also told us that another of its chemicals, DDT, was completely safe. And we now have studies proving that women exposed to DDT in the womb face a quadrupled risk of developing breast cancer.[16] It's never wise to trust a poison manufacturer to confirm the safety of its products.

For many people, one of the most compelling reasons to choose organic or certified non-GMO foods is to keep glyphosate out of their diet.

WHAT ABOUT ANTIBIOTICS?

The most powerful microbe killers of our times are antibiotics. Antibiotic drugs such as penicillin and streptomycin have saved millions of lives from diseases including cholera, tuberculosis, and meningitis. For the right condition, they can be a godsend.

When I was a few months old, I came down with a high fever. Up until that point I had subsisted entirely on breast milk, but although I lived in a relatively unpolluted environment, I'd picked up contamination from somewhere. Before long my fever was raging at 104 degrees, and I was so weak that I was unable to muster even a cry.

I'm grateful that my parents took me to a doctor, who put me on antibiotics. Within hours, my fever was down and my sickness was reversed.

That antibiotic prescription may have saved my life.

I've always been a fan of antibiotics when they're used in their rightful place. But the reality is that they're vastly overprescribed. As many as four out of five Americans are prescribed antibiotics in any given year— and many of these prescriptions are unnecessary.[17]

And there's a dark side to antibiotics. Because they wipe out microbes fairly indiscriminately, they can leave your body's microbial balance damaged, and unless rebuilding methods are employed, some bacterial ecosystems may not recover.

If you've ever taken antibiotics, as almost all of us have, then this is probably a significant factor in the balance of your microbiome today. And it's not one that's addressed adequately, if at all, by most prescribing doctors.

Last year, as I was contemplating taking antibiotics to fight a strep infection, I asked my doctor if he could recommend any protocol for repopulating my body with healthy bacteria. He replied that he didn't learn anything about that in medical school, so he couldn't offer me any advice. "My wife took a nutrition class online," he told me, "so she'd be a better person to ask." It's pretty crazy, if you think about it, that our medical system is so good at destroying a bacterial ecosystem but so ineffective at rebuilding it.

The overuse of antibiotics is fueling the development of antibiotic-resistant bacteria, making these medicines increasingly ineffective at treating the diseases for which they can be so helpful. Many diseases that would have been cured by antibiotics a few short years ago are no longer responding in the same way. In fact, worldwide, antibiotic-resistant bacteria are estimated to be causing more than 700,000 deaths per year.[18] And all projections are that this number could rise dramatically, potentially exceeding 10 million deaths annually by the year 2050.[19]

No wonder the World Health Organization has declared that antibiotic resistance is one of our greatest global threats to health, security, and development.[20]

(The spread of antibiotic-resistant bacteria isn't only being caused by overuse of antibiotics in humans. According to a study in the *Proceedings of the National Academy of Sciences of the United States of America* in 2015, the world uses about 63,000 tons of antibiotics each year to raise cows, chickens, and pigs.[21] That's roughly twice as much as the volume of antibiotics prescribed by doctors globally to fight infections in people. I'll explain this more, and share what you can do to help turn it around, in chapter 29.)

Anytime you're considering taking antibiotics, here are a few questions to ask:

1. Is it necessary? If you don't take the medicine, is it likely that your body will recover naturally? If you don't take it, what are the potential consequences?
2. Will it help? Are you or your doctor sure that the offending organism is bacterial? (Antibiotics are ineffective against viral infections, and yet an estimated 30 percent of antibiotic prescriptions in the United States are for common colds, viral sore throats, bronchitis, and sinus and ear infections not typically helped by antibiotics in the slightest.[22])
3. How will I rebuild afterward? (If you take antbiotics, you should build in a plan for restoring your gut health on the other side. The following pages will give you helpful guidance.)

HOW TO NURTURE THE GOOD GUYS

We know that junk food, lack of fiber, glyphosate, antibiotics, and other toxins can compromise the bacteria upon which your digestion and brain health depend. Is there anything you can do about it?

Yes! There's a lot you can do to nurture a healthy microbiome and support a flourishing collection of beneficial bacteria in your digestive tract.

1. Don't kill the good ones.

When you steer clear of unnecessary antibiotics, glyphosate, and environmental toxins, you help to create the conditions for microbial health. Organic food, anyone?

2. Don't feed the bad ones.

A diverse population of health-promoting flora protects your gut from the less helpful strains. But not all flora are good for you. A diet high in sugar, unhealthy fat, and processed food can feed the very kinds of flora that will cause gas, discomfort, bloating, and chronic inflammation.

3. Feed the good ones.

Probiotics are the so-called "good" microorganisms inside your gastrointestinal tract. They aid in digestion and keep your tummy happy. Like all living things, probiotics must be fed in order to remain active and vibrant.

Prebiotics are the food that probiotics need to thrive. They're a type of plant fiber that humans can't digest and that take up residence inside your large intestine. The more of these prebiotics you feed to your probiotics, the more efficiently they'll do good work inside you.

The simplest way to think of it is this: If you want to nurture good bacteria, eat lots of fiber. Whole plant foods—especially fruits, vegetables, legumes, and whole grains—have the most. As *New York Times* personal health columnist Jane Brody writes, "People interested in fostering a health-promoting array of gut microorganisms should consider shifting from a diet heavily based on meats, carbohydrates, and processed foods to one that emphasizes plants."[23]

If your probiotic bacteria were in charge of the menu, they'd want abundant sources of prebiotic fibers like inulin and oligofructose, as well as pectin, beta-glucans, glucomannan, cellulose, lignin, and fructooligosaccharides (FOS). If you don't know how to pronounce these names, don't worry. Luckily, you don't need a degree in biochemistry to eat good food.

Some top superfoods that provide an abundance of the best microbe-fueling nutrients include gum arabic (sap from the acacia tree, often sold as the supplement acacia fiber), chicory root, Jerusalem artichoke, baobab fruit, dandelion greens, garlic, leek, onion, asparagus, wheat bran, banana, jicama, apples, barley, oats, flaxseed, cocoa, burdock root, yacon root, and seaweed.

4. Eat the good ones.

The word *probiotic* comes from the Greek for "support of life." The two main ways to consume probiotics are in dietary supplements and in fermented foods. Probiotics have been found to be helpful in treating irritable bowel syndrome, diarrhea, colitis, acne, and eczema.[24]

But they don't always work. A lot of people are taking probiotic supplements that are pretty much just a waste of money. The challenge is that the vast majority of probiotic bacteria are active and effective in the lower portions of the gastrointestinal (GI) tract, but to get there, they must survive the corrosive and highly acidic environment of your stomach.

When are the odds the best—on an empty stomach, or with a meal? Researchers attempted to settle this question with a study reported in the journal *Beneficial Microbes* in 2011.[25] (Yes, although it may never rival *People* magazine for newsstand popularity, that really is the name of a journal!) The team built a fake digestive tract with a fake stomach and intestines, but complete with real saliva and digestive enzymes, acid, bile, and other digestive fluids. They put probiotic capsules into this stomach "empty" and with a variety of foods, and tested how many survived the trip.

What did they find? Probiotic bacteria had the highest rates of survival when provided within 30 minutes before or simultaneously with a meal or beverage that contained some fat.

This makes sense. Consuming probiotics with food provides a buffering system for the bacteria, helping to ensure safe passage through the digestive tract. But consuming them after a large meal could slow everybody down, making bacteria more likely to die in the corrosive stomach environment before reaching their intended new home in the lower intestine. So right before, or with, a meal that includes some fat seems the best way to go.

Which Probiotic Supplements Are Best?

There are thousands of probiotic products on the market, with each company or retailer telling you theirs is best. The factors I look at in evaluating a probiotic supplement are:

1. **Price.** No one likes to waste money.
2. **CFUs (colony-forming units).** This is the total count of all the bacteria in the probiotic. There's a huge range, with brands offering anywhere from 1 billion to 100 billion CFUs per dose. The bigger the number, the more beneficial bacteria you get.
3. **Strains.** The total number of different types of bacteria in each probiotic varies greatly. Diversity is good. Every expert has a favorite combination, but the reality is that we know very little about how the various strains interact with the human body. A broad spectrum of different kinds is likely to give you the best odds of success.
4. **Expiration date.** Some probiotic supplements get so old that the bacteria are literally dead by the time they reach the consumer. Check expiration dates.

One probiotic supplement that's also a food is a coconut water kefir made by inner-ēco. It's a naturally effervescent and mildly sweet refrigerated product that provides 50 billion CFUs per tablespoon. I often take a tablespoon with breakfast or dinner. It has the added benefit of being delicious.

What About Fermented Foods?

Fermentation helps to preserve food and creates beneficial enzymes, B vitamins, and numerous strains of probiotics.

Natural fermentation has been shown to preserve nutrients and to break some foods down to a more digestible form. The most studied is kimchi, a traditional Korean food made from fermenting salted cabbage with a variety of vegetables and spices (sometimes salted shrimp or anchovy is included, as well). In addition to, or perhaps in part because of, its probiotic properties, studies have shown that kimchi can help fight cancer, obesity, effects of aging, and constipation while contributing to your immune system, skin health, and brain health.[26]

Other popular fermented foods include sauerkraut, yogurt (which can be made from cow, soy, coconut, or almond milk), kefir, miso, natto (made by boiling and fermenting soybeans with bacteria), beet kvass (a fermented beet drink), vinegar, and kombucha.

Some fermented foods are used in condiments, while others make a tasty snack or topping. Remember not to cook them if you want to preserve the probiotics.

Keep in mind that some probiotic kefirs and yogurts come loaded with added sugar. Even if there are beneficial bacteria in these probiotics, the sugar will feed "bad" bacteria already in your gut. Always check labels for sugar content.

If you want to do your own fermentation, I recommend finding a good book or website to guide you. A book to consider is *Fermented Vegetables* by Christopher and Kirsten Shockey.

Some people using homemade fermented foods are experiencing great benefits.

Like Emily Iaconelli, for example. At the age of 17, after growing up on the modern industrialized diet, Emily developed irritable bowel syndrome, migraines, and emergent arthritis. She suffered from massive bloating and chronic pain, and became resigned to a life of embarrassing pain and urgent bathroom runs.

After 20 years of misery, she joined a Food Revolution Network event I was hosting and decided to turn her kitchen upside down. Emily began enjoying a whole-food, plant-powered diet that featured an abundance of fermented foods, such as kimchi, fermented vegetables, tempeh, homemade almond milk yogurt, and miso. Her fiber consumption went up dramatically, providing abundant nourishment for the probiotics now streaming into her body every day.

The journey was difficult. Emily had to squeeze in all her learning and food preparation while working full-time and raising a two-year-old daughter. But every step she took seemed to give her more energy and stamina, which fueled her actions as well as her determination. Eventually her irritable bowel syndrome, migraines, and emergent arthritis all disappeared. And her daughter, now five, loves to cook and has decided that her favorite food is…broccoli!

WHAT ABOUT KOMBUCHA?

Kombucha is a drink made by fermenting green or black tea with sugar and a SCOBY, which is an acronym for "symbiotic culture of bacteria and yeast." Sometimes herbs, spices, and fruits are added as well. The drink originates from Asia and has been around for centuries, but it's enjoying a booming status in the West now, with annual sales in the U.S. alone exceeding $600 million.[27]

Some people (especially those who are selling it) have touted kombucha as an elixir that can cure everything from arthritis and cancer to digestive problems. But by others, it's been maligned as a highly acidic, often heavily sweetened, and potentially toxic beverage.

What's the truth? Well, here's what we know.

No long-term studies have been completed on the effects of kombucha consumption on humans. One study found that it helped treat stomach ulcers in mice.[28] Another found that it could help rats to detoxify heavy metals.[29] (Poor rats!)

The green or black tea used as a base for kombucha is known for its health benefits. And the probiotics in kombucha are probably beneficial, although most probiotics need to be consumed in proximity to some amount of fat in order to survive the journey through your stomach. The sugar in kombucha is partly digested by the fermentation process, but if the drink tastes sweet, don't be deceived—it is. Some kombuchas are so sweet that their sugar content can rival that of soft drinks.

Personally, I drink kombucha from time to time. There's no doubt it can be tasty. I regard it as a treat because I know it contains sugars, and I'm not totally convinced of its safety or health benefits, so I'm looking forward to further studies.

LISTEN TO YOUR GUT

True gut instincts can provide an essential source of wisdom, clarity, and discernment. Does your gut tighten when you confront danger, or soften in the presence of an epiphany?

Whatever your relationship is with your gut, and however clearly it does or doesn't speak to you, I'd like to invite you to consider a possibility.

What if you didn't think of your gut as being yours alone? What if you conceived of it as being home, also, to trillions of microbes that can tell you what's good for you or let you know when you're hungry (because they are)? When you're in a symbiotic relationship with the community of critters inside you, you can feel pride in feeding the good ones. You can feel gratitude for how they help you digest food, secrete brain-boosting neurotransmitters, and protect you from harm. And you can feel it's your responsibility to protect and work in harmony with them, for your own ultimate well-being along with theirs.

ACTION:

Option 1: Begin eating a fermented food or taking a probiotic supplement daily.

Option 2: Incorporate at least one of the prebiotic vegetables or fruits (such as chicory root, Jerusalem artichoke, dandelion greens, garlic, leek, onion, asparagus, jicama, apple, flaxseed, or burdock root) into your daily diet along with a probiotic.

Option 3: Make your own fermented products. Experiment with sauerkraut, kimchi, a yogurt, or whatever sounds appealing.

CHAPTER 10

Is Breakfast Sabotaging Your Day?

I have a problem with breakfast.

I don't blame the meal itself. My problem is with what our industrialized food industry tells us we should eat every morning.

Recently, I took my kids on a road trip. We traveled across a few states, visiting national parks (my idea) and going to country music concerts (their idea). In Utah, we stayed in a hotel that offered a free continental breakfast.

I wasn't expecting much. But even so, I found it fairly disheartening. The hotel's idea of breakfast was fried bacon (no doubt the product of factory farms), white-flour pancakes smothered in "maple-flavored" high-fructose corn syrup, sugary cereal with milk, and pastries.

No offense to anyone who might enjoy those foods. A lot of our fellow hotel guests seemed happy enough. But this wasn't what I wanted to feed my kids. And I'm thankful it wasn't what they wanted, either. River suggested we head to the nearest natural-foods store to get some real food.

No more free hotel breakfasts for us.

As we continued our journey into Colorado, a question kept burning in me: Why do so many people think it's normal to start the day with an overdose of sugar, white flour, and fried meat? What would happen if we started the day off right, with vegetables and wholesome foods? Is it possible that days would go better if brains had nourishment from the get-go?

SO WHAT'S THE SOLUTION?

Some people need a filling meal by 7 a.m. in order to have clarity to meet their day. Others don't start to get hungry until noon. Every one of us has a unique metabolism, and sometimes what feels right on one day will feel very different on another day.

If you engage in a lot of sports or physical activity, you're more likely to need a good dose of calories in the morning. But if your body starts the day slowly, or at a desk, then you might feel better if you eat lightly. When I eat late at night, I don't usually wake up hungry the next morning. My stomach seems to gravitate toward having at least 12 hours off, and the clock starts ticking whenever I close up the culinary shop at night.

Listen to your body and see what you learn. Here are four very different approaches to breakfast on the Food Revolution Diet Plan.

The Smoothie

While many commercial smoothies come packed with sugar, you can create your own smoothie with green vegetables; nuts and seeds; avocado, coconut, or other healthy fats; and enough bananas, berries, or other fruits to make it tasty as well as nutritious.

Blending fruits and vegetables can enable you to absorb a lot of nutrients more quickly than if you ate the foods whole. If you want to suffuse your body with large amounts of phytonutrients, and to maximize your nutrient intake from vegetables and fruits, then a blender can be a powerful partner.

Want extra nutrition boosters? Presoak chia and/or flax seeds to make a paste, which you can keep in the fridge. Incorporate 2 to 3 tablespoons of this paste, or of ground chia and flax seeds, into smoothies. Try adding turmeric, tamarind, chopped ginger, or a splash of lemon or lime juice to your smoothies as well.

When you have your ingredients on hand, you can prepare your morning treat in minutes. A classic build-your-own-smoothie recipe is on page 279. This blueprint will allow you to create a custom blend. Chocolate lover? Add cacao powder and frozen pitted cherries. Looking to boost your protein intake? A scoop of hemp seeds will do the trick. Need something sweet? Add a few pitted Medjool dates or a banana to satisfy your craving naturally.

A word of caution: When you blend food, you can drink it down fast. When your smoothie is full of veggies, it can provide rapidly absorbed nourishment. But guzzling sweet smoothies can give you more calories than you might want and can spike blood sugar in a hurry. Adding whole-food-based fats (like nuts, seeds, or avocado) will help to slow digestion. But diabetics and prediabetics may still need to be careful and keep their smoothies' fruit content low.

The Presoak

A couple of nights each week, I like to soak my next morning's breakfast in the fridge. I'll drop a base of ½ cup of oats or 6 tablespoons of chia seeds into 2 cups of soy or nut milk. Then I add spices, vanilla, fresh or frozen berries, raisins or other small dried fruits, chopped nuts or seeds, and if I'm feeling decadent, a couple of teaspoons of maple syrup. My nutrient-rich feast is ready to grab and go.

The Classic

Some people like an old-fashioned, hearty breakfast. Here are tips for a healthier version: If you like bagels or toast, try sprouted whole-grain options, and serve them toasted with avocado, salt, lemon juice, and a dash of your favorite spices. Try porridge with nuts and seeds for healthy fat, and make the main sweetener bananas, other fresh or dried fruit, or 100 percent fruit-sweetened jam. If you like a scramble, go for tofu (or pasture-raised eggs if that's your preference) and include plenty of veggies. If you're big on pancakes, make some with whole-grain or almond flour, your favorite form of milk, and some nuts, and garnish with berries or bananas (you can even add fruit to the batter). If you want cold cereal, look for options with a low ratio of sugar to overall calories. Some granolas and mueslis are high in nuts and seeds, while others are packed with sugar. Read labels and practice discernment. For a little more sweetness, toss in a few berries or slices of apple.

The Regular Meal

I have a confession to make. I hope you don't hate me for it.

Often, for breakfast, I eat leftovers from dinner.

I'm not against traditional breakfasts. It's just that sometimes dinner was really good! I've never quite understood why so many people think breakfasts should be so different from other meals, when the human body's needs for nourishment are not fundamentally all that different in the morning.

So there you have it. If the idea of eating a warm "cheezy" broccoli casserole or a sweet potato with tofu chive spread for breakfast grosses you out, don't do it. But if hearing it from me gives you permission to enjoy a delicious meal that's a little outside the box, consider yourself liberated!

ACTION:

Option 1: Concoct a healthier version of a classic breakfast. You might sweeten porridge or pancakes with fruit or berries, eat 100 percent whole-grain bagels or toast, or include a few vegetables as a main or side dish.

Option 2: Make a green smoothie, combining green vegetables, nuts or seeds, and some lemon, tamarind, and/or ginger for extra flavor. Use just enough fruit to make it tasty. (Hint: When it comes to adding sweetness to a smoothie, bananas and frozen mango are especially potent.)

Option 3: Try my "regular meal" option. It might sound weird, but seriously, give it a try! See what happens if you eat a nice plate of vegetables with some spicy beans and greens, a piece of lentil-walnut loaf, or a warm bowl of fragrant Indian dal over quinoa. If it doesn't work out, at least you gave it a fair try! And if it does, your concept of breakfast might expand in a way you love.

CHAPTER 11

The World's Best Snacks

In 2007, Kate McGoey-Smith of Calgary, Alberta, faced a brutal diagnosis: idiopathic pulmonary arterial hypertension—a degenerative autoimmune disease that restricts blood flow to the lungs. She found herself beholden to a 20-pound oxygen tank, unable to work. Kate developed insulin-dependent diabetic retinopathy, and eventually went blind. She was placed on a lung transplant monitoring list and told that this might be her only hope of surviving an incurable, progressive, terminal disease.

Kate's three children—then between the ages of 11 and 17—faced the prospect of losing their mother. That's when she came upon the powerful documentary *Forks over Knives*, which gave her a glimmer of hope and inspired Kate and her husband to commit to a whole-foods, plant-based diet that was free of sugar, oil, and salt.

Despite being blind and unable to stand for more than a few minutes at a time, Kate nevertheless taught herself to cook and began an extraordinary journey to radical recovery. She found meals she loved, like Indian chana masala (chickpeas cooked with tomato and onions) and Chinese stir-fried veggies cooked in no-salt veggie broth. Seeking to improve her health, Kate snacked on steamed greens sprinkled with flavored vinegar six times each day.

Kate lost—and has kept off—120 pounds. Her risk of heart failure has plummeted as she's reversed her severe right-sided heart failure and her neuropathy. She no longer needs a lung transplant. After five years of blindness, her eyesight has been restored. And she is no longer considered a diabetic who needs insulin injections. As a result of a combination of adverse drug reactions and her prior state of diabetes, though, Kate still suffers from late-stage kidney failure, with only 12 percent function. But despite a bleak prognosis, her doctors have been utterly confounded that, for the last five years, her kidney deterioration appears to have been arrested, and she hasn't needed dialysis. All the changes Kate has made since 2007 sent out ripples of inspiration in her family. Her teenage son lost 70 pounds and developed significantly more confidence. Her husband, too, has experienced radical positive changes, including reversal of his type 2 diabetes.

Despite the fact that she's living a miracle, Kate's level of kidney failure makes her constantly aware of her mortality. She thinks a lot about what she'll be able to give to her kids, and expects that she won't be able to provide them much financially when her time comes. She told me: "Many people don't have the money to leave their kids a legacy of wealth. Certainly that's the case for me. But everyone, regardless of economic background, can leave their kids something much more important, which is a living legacy of health. And the truth is, that's worth far more."

Kate's passion is helping other people to implement the changes that have made such a profound difference in her life. Grateful to be alive at all, she's eager to share the blessing of health as widely as possible and founded forksmart.org, a nutritional coaching program. She writes, speaks, and acts as a mentor for aspiring healthy eaters.

When I start to feel sorry for myself, or frustrated if things don't go the way I want, I remember Kate. There she was—blind, diabetic, 120 pounds overweight, barely able to breathe or stand—teaching herself to cook vegetable stir-fries. Suddenly my gripes seem pretty small.

Every one of us who can walk, see, or move through life, choosing what we eat while blessed with knowledge about the healing power of healthy foods, is truly privileged.

ONE STEP AT A TIME

The journey of a thousand miles, the old saying goes, starts with a single step. Over the course of a lifetime, steps add up to shape destiny, for good or ill. Of all the small steps we take, the cumulative impact of snacks may be the most deceivingly significant.

I have a friend who eats carefully for breakfast, lunch, and dinner, and then figures it's okay to cheat a little around snack time. She has a point. After all, it's what you do most of the time that matters. A dough-nut now and then won't kill anyone whose overall dietary pattern is sound.

But the trouble is, many people snack so much that the "exception" becomes the norm. One five-ounce package of my personal nemesis, potato chips, for example, can deliver more than 750 calories—about a third of the *total* daily recommended calories for an average person.

We may not all want to eat steamed greens with vinegar six times each day, as Kate McGoey-Smith did (although it certainly worked out well for her!). But we need to find snack foods that pack a health-giving punch.

FRUITS

Fruits provide a source of vitamins and minerals as well as dietary fiber, antioxidants, and other nutrients. Fruits are good for your arter-ies, and they can improve digestion and help fight cancer, obesity, and (despite their high sugar content) even type 2 diabetes. And middle-aged men take note: Fruit has even been found to promote healthy hair growth![1]

Since it can be very sweet, you might think that fruit would cause unstable blood sugar levels. But for most people this isn't a problem, because the sugars in fruit come with fiber and other nutrients that slow down digestion and enable your body to regulate the influx of sugar effectively. Fruit juice, however, is another story. By separating out and throwing away the fiber-rich pulp, we reduce the juice to essentially a refined product that may be linked with blood sugar instability and other problems. For most people, a little juice won't do any major damage. Just keep in mind that eating whole fruit is where the real benefits lie. Next time you want a snack, grab an apple, pear, banana, orange, nectarine, pluot, mango, or peach. Or try a handful of berries.

BERRIES

Berries are one of my favorite superfoods. Perhaps it's because I grew up on a little island in Canada, and every summer I would go berry picking right outside our front door. I picked (and gorged on) wild blackberries, thimbleberries, and salal berries—and I loved them all.

When they're in season, berries are fabulous fresh (if you can forage for them or afford them). Out of season, you can find them, often more affordably, frozen or even dried. Add them to salads, breakfast cereals, or smoothies—or simply eat them by the handful.

Berries aren't just delicious; they also have a stunning ability to support your brain. In 2012, researchers from Harvard concluded that women who consumed at least one serving of blueberries or two servings of strawberries per week showed substantially slower rates of cognitive decline.[2]

Another study published in *Annals of Neurology* analyzed data from 16,000 women with an average age of 74.[3] Those with the highest levels of blueberry consumption delayed their cognitive aging by as much as two and a half years.

The cost of treating Alzheimer's is fast approaching $1 trillion worldwide.[4] About one-third of people aged 85 or older have contracted this devastating ailment.

One of them was my own grandma Irma, who developed Alzheimer's in her eighties. She'd always had a keen intellect and a stunning capacity for sarcasm. She possessed an extraordinary ability to remember, in lucid detail, every mistake anyone in the family had ever made. But by the end of her life, she could no longer even remember our names.

I wish I could go back in time and tell my grandma about berries, and all the other things we've learned about how to prevent dementia. I'll never be able to go back, but at least I can move forward and share this message with you.

Many foods have been found to help prevent Alzheimer's—including greens, legumes, and whole grains. But berries definitely deserve to be high on the list.

And they're good for your heart and your blood sugar balance, too. A 20-year Harvard study of 93,600 women, published in the journal

Circulation in 2013, found that those who ate the most berries were significantly less likely to suffer from cardiovascular disease or type 2 diabetes.[5]

Berries of all types bring you critical minerals, vitamins, antioxidants, flavonoids, polyphenols, and a host of other important phytonutrients that are good for your brain, heart, and overall health.

But what if you want something a bit more filling than fruit or berries? What if you want a snack that will give you a sustained lift of energy, that can last for days or even weeks without refrigeration, and that you can take anywhere without getting squished? It might be a good time for some...

NUTS

Have you ever looked at a walnut encased in its shell and marveled at the fact that if it were planted, it could sprout into a tree that would live for more than a hundred years and produce tens of thousands of nuts, each of which could in turn reproduce into a new tree?

In 2016, an archeological dig in Israel found evidence that nuts formed a major part of human diets 780,000 years ago.[6] Archaeologists discovered seven varieties, along with stone tools to crack them open. These stone tools, called "nutting stones," are similar to those found in North America and Europe, which archeologists date back 4,000 to 8,000 years.

Many of us munch on walnuts, almonds, pecans, Brazil nuts, pistachios, cashews, macadamia nuts, and hazelnuts, plus an honorary nut we call peanuts (even though peanuts are technically legumes). Sometimes we enjoy them with a sprinkling of salt; in a trail mix, nut loaf, or casserole; blended into nut milk; added to smoothies; prepared into nut "cheezes"; or even ground and made into pie crusts.

You can make your own nut butters in a blender or food processor and get creative with complementary accents. Homemade peanut butter is delicious, but add a dash of cinnamon for a new spin on an old favorite. Or fold cacao powder into your next batch of homemade almond butter.

We're only beginning to appreciate the benefits that nuts offer. They're rich in high-quality protein, fiber, minerals, tocopherols, phytosterols, vitamin E, vitamin B_6, folate, and phenolic compounds. Epidemiologic studies have linked nut consumption with reduced rates of heart disease, gallstones, and obesity, as well as beneficial effects on hypertension and inflammation.[7] Recent studies also indicate that nut consumption can help to prevent type 2 diabetes.[8]

One study involving more than 9,000 North Americans found that those who ate nuts at least five times per week gained, on average, an extra two years of life expectancy.[9] The nut eaters also experienced a 50 percent reduction in rates of heart disease risk.

That's not all. A clinical study published in the *International Journal of Impotence Research* looked at what happened to men with erectile dysfunction who ate three to four handfuls of pistachios a day for three weeks. These men experienced a significant improvement in blood flow through the genital area and significantly firmer erections. The researchers concluded that three weeks of pistachios "resulted in a significant improvement in erectile function...without any side effects."[10]

Each year, Pfizer makes more than $1.5 billion selling Viagra.[11] The company fears competition from rival drugs like Cialis and Levitra. Perhaps it should also be a bit worried about competition from pistachio farmers!

What About Seeds?

From sesame to sunflower to pumpkin, seeds are delicious and offer many of the same health benefits as nuts. And some seeds, especially chia and flax seeds, offer an abundance of a bonus nutrient—alpha-linolenic acid (ALA), one of the omega-3 fatty acids critical to your brain and cardiovascular health.

Any Downsides?

Surprisingly enough, considering how dense they are in calories, studies find a correlation between eating more nuts and weight loss. At least to a point. But keep in mind that an ounce of almonds (about 23 nuts), for instance, has 163 calories. If weight loss is a goal of yours, you might want to limit your nut consumption to no more than one serving (around ¼ cup) per day.

Nuts also have phytates and tannins that can cause gas or bloating for some people. If you find that happening, scale back to a serving size that works for you, or try soaking or sprouting nuts for a couple of days and storing them in the fridge, which will generally make them easier to digest.

Nut Sprouting and Soaking Guide

- Almonds: Soak for 8–12 hours. Sprout by leaving in a jar and rinsing every morning and evening for 2 or 3 days.
- Brazil nuts: Soak for 3 hours. Do not sprout.
- Cashews: Soak for 2–3 hours. Do not sprout.
- Hazelnuts: Soak for 8 hours. Do not sprout.
- Macadamias: Soak for 2 hours. Do not sprout.
- Pecans: Soak for 6 hours. Do not sprout.
- Pistachios: Soak for 8 hours. Do not sprout.
- Walnuts: Soak for 4 hours. Do not sprout.

Roasted, chopped, and ground nuts go rancid more quickly than whole and raw ones. Rancid oils are pro-inflammatory and can even be carcinogenic, so it's best to eat nuts fairly quickly or to store them in the refrigerator.

If nuts have been flavored, check the list of ingredients to see how much oil, salt, spices, sugar, or whatever else was added. And if you're allergic to nuts, as about 1 in every 200 people is, then of course, don't eat them.[12]

ACTION:

Option 1: Make fresh or frozen fruits or berries your go-to snack for the next few days.

Option 2: Make up 10 bags (or travel-ready containers) of dried-fruit-and-nut trail mix, and keep them handy as grab-and-go snacks.

Option 3: Get a dedicated coffee grinder to use exclusively for grinding flaxseed and/or chia seeds. Store a combined flax-chia powder in the fridge, and sprinkle it on porridge, casseroles, and soups.

CHAPTER 12

How to LOVE Eating Vegetables

I remember when our teenage sons went to summer camp for the first time. I was excited for them, but I was also nervous. They'd been home-schooled, and had grown up in a relatively protected environment.

A week later, when they got home, I asked Bodhi how camp had been.

· "I had a great time," he said. "It was so fun! But the only trouble was the food."

I felt a bolt of fear. Was he about to reveal a newfound taste for Ding Dongs and bacon?

"They didn't serve enough vegetables," Bodhi complained. "I really missed them. Could we have a big pot of vegetables for dinner?"

I was proud of him, because he'd had a great time at camp even though the food wasn't what he was used to. And I was proud of him for taking action when he got home by asking for a big pot of vegetables.

This didn't happen overnight. It took time, patience, and creativity to find out which vegetables, and which sauces, worked for our kids. And it's a never-ending effort that continues to this day.

Vegan chef and wellness professional Lauren Kretzer advises us never to assume that someone won't enjoy vegetables. If you deliver them with pushiness or timidity, they're more likely to be met with scorn. But if you share them with the same confidence and keenness that many people bring to a chocolate cake or a plate of piping-hot french fries, you might be amazed how contagious your enthusiasm can be. If your family doesn't like steamed broccoli, try roasting it. If you encounter resistance to yellow peppers, you might try red ones with coriander–jalapeño hummus.

Creativity and playfulness go a long way in making new traditions appealing.

It's worth the effort, because there's a direct link between how many green veggies you eat and your chances of steering clear of cancer, heart disease, type 2 diabetes, dementia, osteoporosis, and nearly every other major illness of our times. It seems as if every day another study shows the extraordinary power of nutrient dynamos such as broccoli, bok choy, brussels sprouts, Swiss chard, cabbage, collards, mustard greens, kale, beet greens, spinach, and dark greens of every kind.

For one example, let's look at mental decline in the elderly. In 2015, researchers at Rush University in Chicago evaluated the diet and mental function of 950 people with an average age of 81. After adjusting for variables such as education, exercise, and family history of dementia, the researchers found that participants who ate leafy green vegetables, such as spinach and kale, once or twice per day experienced significantly less cognitive decline than those who didn't.[1]

How much less? **The participants who ate greens regularly halted their mental decline by an average of 11 years.**

Eating greens has been linked to bone health, sharper eyesight, and even to muscle strength. At first I thought that latter point was going too far. Greens are potent, but I hardly associate them with bulging muscles. Nevertheless, Swedish researchers have found that spinach can indeed boost muscle potency.[2] Popeye may have been onto something after all!

I could go on and on, but I'm sure you don't need another lecture on why it's important to eat your greens. We all know it, and we've all known it for a long time. But there's a world of difference between knowing something and doing it. The honest truth is that most people just don't much like the taste of greens.

A lot of people think it would be nice if doughnuts and french fries were good for you, while it was Swiss chard that was carcinogenic. But that's not how it is. And no matter how much you might think you love doughnuts and french fries, they'll never love you back. But Swiss chard will.

The more your body gets used to greens, the more you'll enjoy them. Here are 12 of the top tips that have helped a lot of people enjoy greens and other vegetables.

1. ## Cut Them Up Playfully

     Studies have found that kids (and some adults!) respond differently to foods depending on how they're sliced and prepared.[3] And when vegetables have been cut into appealing shapes, like stars or cartoon characters, that can help, too. Some parents even give vegetables fun names, like calling broccoli florets "trees."

     As healthy-parenting expert Emily Honeycutt reminds us, "Kids learn through play. We develop habits by creating habit loops—building associations with positive or negative emotions. The more positive emotions we associate with vegetables throughout our childhood, the more likely we are to continue those healthy habits throughout our lives."[4]

2. ## Cook Creatively

     Cook vegetables in a variety of ways. Grill asparagus with lemon, bake squash and serve it as boats filled with quinoa or a stir-fry, or roast cauliflower "steaks." Want something simpler? My mom, Deo, makes some of the best greens I've ever tasted. (You'll find her easy recipe on page 309.) In brief: She cuts kale into thin strips and sautés the strips with garlic and onion in coconut or olive oil, and then steam-cooks it with a little soy sauce. Delicious!

3. ## Give It a Whirl

     Make a soup by puréeing steamed veggies in a blender with your favorite herbs and spices (many people especially love ginger and garlic). If you want a thicker or creamier texture, you can add white beans, potatoes, cashews, or a coconut or nut milk.

4. ## Add Them to Everything

     You can add veggies to pasta sauce, pizza, lasagna, casseroles, and chili, or to cooked quinoa, brown rice, or barley. Chop up fresh vegetables like spinach, cucumbers, mushrooms, peas, or kale and toss them into whatever you're cooking. You can even blend your veggies so they effectively become part of the base.

5. **Feature Them**

Pour tomato sauce over cooked chopped vegetables like onions, courgette, mushrooms, and leafy greens. Or if you want to get fancier, try a spiral slicer or a mandoline, or even a simple vegetable peeler, to make fun noodle shapes out of courgette, spaghetti squash, or aubergine. Don't limit vegetables to a side dish or a side salad. See what happens if you make them into the main event. Some chefs even use courgette or avocado as a base for desserts.

6. **Grow Them**

Studies find that when children (or adults!) grow vegetables, they're more likely to eat them. Plant a few seeds in the yard or in a container inside your window. Water as needed, and watch the miracle of life unfold. Gardening is a great way to enjoy the freshest, healthiest possible food, and it builds a strong relationship with produce that sets up your family to enjoy it more. You'll find out more about growing your own food in chapter 27.

7. **Dehydrate Kale Chips**

Instead of reaching for potato or corn chips, you can make your own kale chips with a dehydrator, or use your oven on a low setting, like 200 or 250°F. Destem the kale, marinate it in lemon juice and seasonings, and then dehydrate or bake it. The flavor and crunchy texture can be intoxicating!

8. **Make a Slaw**

With a food processor or by hand, shred the tough "winter veggies" like cabbage and carrots into an easy-to-enjoy slaw. Fold in some raisins and top it with your favorite dressings. It's easy to plop slaw into a container and grab it when you're on the go.

9. **Marinate Yumminess**

Marinate your favorite vegetables, chopped, for a few hours to soften and flavor them before cooking. For the marinade, I like a mix of olive oil, garlic, ginger, and soy sauce. You can marinate mushrooms, broccoli, string beans, asparagus, collards, and lots more. You can enjoy some marinated vegetables raw. Or if you like, you can roast, grill, bake, or sauté them—or add them to a stir-fry.

10. **Wrap It Up**

Simply wrap veggies up in a lettuce leaf (or a steamed leaf of collard greens or cabbage) or a tortilla and add your favorite sauces, salsa, or spices.

11. **Slice and Dip**

You're a lot more likely to reach for the veggies instead of the chips if they're already in snackable form. When you get home from a shopping trip, wash and cut some snacking vegetables and store them in the fridge for easy access. You can also make your own veggie dips (like the Roasted Red Pepper Hummus on page 287) for when the snacking urge strikes!

12. **Steam Away**

Probably the best way to eat abundant vegetables is to steam a pot of them. Our family does this frequently. We like broccoli, kale, collards, cabbage, onions, carrots, courgette, and Swiss chard. Our kids love eating with their fingers, so we leave big chunks, including whole leaves and carrots. We often keep sauces for dressing or dipping on hand.

SEASONING

If vegetables, or any other food, still seem a little plain to you, there's one simple way to add flavor and even *more* nutrition. Spice it up! More on that in the next chapter.

ACTION:

Option 1: Add chopped or blended green vegetables to a recipe or dish that wouldn't normally include them—such as a pasta sauce, casserole, or grain dish.

Option 2: Make vegetables the "main dish" for a meal. Serve them with a sauce, or grill them with a marinade. Treat them as the centerpiece, because when it comes to nutritional value, that's what they are.

Option 3: Eat at least a pound of green vegetables every day for the next week. You can enjoy them in smoothies, soups, steamed, grilled, stir-fried, raw, baked… get creative!

CHAPTER 13

The Healthiest Way to Add Flavor

Every culture is defined, in part, by the spices used in its cuisine. In India, there's cardamom and cumin. In Italy, there's basil and oregano. In Mexico, there's chili, garlic, and coriander. In Thailand, there's lemongrass, sweet basil, and galangal. And in North America, there's a bit of everything in the culinary melting pot. But what is North America most known for adding to the mix? Salt, sugar, and fat.

Not that North Americans don't use spices. They're just not what North American cuisine is typically known for. And speaking as a North American, I think that's a shame.

Fortunately, you don't have to live in Thailand to enjoy kaffir lime leaves, or in Mexico to partake of green chilies. Herbs and spices travel the globe. And they don't just bring wonderful, mouthwatering bursts of flavor. They also bring stunning levels of nutrition.

Cooking with herbs and spices is an art form. Knowing which ones are especially good for you, on the other hand, is science.

TURMERIC

Turmeric is a flavorful addition to sauces, curries, stir-fries, and casseroles. Popular in India for more than 5,000 years, it's widely thought to be one of the primary reasons that country has one of the world's lowest rates of Alzheimer's disease.[1]

Turmeric is known for its bright orange color. In fact, it's sometimes used as a coloring agent. The orange comes from a polyphenol called curcumin, which is something of a miracle compound.

Hundreds of studies have demonstrated that curcumin may help prevent or even reverse Alzheimer's and other forms of dementia, reduce unhealthy levels of inflammation, protect against heavy metal toxicity, and even lower heart disease risk.[2]

The average daily intake of curcumin in India is thought to be about 125 mg—the amount found in about a half-teaspoon of turmeric powder.[3] Research has found low rates of certain types of cancer in countries where people eat 100 to 200 mg of curcumin per day over long periods of time.[4]

If a half-teaspoon of turmeric seems like a lot, you might consider a curcumin supplement. My personal favorite (made by a company that also supports Food Revolution Network) contains a potent absorption-boosting breakthrough, and is available at turmeric4health.com. You'll get better curcumin absorption if you combine turmeric with some black pepper and/or a bit of (healthy) fat.

GARLIC

Garlic can be chopped, minced, blended, or eaten as a powder. It's delicious in pasta sauces, soups, and almost any savory dish. People at the annual garlic festival in Gilroy, California, have even been known to make garlic ice cream, though I can't say I recommend it!

Garlic is known for helping to ward off the bad guys. But instead of hanging it over your doorway to scare away vampires, you can eat it to fight off certain cancers.

Researchers studied 41,387 Iowa women, tracking their consumption of 127 foods over a five-year period.[5] The food found to be most highly associated with a statistically significant decrease in colon cancer was garlic. Women with the highest amounts of garlic in their diets had a 50 percent lower risk of certain colon cancers than women who ate the least.

Another study of 5,000 men and women, conducted in China over a five-year period, found that a garlic extract was linked to a 52 percent reduction in stomach cancer rates, compared to a placebo.[6]

Garlic has been rumored to help fight colds and flus. But is this folklore backed up by real-world science? A team of researchers studied 146 participants, giving half of them a garlic tablet and half a placebo tablet, every day for three months. The people who took the placebo reported cumulatively catching 65 colds. The people who took the garlic reported only 24. And for those garlic-takers who did catch a cold, the symptoms ended 20 percent sooner.[7]

GINGER

Ginger is one of my favorite spices. It has a refreshing, clean, invigorating flavor. I love it in soups, stir-fries, casseroles, salad dressings, smoothies, stews, and desserts. If you like, you can mix ginger powder or ginger tea with sparkling water and stevia for a healthy homemade ginger ale.

Ginger can be used to treat stomach problems, including motion sickness, morning sickness, colic, upset stomach, irritable bowel syndrome, gas, diarrhea, nausea, and loss of appetite. It has potent anti-inflammatory properties, and some people find it very effective in relieving pain caused by rheumatoid arthritis, osteoarthritis, and menstrual cramps.

As if all that weren't enough, ginger has also been found to be extraordinarily effective in the treatment of migraines.

If you've ever suffered from a migraine, you know that it's way more than a headache. Migraines make normal activities impossible for an estimated one billion people worldwide. And migraines are responsible for billions of dollars in health care costs.

But could a natural remedy like ginger really work as well as drugs, with fewer side effects?

In 2014, a double-blind randomized controlled clinical trial was published in *Phytotherapy Research*.[8] Researchers studied 100 people experiencing moderate to severe pain from migraines. Half the study participants were given one-eighth of a teaspoon of powdered ginger, and half were given a standard dose of sumatriptan, also known as Imitrex—one of the top-selling, billion-dollar drugs in the treatment of migraines.

The results? Both worked equally fast. Most participants started out with moderate or severe pain. After taking either the drug or ginger, they were either in mild pain or completely pain-free. The same proportion of migraine sufferers reported satisfaction with the results, whether they took sumatriptan or ginger. But with ginger, there were substantially fewer negative side effects. With sumatriptan, some people reported dizziness, a sedative effect, vertigo, and heartburn. The only adverse side effect for ginger was that two of the ginger-taking participants reported an upset stomach.

If you want to try the natural remedy, mix 1/8 teaspoon powdered ginger in water at the first sign of a migraine. Drink it, and see if your migraine lessens or goes away within half an hour.

Compared to sumatriptan, ginger not only spares you side effects—it also comes at about 1/3,000th the price. And it just might do the job.

CINNAMON

Cinnamon is one of the most popular spices in the world. It's made from the inner bark of a genus of tree called cinnamomum. When strips of it dry, they curl into rolls, called cinnamon sticks. The sticks can also be ground to form a powder. This mild-mannered, delectable spice can flavor drinks, baked goods, porridge, stir-fries, and dishes both savory and sweet.

For thousands of years, cinnamon has also been prized for its potent medicinal properties. It's loaded with polyphenols and other antioxidants. Cinnamon is an anti-inflammatory, antidiabetic, antimicrobial, anticancer, lipid-lowering, and cardiovascular-disease-lowering superstar.[9]

Whoever knew that such a sweet spice could be so potent a healing force!

HOT PEPPERS

Hot peppers look a lot like regular peppers, but with one major difference. They contain a compound known as capsaicin, which is colorless and odorless—but definitely not flavorless! Capsaicin is so intensely spicy that many people can tolerate hot peppers only in small amounts.

The capsaicin that brings peppers their heat, it turns out, is also a powerful medicine. Chili peppers aid digestion by promoting salivation, boosting the stomach's defense against infections, increasing digestive fluid production, and helping to deliver enzymes to the stomach.[10]

In a 2017 study conducted on mice, researchers found that the capsaicin in hot peppers was able to alter the composition of gut bacteria, promoting more beneficial strains.[11] This in turn led to lower levels of chronic inflammation and obesity.

In another study, 16,179 human participants were tracked for an average of more than 15 years.[12] After factoring out demographic, lifestyle, and clinical characteristics, the people who consumed hot peppers had a 13 percent lower rate of mortality over the course of the study. Put in plain English, that means people who ate more hot peppers were more likely to live longer.

There are many varieties of hot peppers, and their level of capsaicin ranges from mild to intense. Some people love the spiciness, but others, especially children, may not. Instead of mixing hot pepper into a whole dish, you can arrange it on top or serve it separately. A word to the wise: When you chop hot peppers, be careful to wash your knife, cutting board, and hands with soap afterward, and be sure not to touch your eyes before you've washed your hands. I've learned from personal experience that capsaicin can burn eyes (and other sensitive parts of the body!).

THERE ARE SO MANY MORE

Turmeric, garlic, ginger, cinnamon, and hot peppers barely scratch the surface in the wonderful world of spices. Your spice cabinet is a virtual pharmacy of medicinal compounds. Nutmeg, cloves, basil, dill, oregano, thyme, sage, parsley, fennel, and many other herbs and spices contain substances that could help fight cancer and heart disease, reduce inflammation, stabilize your blood sugar, fend off dementia, and add culinary delight to your menu.

ACTION:

Option 1: Enjoy at least one herb or spice that isn't normally in your repertoire.

Option 2: For one day, try using little or no sugar, salt, or added fats in your foods—season them with spices instead.

Option 3: Open up your spice rack and smell or taste every spice in it. Get rid of any that are old or that you don't care for. Put new ones on your shopping list, and find recipes that incorporate any new spices you'd like to try.

CHAPTER 14

Enjoy Healthy and Delicious Pleasures

Recently, I was preparing to speak at a conference. As I walked through the lobby, I came upon a woman scarfing down a chocolate bar. Her face reddened as she mumbled, "I had this in my pocket, and I figured I'd better eat it now—before I hear what you have to say."

She believed that I'd judge her.

When I got up onstage to begin my talk, I told the audience what had just happened, and asked, "How'd you like to be the guy everyone thinks is going to take away their chocolate?"

The audience laughed nervously. I'd struck a nerve.

"Well," I went on, with a smile, "let's get one thing straight. I love chocolate. I especially love organic, fair-trade dark chocolate. And I love pleasure—especially healthy pleasure."

The relief on many faces was visible.

I say that life is too short for misery. You aren't just meant to survive. You are meant to thrive.

We're going to look at four foods that might put pleasure and wellness on the same page, but each has incurred some level of controversy. So let's get the real scoop, and you can decide if and how you may want to incorporate these into your life.

COFFEE

If you greet the morning with the aroma of freshly brewing coffee, you're enjoying a pleasure shared by billions of people.

Until recently, you wouldn't have expected to see coffee listed as a health food. For decades we've been advised to drink less of it. But it turns out that much of that advice is debatable.

Of course, what's done to coffee has a big impact on the results it brings. Many coffee shops add sugar, milk, high-fructose corn syrup, artificial flavorings, and other chemicals. Just because coffee is linked to health benefits doesn't mean that you should guzzle the Salted Caramel Mocha at Starbucks—which actually has more sugar than an 8-ounce bottle of Coke.[1]

And there's no question that coffee isn't for everyone. I drink it only rarely, because while I enjoy the taste as well as the "buzz" it brings, I find that a few hours later, I feel jittery, anxious, and even a bit cranky. But I've been enormously impressed with the research, which tells us that for many people, coffee can confer significant benefits. It's often found to be good for mood, reaction time, and general mental function.[2] Coffee's also a vasodilator. This means that it causes blood vessels to expand, which is good for your circulation. And it seems to have a particular effect on the blood vessels that feed your brain—making it an ally in the fight against all forms of dementia.

The Cardiovascular Risk Factors, Aging and Dementia study tracked more than 1,500 randomly selected Finnish people for 21 years, examining a broad range of diet and lifestyle choices and how they correlated with health outcomes.[3] The study found that when, at midlife, people drank three to five small cups of coffee per day (which sounds like a lot to me!), then as they grew older they had, compared to non–coffee drinkers, a 65 percent decreased risk of dementia.

In another study, 34,670 women in Sweden were tracked for more than 10 years.[4] Those who drank no coffee were at elevated risk of stroke, while the women who drank at least a cup per day reduced their risk of stroke by 22 to 25 percent.

Based on these and dozens of other studies, it seems clear that coffee can protect against dementia and stroke. Both of those relate to the brain, and we know that coffee stimulates brain activity. But what about cancer? Does coffee fight cancer? Or does it, as some media reports have implied, actually cause it?

In 2018, a judge in the state of California ruled that Starbucks and other coffee chains needed to post warnings because their brews may contain a chemical that's been linked to cancer.[5] The target of the ruling was acrylamide, a potential carcinogen that's formed when foods containing both starches and the amino acid asparagine are cooked at high temperatures.[6] Acrylamide is a by-product of the coffee-roasting process. It's also found in breads and crackers, canned black olives, prune juice, and even breakfast cereals. The highest levels are found in french fries and potato chips.

So is the acrylamide in coffee a serious concern? Unlikely. If we look at the real world, outside of courtrooms and lab theories, I've never heard of a single study that found elevated risk of cancer in people who drank more coffee. To the contrary, according to one study, consumption of coffee could cut mouth and throat cancer risk by 50 percent.[7] Other studies have found that coffee reduces the risk of many types of cancer—including uterine, prostate, brain, breast, liver, lung, and skin cancers.[8]

We don't know for certain if the acrylamide in coffee poses health risks. But we do know that coffee is associated with broad health benefits in large numbers of people. Avoiding coffee altogether on account of acrylamide strikes me as a bit like avoiding the outdoors because sunshine can cause cancer. It's true that some danger exists. But your health would surely suffer if you spent your whole life indoors as a result.

The documented health benefits of coffee consumption are considerable and widespread. This bean has even been linked with decreased risk of type 2 diabetes.[9] And for those who already have type 2 diabetes, coffee can prolong life expectancy. One study of nearly 4,000 type 2 diabetics found that those who drank coffee were 30 percent more likely to still be alive after being tracked for 20 years.[10]

Caffeine is the most widely appreciated compound in coffee, but it makes up only about 1 to 2 percent of the bean. Coffee also contains an abundance of antioxidants, which help prevent the damaging effects of oxidation on cells throughout your body, thus lowering your risk of cancer.[11]

Here's a stunning reality: Coffee, by a wide margin, is the number one antioxidant in the American diet!

We know that the average American's diet is woefully deficient in antioxidants. But one thing we don't know is how beneficial coffee might be for people who are already eating an abundant amount of antioxidant-rich fruits and vegetables. If your body isn't antioxidant-starved, it's possible that the net benefits of coffee will be less dramatic because your diet's already healthier than the norm.

Since the studies on the health effects of coffee have been done on people eating, for the most part, the modern industrialized diet, we don't really know whether it confers a similar level of benefit for a population of already healthy eaters.

Isn't Caffeine a Problem?

Coffee isn't for everybody. Caffeine makes some people feel relaxed, but it makes others get stressed out. And it can become addictive. Many consistent coffee drinkers find that if they miss more than a day or two, they get headaches and feel miserable.

If you tend to be lethargic, coffee can make life brighter. For many people, it feels like an on switch to start their day. But if you tend to be hyperstimulated easily, with your adrenals on overdrive, coffee might ultimately add more agitation than joy.

And here's something to watch out for: Caffeine may be harmful to fetuses and infants. Most women avoid it during pregnancy, and for good reason. Many official recommendations are that if you're pregnant or breastfeeding, you should consume no more than two cups per day. And honestly, if I were pregnant (though barring a medical miracle, that's highly unlikely to ever happen!), I'd consume none at all.

Caffeine content can vary by roast type. The darker the roast, the less caffeine there typically is. Light roasts usually contain the most caffeine.

If you'd prefer to skip caffeine, opt for decaf. We don't have a lot of studies on the health effects of decaffeinated coffee, but we know it has about 75 percent of the antioxidants of the caffeinated version.[12] While many decaffeination methods involve use of solvents like methylene chloride or ethyl acetate, the Swiss Water Process is a more environmentally friendly and chemical-free method.[13]

Why Fair Trade Matters

Because coffee accounts for almost half the total exports from tropical countries, coffee production has a massive impact on the lives and livelihoods of hundreds of millions of families and farmers.[14] Many of them are living in abject poverty.

Therefore the kinds of coffee we choose have a profound impact on the kind of world we shape for future generations. If you want a healthier and more sustainable world, then fair-trade, shade-grown (coffee grown under the shade of trees means less deforestation and a more sustainable habitat for birds and wildlife), and organic coffee are the types to reach for.

How to Enjoy Coffee

Enjoy your coffee black, or add coconut and/or organic soy or other milk. If you want to add some bonus flavor, mix in cocoa, cinnamon, or vanilla. To add sweetness, try a pinch of stevia or a splash of maple syrup.

If you're concerned about acidity, try cold-brewing, which drops the acidity level by approximately two-thirds.[15] Many people just like the cold-brewing flavor. You can make it yourself, to whatever strength you desire. If you like your coffee very strong, you can put ½ cup of ground coffee in a mason jar with 3 cups of filtered water and let it sit in the fridge at least 12 hours. Filter it as you would any coffee, and voilà— cold-brewed coffee. It stores well in the fridge, and you can also leave it at room temperature for a couple of hours, or add some hot water if you want to warm it up.

HOW A CUP OF TEA CAN CHANGE YOUR LIFE

I love sitting down for a warm cup of tea. Something about the warmth in my hand and in my belly brings me a sense of relaxation and comfort.

The story of tea begins in China.[16] According to legend, in 2737 BC, the Chinese emperor Shen Nung, a renowned herbalist, was sitting beneath a tree while his servant boiled drinking water. Some leaves from the tree blew into the water, and Shen Nung decided to try the infusion his servant had accidentally created. And thus the emperor enjoyed the first teatime in the history of the world.

It would take another several thousand years before tea became the national drink of China—around 700 AD.

Today, next to water, tea is the most widely consumed beverage in the world. (Yes, even ahead of Coca-Cola.) Yet we're only now discovering how powerful it really is.

Here I mean tea as in the green leaves of the *Camellia sinensis* plant— not herbal teas, like peppermint, rooibos, or chamomile, which have their own distinct health-giving properties.

There are four types of tea: white, green, oolong, and black. All of these can be derived from the same plant. Of the four types of tea, white and green are the least processed. They have the highest levels of antioxidants and the lowest levels of caffeine.

Researchers have known for years that rates of prostate cancer are considerably lower in many Asian countries than in other parts of the world. Many scientists believe this is because of the high consumption of plant foods among Asian populations. But some also think that the consumption of green tea—the most popular tea in Japan, China, and other Asian countries—plays a role.[17]

Like coffee, tea is high in antioxidants, which may help protect against a broad range of cancers, including cancers of the breast (one study found that three cups of tea per day reduced the risk of breast cancer by one-third), colon, skin, lung, esophagus, stomach, small intestine, pancreas, and liver.[18]

Green tea also contains catechins, which increase the body's ability to burn fat as a fuel, leading to improved muscle endurance.[19] And it's been found to help fight osteoporosis by enhancing bone strength.[20]

Studies have also found that drinking all types of tea can help protect against cardiovascular disease and may reduce the risk of heart attack.[21] What's more, studies have linked consumption of tea with reduced rates of Alzheimer's, obesity, arthritis, type 2 diabetes, and even malaria.[22]

Of course, unless it's been decaffeinated, tea has caffeine (more in black and oolong than in green or white). As with coffee, listen to your body and use your best judgment.

Also keep in mind that many bottled tea products are mostly sugar water. For example, Lipton's Lemon Iced Tea contains 31 grams of added sugar.[23] When you brew your own, you save money and have complete control over the ingredients. Try it plain, or with a squeeze of lemon and/or a dab of honey or other sweetener.

RED WINE

In 2014, my mother-in-law, Diane, died of primary biliary cirrhosis— an autoimmune disease that attacks the liver and that's heightened by alcohol consumption. Diane gave up alcohol completely once she was diagnosed. But by then, sadly, it was too late.

So, for me, any discussion of red wine needs to start with a few sobering facts about alcohol. It is, by almost any measure, the most destructive drug on the planet. According to the World Health Organization, harmful use of alcohol results in the deaths of 2.5 million people annually, and it causes illness and injury to millions more.[24] In addition to being a cause of countless injuries and car accidents, alcohol abuse is a leading driver of cancer, cardiovascular diseases, and as our family knows all too well, liver cirrhosis.

There is evidence that even moderate alcohol use may increase risk of breast cancer.[25]

Why, then, would I suggest that red wine could be considered a healthy pleasure? Because many people around the world enjoy positive social connection (which is good for your health) and relaxing meals (also good for your health) while sharing a glass of wine. And while there's nothing healthful about alcohol, there's a lot more than alcohol in red wine.

It is, after all, made from red grapes—and they contain many potent phytonutrients, which help the body resist cataracts, Alzheimer's disease, macular degeneration, and heart disease.[26]

Studies have shown that modest red wine consumption (limited to a glass or less per day) may help prevent dental cavities by getting rid of damaging bacteria on the teeth, may cut the risk of nonalcoholic fatty liver disease in half among those who are at risk of the condition, may lower the risk of depression, and might even reduce the risk of dementia.[27]

The skin of red grapes is a particularly rich source of an antioxidant called resveratrol.[28] (Resveratrol is also found in smaller amounts in blueberries, raspberries, blackberries, pistachios, and peanuts.[29])

Researchers at the MD Anderson Center at the University of Texas have researched resveratrol and shown that it could be a potent force to prevent cancer, and it may also improve success rates with chemotherapy.[30] This may be why a 2004 study conducted by the Fred Hutchinson Cancer Research Center found that consumption of moderate amounts of red wine was linked to a 50 percent reduction in rates of prostate cancer for men.[31]

It turns out that how grapes are grown matters, too. Resveratrol is produced as a protectant against potential invaders like molds and fungi. When modern pesticides and fungicides are applied, less resveratrol is required to protect the plant—so less may be produced. That's why resveratrol levels seem highest in organically grown red grapes.[32]

Would you get most of these same benefits from drinking red grape juice or eating handfuls of red table grapes? Apparently, yes! A growing body of research has found that eating red grapes, or drinking red grape juice, may provide many of the same benefits as red wine (and possibly even more), without the alcohol.[33] I find red grape juice intensely sweet, but love mixing it with sparkling water for a kind of resveratrol-infused soda.

If you do well with small amounts of alcohol and find that it adds pleasure to your life without causing problems, then red wine is a wise choice. But eating red table grapes may be an even better one. And always remember that some people are chemically susceptible to alcoholism. For them, any amount of alcohol is too much. Always respect and support the sobriety of anyone, including yourself, who has this susceptibility.

CHOCOLATE

For several centuries in premodern Latin America, cacao beans were considered valuable enough to be used as currency.[34] Both the Mayans and the Aztecs believed the cacao bean had magical properties, suitable for use in the most sacred rituals of birth, marriage, and death.

More recently chocolate has been vilified, with many so-called experts considering it a junk food or saying it causes acne. When it's paired with large amounts of sugar, cow's milk, and chemicals, the final product has substantial drawbacks. But that's not the chocolate's fault.

Modern science is proving that the Mayans and the Aztecs were onto something.

The Guna people of the San Blas Islands, off the coast of Panama, have loved cocoa for thousands of years, and to this day, cocoa beverages remain central in their diet. An *International Journal of Medical Science* article reported that despite intense poverty, the Guna who keep drinking cocoa in their home islands enjoy much lower death rates from heart attacks, strokes, diabetes, and cancer than those who give up their beloved drink when they move to mainland cities and suburbs.[35]

Of course, the amount of cocoa the Guna drink isn't the only thing that typically changes when they move to the city, with its stress, environmental pollution, and shift in dietary patterns. But I still think it's pretty remarkable that heart disease rates among the cocoa-drinking Guna are a full nine times less than they are for mainland Panamanians.[36]

Many scientists believe that the traditionally living Guna owe their expanded heart health and longevity in part to the cocoa beverage they drink so generously, which supplies them with abundant cardiovascular-system-boosting flavanols.[37]

Scientists are learning that chocolate is also a plentiful source of antioxidants, including some of the same polyphenols renowned in red wine and green tea.[38] These substances reduce the ongoing cellular and arterial damage caused by oxidative reactions. In layman's terms, they help fight cancer and heart disease.

In a study of 1,000 heart attack survivors, published by Stockholm's Karolinska Institutet in 2009, patients who ate dark chocolate several times per week cut their risk of dying from heart disease threefold compared to those who didn't eat chocolate at all.[39]

What's more, chocolate has long been celebrated for its remarkable effects on the human mood. It's high in a number of compounds linked to mood elevation, stress reduction, and even to enhanced feelings of love and euphoria.[40] No wonder so many people delight in chocolate hearts on Valentine's Day.

What Are Cocoa, Cacao, and Chocolate?

The cacao tree produces inedible pods, inside of which are the precious cacao beans. The outsides of these cacao beans have a soft and fatty whitish coating, which we call cacao butter, while the harder, dark brown bean itself is used to make cacao powder. Cocoa is cacao that's been exposed to high heat and roasted during processing. Chocolate can be made using any combination of cocoa and cacao, although cocoa (which has been roasted) is far more common. Cocoa and cacao can be used interchangeably in most baking recipes, smoothies, cookies, and treats, or for stirring into coffee for a homemade mocha.

Cacao has a higher antioxidant content than cocoa, but most of the studies that have found chocolate to be beneficial have been based on cocoa, since it's far more widely used.

Both cocoa and cacao have a bitter flavor, which is why most chocolate today is sweetened. If you're choosing between different kinds of chocolate, remember that in general, the higher the percentage of actual chocolate, and the lower your selection is in sugars, milk, or other additives, the more healthful it will be. There is evidence that combining chocolate with cow's milk, as is done to make milk chocolate, undermines the health values.[41]

Most of the major brands pump their candies full of sugar, emulsifiers, artificial sweeteners, and other chemicals. In general, more natural and smaller-scale brands offer better and safer chocolates. Personally, I look for dark (dairy-free) chocolate that contains at least 65 percent cacao or cocoa content.

The Shadow Side of Chocolate: Child Slavery

Much of the world's chocolate comes from West Africa.[42] Many of the farmers in this region have very low income and can't afford to pay their workers much. The result is that labor conditions on West African cacao farms are notoriously deplorable, and child labor is used widely. A report from Tulane University in 2015 stated that there is evidence of child trafficking for forced labor in the farming of cacao, and that at least 1.5 million children are currently subjected to hazardous and potentially illegal working conditions—primarily in Ghana and the Ivory Coast.[43]

Most of the West African cacao is purchased by huge companies like Hershey, Nestlé, Mars, and Cadbury.

If you want to be sure your chocolate is slavery-free, the top thing to look for is a fair-trade certification. This means that the farmer was paid a living wage, and farmers paid living wages almost never resort to child slavery. Another option is to stick to chocolate from Central and South America, where slavery is fairly nonexistent. Organic chocolate is almost exclusively grown in Central and South America, and therefore also most likely slavery-free.

When I first told my son River about child slavery in the chocolate industry, his jaw dropped. He'd heard about my work for a Food Revolution but had so far shown little direct interest. But when he learned about kids being ripped away from their families and forced into slavery, suddenly he could relate. The injustice of it all brought him almost to tears.

For the first time in his young life, he asked me how he could help.

ACTION:

Option 1: Look at labels for coffee and chocolate, and choose organic and/or fair trade. When you choose consciously, you support a world in which children can go to school instead of being forced into labor. More and more chocolatiers are selling ethically made chocolate. They deserve our support.

Option 2: Make unsweetened green tea, white tea, or coffee into a daily habit.

Option 3: Educate your children, grandchildren, nieces, nephews, friends, and family about why ethical sourcing matters. Urge everyone you know to support organic and fair-trade certified foods—especially chocolate, coffee, bananas, and other foods that come from tropical countries.

CHAPTER 15

Get the Goods on Grains and Gluten

For thousands of years, grains have enabled entire civilizations to weather harsh winters, stave off famine in times of poor harvest, travel long distances without going hungry, and feed an ever-expanding population.

Grains continue to play a fundamental role in feeding the world. Out of more than 50,000 edible plants, just three—rice, corn, and wheat—provide almost two-thirds of humanity's food energy intake today.[1]

Yet in spite of, or perhaps because of, the huge role they play in feeding the world, grains are no stranger to controversy. On the one hand, numerous health organizations—from the American Heart Association and the Mayo Clinic to Public Health England—endorse whole grains to help fight heart disease, type 2 diabetes, cancer, cardiovascular disease, and even obesity.[2]

But not everything is peachy in grain land.

Paleo diet proponents remind us that humans didn't begin eating significant amounts of grains until the advent of agriculture.[3] We didn't evolve to digest them, these advocates say, and when we do eat them, our bodies can revolt—leading to celiac disease, gluten intolerance, autoimmune disease, and other serious problems.

Antigrain spokespeople remind us that grains are high in phytic acid, which can bind with minerals like calcium, copper, iron, magnesium, and zinc, preventing optimal absorption.

And then there's gluten, which is found in barley, rye, and wheat. Although only about 1 percent of humans have celiac disease, many more shows signs of gluten intolerance, with symptoms such as head-aches, joint pain, skin problems, seizures, mental disorders, and digestive problems.

WHAT'S GOING ON HERE?

Why would government bodies and medical experts advocate eating more whole grains if they can cause so many problems? And if they're good for us, why are some people vehemently opposed to them?

Part of the problem we face with grains is what's being done to them.

Most of the grains grown in the world today are sprayed with pesticides. The corn is usually genetically engineered and sprayed with glyphosate (as we touched on earlier, this herbicide is an endocrine disruptor, antibiotic, and probable carcinogen). The wheat, unless it's grown organically, may also be sprayed with glyphosate, which is used as a desiccant to dry out the crop prior to harvest. (This alone is a very good reason to avoid nonorganic corn and wheat.)

And then there's what happens after harvest.

Grains are grass seeds, composed primarily of three parts. There's the bran, which is the fiber-packed outside of the seed. There's the germ, which is the nutrient-dense core. And there's the endosperm—the white part in between. To turn a whole grain into white flour, the grain must first be milled, and then it must be strained to remove the bran and the germ.

The vast majority of the grains eaten by humans today have had their bran and germ removed.

The trouble is that most of the vitamins, minerals, healthy oils, and fiber in grains are found in the bran and the germ. Nutritionally speaking, refining flour means removing the best part.

Refined starches, including white bread, white rice, white pasta, and anything made with white flour, act a lot like sugar once you digest them.[4] Whole grains are richer in fiber and generally cause a slower, steadier rise in blood sugar.

White flour shows up in breads, cereals, pasta, pizza, and baked goods. And buyer beware: Many of the breads with claims like "made with whole grains" on the label include at least some, if not mostly, white flour. Check the ingredients list. If "wheat flour" appears first, with "whole wheat flour" or other grains farther down the list, you can know that your "whole grain" or "multigrain" bread consists of predominantly white flour.

Even the most die-hard grain lovers have to face the facts. Most of the grains eaten in the industrialized world have been refined in ways that make them drivers of obesity, heart disease, type 2 diabetes, and even cancer.

We turn our wheat into white flour for bread and cakes. We turn our corn into high-fructose corn syrup and Doritos. And we turn our rice into Uncle Ben's and Minute White.

What's more, many commercial bread products come with quite a laundry list of ingredients. In my local supermarket, I can buy Sara Lee "100% Whole Wheat" bread. That sounds healthy, but in addition to whole wheat flour, water, and yeast, which is really all you need to make bread, the label tells us of sugar, wheat gluten, soybean oil, calcium propionate, datem, monoglycerides, calcium sulfate, monocalcium phosphate, potassium iodate, cornflour, and other laboratory-derived compounds.

I'm reminded of the saying: "The whiter your bread, the sooner you're dead."

WHAT WHOLE GRAINS CAN DO FOR YOU

To put it bluntly, processed and refined grains aren't good for anyone. But for many people, *whole grains* are another story.

Whole grains are rich in fiber, vitamins, minerals, and antioxidants. They've been linked to lower risk of age-related illnesses, including cardiovascular disease and gum disease.[5] And many whole grains have been linked to a reduction in cancer risk. According to one meta-analysis of studies, consumption of an average of approximately six ounces of whole grains per day reduced colorectal cancer risk by 21 percent.[6]

Now, consider for a moment that 1.4 million people will be diagnosed with colorectal cancer worldwide this year. What we're seeing is that if the average human ate just six ounces of whole grains per day, in one year we might be able to prevent 294,000 cases of colorectal cancer.

And there's more. In 2015, researchers at Harvard's T.H. Chan School of Public Health announced the results of a 14-year-long study involving 367,000 people.[7] The researchers concluded that eating a bowl of quinoa per day may lower your risk of premature death from diseases like cancer, heart disease, respiratory disease, and diabetes by 17 percent. But it wasn't just quinoa that was beneficial. High whole-grain consumption in general was associated with an 11 percent reduction in respiratory disease, a 48 percent reduction in rates of type 2 diabetes, and a 15 percent reduction in risk of all forms of cancer.

Okay, you might be thinking, that's all well and good. But what about all the people who are cutting out carbs and losing weight? A lot of them are giving up grains. Are we supposed to ignore their obvious results?

Here's the thing to remember: People who eat whole grains and people who eat no grains usually have one thing in common. They're steering clear of sugar, refined flour, and other processed carbohydrates. And when you do that, chances are good that you'll lose unwanted pounds.

WHAT ABOUT GLUTEN?

Hundreds of millions of people worldwide have jumped on the gluten-free train. In 2013, up to one-third of Americans and large numbers in Europe reportedly preferred gluten-free foods.[8] There are now gluten-free chips, gluten-free dips, gluten-free soups, and gluten-free stews; there are gluten-free breads, croutons, pretzels, and beer. There's gluten-free artisanal fusilli and penne from Italy. Companies offer gluten-free cheese sticks, fish sticks, and bread sticks.

Amazingly enough, I've seen gluten-free bottled water for sale. Seriously.

But is this hoopla justified? Is there a downside? Let's take a look.

Celiac disease is a genetic condition affecting about 1 percent of the world population. An additional portion of humanity (by some estimates about 6 percent, by others as high as 25 percent) is gluten-intolerant.[9] These people don't have a celiac diagnosis, but they may still have symptoms linked to consumption of gluten products, such as autoimmune disease, joint pain, headaches, or sustained gastrointestinal distress. If you have celiac disease or gluten sensitivity, avoiding gluten is a good idea.

In fact, if you're facing any of the symptoms often pinned on gluten intolerance, going gluten-free for three to six months and seeing how it impacts your symptoms could be a worthwhile experiment.

Overblown phenomenon or not, there are definitely some people who are allergic to gluten, and whose health improves when they remove it from their diet.

But that doesn't mean that going gluten-free is right for everyone. A 2015 study published in the journal *Digestion* found that 86 percent of individuals who believed they were gluten-sensitive might be mistaken.[10] The study's authors concluded that self-perceived gluten-related symptoms are rarely indicative of the presence of nonceliac gluten sensitivity. So a whole lot of people might be avoiding gluten for no good reason.

And there's a shadow side to the gluten-free craze. If you aren't sensitive or allergic to gluten, going gluten-free could mean missing out on valuable nutrition. Researchers have found that the bran in whole wheat contains a critical prebiotic fiber that boosts bifidobacteria content within the gut, helping to relieve many gastrointestinal issues.[11]

Gluten itself has also been found to boost immune function. In a 2005 study, after less than a week on added gluten protein, subjects experienced significantly increased natural "killer cell" activity, which could be expected to improve their body's ability to fight cancer and viral infections.[12] Yet another study found that high-gluten bread lowered triglyceride levels more effectively than regular gluten bread.[13] And gluten is, itself, a protein—making wheat one of the highest-protein grains in the world. If you're not allergic to it, gluten could actually be beneficial to your overall dietary pattern.

What's more, many gluten-free products on the market today are packed with refined flours and chemicals. For someone who isn't gluten-intolerant, replacing organic sprouted whole-grain bread with bread made from tapioca and potato starch may be a step in the wrong direction.

The irony is that millions of people are eating gluten-free breads and other products because they think they're doing their health a favor. But unless they are, in fact, gluten-intolerant or gluten-sensitive, the truth may be the opposite.

MY WHOLE-GRAIN ADVICE

I love millet, amaranth, buckwheat, corn, teff, and many other grains. My personal favorite is quinoa, which is high in antioxidants and contains all nine essential amino acids. Just be sure to soak it or rinse it before you cook it, because doing so will remove bitter compounds.

Most whole grains can be soaked for 24 to 48 hours before cooking (pouring off the water twice daily) to activate their germination process and make their nutrients more bioavailable. This has also been found to reduce phytate content by 50 to 75 percent, which will help you get more value from the vitamins and minerals in your diet. As mentioned earlier, phytic acid can bind minerals in the gut, reducing your body's ability to absorb them.[14] Phytates aren't all bad—they also have properties that aid in the prevention of cancer, cardiovascular disease, kidney disease, and other illnesses. But when you soak whole grains, you still get some—just less—which is probably a good thing.

If you're going to eat flour products, make sure they're 100 percent whole grain. Read legally mandated ingredient lists, not just front-of-package claims. If you see any reference to wheat flour, and you don't see "whole grain" or "whole wheat," then you can assume it's white (refined) flour. And sprouted-grain breads will digest more slowly and are therefore easier on your blood sugar balance.

When it comes to rice, especially brown rice, I have some sad news. Rice is a staple for billions of people. Unfortunately, most of the rice eaten in the world today (including all basmati, wild, black, brown, and white, as well as conventional and organic) is often contaminated with disturbing amounts of arsenic. Sadly, brown rice is especially problematic because the arsenic tends to concentrate in its outer hull. For this reason, my suggestion is to eat rice once a week or less. You can get a full report on arsenic in rice and how to protect yourself, at 31dayfoodrevolution.com/arsenic.

ACTION:

Option 1: Perform an audit. Where and how do processed grains sneak into your life? Do you eat any breads or bagels that include white (not 100 percent whole wheat) flour? What about semolina or other kinds of pasta? White rice? When you have accurate information, you can make an informed decision. Do you want to cut out the bad stuff?

Option 2: Prepare a recipe featuring a whole grain you don't normally eat, such as quinoa, teff, amaranth, millet, or buckwheat. Make sure to season it with a tasty sauce, stir-fry, or set of seasonings, unless you know you like your foods plain. If you treat it right, you just might make a new friend for life.

Option 3: Soak whole grains before you cook them. Soak 2 cups in water overnight; then rinse well in a sieve. When you cook your grain, see if you can taste the difference.

CHAPTER 16

Legumes for Long Life

The legume family includes thousands of colorful varieties of beans, peas, lentils, and even peanuts. They grow in pods, and like nuts and seeds, each legume has the potential to sprout into a new plant.

Beans are sometimes called the "poor man's meat," as if eating them somehow makes you second-class. But I don't see why the fact that beans are affordable should count against them, or against the people smart enough to eat them. A whole lot of bean eaters are a little richer because they've been well nourished without having to break the bank.

Really, that should make the bean counters happy.

If there were an Olympics for the food group doing the most good for the most people, legumes would stand an excellent chance of winning gold. They're a critical source of protein for billions of people—providing an estimated 33 percent of the world's total protein intake.[1] A half-cup of beans can provide 21 grams of protein. They're also one of the leading sources of fiber in the human diet. A single half-cup serving of cooked kidney beans provides more than 7 grams of dietary fiber—half what the average American gets, from all sources, in a day![2] (While the average American gets about 15 grams of fiber per day, most dietary guidelines recommend getting a minimum of 25 to 30.)

Legumes are also a rich source of vitamins and minerals, including folate, iron, magnesium, potassium, and choline.

As if that weren't enough, legumes turn out to be potent cancer fighters, too. In an eight-year study in Uruguay involving more than 3,539 cancer cases and 2,032 hospital controls, scientists found that the highest rates of bean and lentil consumption were associated with a 25 percent reduction in overall rates of cancers of the kidney and the entire digestive tract—including mouth, stomach, colon, and rectum.[3]

What is it about legumes that might help with cancer prevention?

For one thing, people who eat more legumes are likely to eat less of the stuff we know can cause cancer—like processed foods and, especially, processed meats.[4] But that's not the whole story. Most legumes are also outstanding sources of phytochemicals, including triterpenoids, flavonoids, inositol, protease inhibitors, and sterols, as well as lignans and saponins.[5]

THE BEST WAY TO PREDICT HOW LONG YOU'LL LIVE

In 2004, researchers from Japan, Sweden, Greece, and Australia teamed up for a fascinating study.[6] They wanted to see if there was any one food group that was consistently linked with a longer life span in every nation and group. And they found one.

Legumes.

Whether it was the Swedes dining on brown beans and peas, the Japanese eating soy, or Mediterraneans enjoying chickpeas, lentils, and white beans, one thing was clear: The more legumes people ate, the longer they lived. As the researchers looked at data across all the populations combined, legumes showed up with the most plausible, consistent, and statistically significant results. Over the course of the study, every 20-gram (two-tablespoon) increase in daily legume consumption was correlated with an 8 percent reduction in risk of death.

TIPS FOR TOOT-FREE BEANS

The offending compounds in beans and other legumes most likely to cause gas are the oligosaccharides that can't be broken down before they reach the colon. Because these oligosaccharides arrive in the colon relatively undigested, they are fermented by bacteria, which can result in intestinal gas.

The good news is, there are ways to greatly reduce the effects of the offending oligosaccharides and to diminish or eradicate the flatulence problem. Start by soaking your legumes well, rinsing them every 12 or so hours. For beans, I suggest soaking for 48 hours. For lentils and split peas, 8 to 12 hours will do.

Each time you rinse your legumes, more oligosaccharides will wash away. Over the course of a couple of days, legumes can begin to germinate, which changes their composition and increases digestibility.

Rinse your legumes one final time before putting them in a pressure cooker and covering them with plenty of fresh water (it should reach one or two inches—three to five centimeters—above the legumes themselves). It helps if you also add a piece of kombu, about four inches (ten centimeters) long, to the pot. (Kombu is an edible seaweed that has a unique ability to neutralize any remaining gas-producing compounds in beans.)

Cook your legumes until they're soft—and enjoy them!

One of the advantages of soaking legumes is that, just like with grains, soaking and rinsing can reduce the level of phytate, which may help your body better absorb vitamins and minerals.[7]

THE LECTIN CONTROVERSY

Lectins are a type of protein found in many plant foods. Beans and other legumes are among the main sources of lectins in the human diet—though some are also found in grains, dairy products, seafood, and plants in the nightshade family.

A recent brouhaha over lectins has been fueled in no small part by Steven Gundry, MD, author of *The Plant Paradox*. On his website, Dr. Gundry states, "I believe lectins are the #1 Biggest Danger in the American Diet." Lectins in plants, he explains, are a defense against microorganisms, pests, and insects.[8] He tells us that "plants are literally declaring war on our bodies—dropping little bombs that wreak havoc on our intestines and immune systems."

But if these "little bombs" were really the biggest danger in the modern diet, then why would the longest-lived, healthiest people in the world—those living in Dan Buettner's Blue Zones—tend to subsist on legume-rich plant-based diets that include an abundance of lectins?[9]

Dr. Gundry warns against grains of all kinds (especially whole wheat), beans and other legumes, nuts, and certain fruits and vegetables (especially aubergine, tomatoes, potatoes, and peppers), in addition to dairy and eggs.[10] And yet, these recommendations appear to contradict the findings of the vast majority of the epidemiological studies ever conducted on humans. We're faced with epidemic rates of disease that many experts believe are clearly linked to an abundance of low-nutrient, low-fiber, sugar-enhanced, heavily processed, and meat-centered foods—and Dr. Gundry is declaring war on legumes, grains, and many fruits and vegetables?

But that doesn't leave Dr. Gundry's ideas completely out in the cold. There are many different kinds of lectins, and they don't all have the same effects. Some may, in sufficient quantity, cause digestive issues, ranging from gas to leaky gut, along with other long-term health problems.[11] And one, phytohemagglutinin (found in raw kidney beans) is known to be poisonous to humans. This is why eating as few as four or five raw kidney beans can cause abdominal pain, vomiting, and diarrhea.[12]

Importantly, most lectins are destroyed by adequate cooking.

This is why it's always a good idea to eat your kidney beans, and really all legumes, well cooked. If you soak legumes before cooking, and then cook them well—ideally with a pressure cooker—you'll wind up with a virtually lectin-free food. In case you're wondering, canned beans are always pressure cooked.

WHAT ABOUT SOY?

The most widely eaten (and controversial) legume in the world today is soy. It's exceptionally high in protein, and it provides many other valuable nutrients, including manganese, phosphorus, iron, fiber, vitamin B_2, magnesium, vitamin K, and potassium.

In many parts of Asia, significant soy consumption has long been associated with good health. For example, the elders of Okinawa have been shown to be the healthiest and longest-lived people in the world. This was demonstrated conclusively in the renowned Okinawa Centenarian Study, a 25-year study sponsored by the Japanese Ministry of Health, Labour and Welfare.[13]

Researchers analyzed the diet and health profiles of Okinawan elders and compared them to elder populations globally. They concluded that high soy consumption is one of the main reasons Okinawans are at extremely low risk for hormone-dependent cancers, including cancers of the breast, prostate, ovaries, and colon. Compared to North Americans, traditional Okinawans have a staggering 80 percent less breast cancer and prostate cancer, and less than half the ovarian cancer and colon cancer.

This enormously reduced cancer risk arises in part, the study's authors say, from the Okinawans' large consumption of isoflavones from soy. (Isoflavones are phytoestrogens that keep estrogen levels under control. They can act like a weak estrogen when body estrogen levels are low, and they can also inhibit estrogen's effects when body estrogen levels are high.[14] They help the body to sustain a healthy balance.) This is an important finding. The lowest cancer rates in the world are found in the Okinawans who consume the most unprocessed soy (especially edamame, tempeh, miso, natto, and tofu).

Other studies have confirmed the link between unprocessed soy consumption and reduced cancer risk. The Japan Public Health Center-Based Prospective Study on Cancer and Cardiovascular Diseases found the lowest breast cancer rates in those prefectures where women ate the most soy products. And a huge study published in the *Journal of the National Cancer Institute* in 2003 found that women with a high intake of soy reduced their risk of breast cancer by 54 percent compared to women with a low intake of soy.[15]

What about for people who already have, or have had, cancer? Is soy beneficial for them, too?

In a study of 6,235 American and Canadian women who had breast cancer, researchers from Tufts University found a 21 percent reduction in all-cause mortality among those who ate the most soy.[16]

But Isn't Soy Dangerous?

There are also prominent voices claiming that soy is dangerous. For instance, writing for the Weston A. Price Foundation, vociferous soy critics Sally Fallon and Mary Enig have stated that soy fuels Alzheimer's, throws off hormonal balance, and is "poisonous."[17] Other critics have claimed that soy can damage thyroid function and lead to hypothyroidism.

Let's look at each of these concerns:

Alzheimer's Disease

For anything as complex and slow-developing as Alzheimer's, it's difficult to pinpoint with certainty how various lifestyle factors interact. And there have been many different studies, not all of which seem to point in the same direction. But on the whole, the bulk of the data seems to tell us that soy can be good for brain health. For example, although they are rising with the increasing prevalence of industrialized foods, we know that dementia rates have traditionally been lower in Asian countries (where soy intake tends to be high) than in Western countries.[18] We know that the Okinawans, with their considerable intake of tofu and other soy products, have the best elderly cognition of any peoples in the world. And we know that in the United States, Seventh-day Adventists, many of whom consume abundant soy foods their whole lives, have substantially less dementia in old age than the general population.[19]

In a clinical study published in the journal *Psychopharmacology* in 2001, young adult men and women who ate a high-soy diet experienced substantial improvements in short-term and long-term memory, and in mental flexibility.[20]

I've seen a significant body of evidence linking unprocessed soy foods with positive brain health outcomes. There have also been a few studies that appeared to point in the opposite direction.[21] So at this point I think the preponderance of evidence is in favor of soy, but we need more research to feel certain.

Hormonal Balance

Some people believe that the phytoestrogens in soy lower fertility rates for men and for women, and cause men to produce less testosterone. But there's not much evidence to support these claims. The phytoestrogens in soy are relatively weak, and have actually been found to block harmful estrogenic effects.[22] This might be one of the reasons that studies have shown soy to be beneficial in preventing and reversing hormone-dependent cancers, especially in women.

A large-scale study at a Boston fertility center showed that female consumption of soy improved birth rates for couples undergoing fertility treatment.[23] Meanwhile, for men, a study at Harvard University found men's soy intake had no net impact one way or the other on the clinical outcomes for fertility.[24]

What about male testosterone levels? Do the isoflavones and the phytoestrogens in soy have an impact? A 2010 meta-analysis of 15 placebo-controlled studies concluded that "neither soy foods nor isoflavone supplements alter the measures of bioavailable testosterone concentrations in men."[25] Studies have also found that isoflavone supplementation has no effect on sperm concentration, count, or mobility, and that it leads to no observable changes in testicular or ejaculate volume. So if you're a man who's looking to produce as much sperm as possible, it seems that it doesn't really matter how much soy you eat. But if you're a man or a woman who wants to avoid cancer, then it looks like soy is your friend.

Thyroid Function

Some studies have shown that soy may suppress thyroid function in predisposed individuals—especially for people who have an underactive thyroid gland. But a meta-analysis of 14 studies found no significant adverse effects of soybean consumption on thyroid function in healthy adults.[26] What then to do? This is another place where it's important to listen to what your body is telling you. And if you have thyroid problems, you may want to eat little or no soy.

The Shadow Side of Soy

While I don't find myself agreeing much with soy's harshest critics, some things about industrialized soy bother me.

Voracious global consumption of soy is a leading force behind destruction of the tropical rain forests. Monocrops often drive small-scale family farmers out of business, and soy is one of the biggest monocrops on the planet.

Where is all this soy going? Surprisingly, the vast majority isn't turning into edamame, tofu, tempeh, or miso. It's not even turning into soy burgers or soy milk. Approximately three-quarters of the world's soy harvest is used as livestock feed.[27] As we'll discuss in chapter 28, it can take up to 12 pounds of feed (such as corn or soy) to create 1 pound of feedlot beef. So, as counterintuitive as it may sound, if you want to save farmland and rain forests from being turned into soy plantations, you might actually be most effective if you eat more tofu and less meat.

Most of the soy crop is genetically engineered so that it can be sprayed with glyphosate (which, as we've discussed, is probably carcinogenic). This is a very good reason to make sure your soy products are organic or certified non-GMO.

And keep in mind that there's a real difference between natural soy products and refined ones. Of the soy eaten directly by humans, most is consumed in the form of soy oil and isolated soy protein, both of which are used in highly processed foods. Soy-based processed foods like fake meat, soy bars, or protein powders usually contain only soy protein isolates, rather than nutrition from the whole soybean. Removing the protein from the rest of the soy affects the nutritional quality and the bio-availability of soy's isoflavones, deprives your body of soy's natural fiber, and gives you a nutritionally inferior food.[28]

To my eyes, the bottom line on soy is this: If you have thyroid problems, you should probably limit your consumption. But it seems that organically grown soy products that are minimally processed (such as tofu, tempeh, edamame, soy milk, and miso) can be a real contribution to a healthy diet. To avoid GMOs, choose organic or certified non-GMO soy products. And if you're concerned about the social and environmental impact of soy production, then the number one action you can take is to eat less industrialized meat (since most of the world's soy crop is fed to livestock). More on that in chapter 28.

ACTION:

Option 1: Add a can of low-sodium beans to your menu today.

Option 2: Soak a cup or two of your favorite legumes in 4 to 8 cups of water. Rinse and resoak them every morning and evening for two days, cook them well with a piece of kombu, and enjoy!

Option 3: *Buy at least four kinds of legumes, one of which you've never eaten before. Make a plan to soak (for 48 hours) and cook one of them each week for the next four weeks. Find legume-featuring recipes that you like—like the recipe for Espresso Black Bean Chili on page 297, or the one for Quickest Black Bean Salad on page 301.*

CHAPTER 17

What About Meat and Dairy?

At the age of 40, Paul Figueroa of Stanton, California, was already taking drugs to try to control his sky-high blood pressure levels when he was diagnosed with gout. His doctor gave him even more medications.

They didn't work.

A year later, Paul suffered a massive heart attack, which resulted in full blockage of his left anterior descending artery and damage to 40 percent of his heart.

Paul shares that the hardest thing he's ever witnessed were the faces of his wife and kids as he was rolled into the catheterization lab. The outcome was unknown, and their worry hit him like a ton of bricks. When he did make it out (three stents later), the first meal offered to him after his catheterization was meatloaf.

But as his cardiologist explained what he'd been through, and the high probability that he could still have more heart attacks in the future, Paul knew that changes were in order. Soon after he left the hospital, Paul and his family watched the documentary *Forks over Knives*.

Previously, Paul's favorite foods had been steaks, burgers, and pizza. But now, with his life on the line, he adopted a whole-foods, plant-centered diet. After about a week of going "cold turkey," there was a moment when Paul felt angry that he had to eat this way. He asked his wife, Monica, why he needed to go to so much trouble and give up foods that he'd previously enjoyed, when his cardiologist's only dietary advice had been to watch his sodium. She reminded him that doctors don't learn about nutrition in medical school, that she and their whole family wanted him alive, and that they were all in it (and eating this new way) together.

Over time, Paul's palate expanded, and he began to enjoy wholesome, plant-based cuisine more than he expected. His taste for vegetables, in particular, changed. He never would have eaten raw carrots or broccoli before, but now he snacked on them with hummus and grew to like pretty much any vegetable (except coriander!).

Within two years, Paul's cholesterol levels and blood pressure returned to normal, and he drastically reduced his risk of heart attack. Paul has gone on hikes he never would have tried before, including trekking up to the Hollywood sign in the city's hills.

Some people might find Paul's story miraculous. And in many ways it is. But it's also, in some respects, almost predictable. Because when people adopt a whole-foods, plant-based diet, their heart health typically improves dramatically.

This is why Dean Ornish, MD, was able to become the first clinician to offer documented proof that heart disease could be halted, or even reversed, simply by changing your lifestyle. One of the cornerstones of his renowned Ornish Program is a plant-centered diet with little or no meat, dairy, or eggs.

In his study of the Blue Zones, Dan Buettner has documented that the populations that have traditionally enjoyed the longest and healthiest lives, with some of the world's lowest rates of cardiovascular disease, all share a number of common dietary factors. They tend to eat large amounts of fruits, vegetables, and other whole plant foods. They usually eat low amounts of sugary and processed foods. And they eat very few, if any, animal products.

This is consistent with the Food Revolution Diet Plan, which focuses on essentially this same set of principles.

Some people get especially passionate on the topic of meat. There are some who feel that it's morally wrong to take the life of an animal for human consumption. And to be honest, having been raised as a vegetarian, I thought that way for a good portion of my life—sometimes to the point of manifesting more than my fair share of dogmatism.

When I was in my late twenties, I became close friends with someone who opened my mind to another perspective. Evon Peter was, at the time, chief of the Neetsaii Gwich'in tribe in Vashraii K'oo (Arctic Village), Alaska. To say that Evon lived "off the grid" would be an understatement. His people are 200 miles from the nearest road, well above the

Arctic Circle. Their diet depends heavily on fish and caribou. Evon told me that his people have loved and revered animals for millennia, and that they depend on them for their survival.

"If you love animals," I asked, "why do you eat them?"

"I do love animals," he answered. "And I eat them. We refer to our-selves as 'the Caribou People.' We would die for the caribou. And they die for us. Our lives are inextricably intertwined, and they have been for thousands of years. If there were no caribou, there would be no Gwich'in. We are part of each other."

When Evon learned about factory farms, he was heavily disheartened. He told me that treating animals in this way went against everything that he and his people stood for.

Yet to him, and for his people, killing animals for food was a neces-sary part of life itself.

Those of us who live with access to stores and summers long enough to grow food are truly blessed. And I, for one, want to make the best use I can of the choices I have.

I also want to respect the diversity of human experiences and life con-texts. There really is no one diet, or one philosophy, that is right for everyone in every circumstance.

But in the modern world, with animals being raised as they are, our food choices have significant ethical and environmental impacts, which we'll explore together more in Part Four. Right now we're focusing on how you nourish your body. So let's look at meat, dairy, and your health.

PROCESSED MEATS

Manufacturers add nitrates and nitrites to processed meats such as cured deli meats, bacon, salami, and sausages to give them color and to pro-long their shelf life. The trouble is that both nitrates and nitrites can form nitrosamines in the body. This can increase your risk of developing cancer.

In 2015, the International Agency for Research on Cancer, the cancer agency of the World Health Organization, released a report on processed meat and cancer.[1] After 22 experts from 10 countries had reviewed more than 800 studies, they decided to classify processed meat as a Group 1 carcinogen—in the same category as asbestos, alcohol, arsenic, and tobacco.

The researchers found that eating 50 grams of processed meat (the equivalent of about four strips of bacon or one hot dog) every day increased the risk of colorectal cancer by 18 percent and bowel cancer by 17 percent.[2]

Other studies have linked consumption of processed meat with higher rates of heart disease and diabetes.[3]

What About Red Meat?

Red meat supplies vitamin B_{12}, which helps make DNA and keeps nerve and red blood cells healthy, and zinc, which keeps the immune system working properly. It provides an abundant source of protein, which helps build bones and muscles, and heme iron, which is easily absorbed by the body.

But red meat also has some significant drawbacks. As we discussed in chapter 1, many people may be getting too much protein. And excess iron can be a serious health problem, as it is often deposited in the liver, heart, and pancreas, where it can cause cirrhosis, liver cancer, cardiac arrhythmias, and diabetes.

When the World Health Organization determined that processed meat was a known carcinogen, it also declared that red meat is "probably carcinogenic to humans," stating that it is linked to cancers of the pancreas and the prostate.[4]

In one of the largest long-term studies on diet and health ever conducted, a research team led by Dr. Frank Hu of the Harvard School of Public Health examined the reported diets and health outcomes of 37,000 men and 83,000 women over the course of several decades.[5] All the participants were free of cardiovascular disease and cancer at the start of the study. Almost 24,000 participants died during the study, including about 5,900 from cardiovascular disease and about 9,500 from cancer.

The team's report, published in the *Archives of Internal Medicine* in 2012, concluded that those who consumed the highest levels of red meat had the highest overall risk of death, as well as the highest rates of mortality from cancer and cardiovascular disease. After adjusting for other risk factors (such as smoking, exercise levels, and economic background), the researchers calculated that one additional serving per day of unprocessed red meat over the course of the study raised the risk of total mortality during the period of the study by 13 percent. An extra serving of processed red meat (such as bacon, hot dogs, sausage, or salami) per day raised risk of death by 20 percent.

The majority of the meat and dairy products produced in the United States and other developed nations today comes from what most consumers refer to as factory farms. The industry calls them concentrated animal feeding operations (CAFOs). These large-scale facilities confine animals in close quarters and feed them a totally unnatural diet. The animals are unable to exercise as they normally would, and many never see the sun or a blade of grass in their entire lives.

Modern meat is totally different, from a nutritional standpoint, from the wild game that our Paleolithic ancestors hunted, and completely unlike the caribou that the Neetsaii Gwich'in tribe depends on to survive in northern Alaska. Three ounces of lean beef from a CAFO, for example, contains 15 grams of fat, while the same amount of wild venison contains only 3 grams.[6]

Meat, dairy, and eggs that are pasture-raised and grass-fed have some health benefits that CAFO-sourced animal products do not. They tend to be lower in fat and to have more conjugated linoleic acid (a type of fat thought to reduce heart disease and cancer risks), more omega-3 fatty acids (though still very little), and more antioxidant vitamins, such as vitamin E.[7] Plus they don't come laced with artificial hormones and antibiotics.

So far, I'm not aware of any long-term studies that have looked at the health outcomes for humans who ate pasture-raised animal products and compared them to humans who ate comparable amounts of factory-farmed ones. But many studies have shown us clearly that consumption of meat, at least as it is mass-produced today, is linked with major negative health impacts for large numbers of people.

Some people fear that if they drop meat out of their diet, their culinary life will take a downturn. But the reality is that for many people, going plant-based can open up new vistas of flavor and be even more exciting than a meat-based diet. In the modern industrialized diet, food too often relies on things like salt, fat, and sugar to provide flavor. But in the whole-foods, plant-based world, things like spicy chilies, fresh herbs, exotic spices, and citrus are used to make food satisfying and interesting. And for those looking for that "meaty" texture, there are an abundance of options, from tofu and tempeh to jackfruit, mushrooms, and even aubergine, that can provide a delightfully pleasant "mouthfeel" to complement savory flavors.

What About Cultured Meat?

Cultured meat takes the cells of meat and cultures them on a growth medium. The result is a laboratory product that looks, tastes, and presumably digests just like the real thing—but with the potential for dramatically lower environmental impact, and no animal cruelty. In theory, at least from an environmental and ethical standpoint, this sounds promising. But the trouble is, if meat isn't especially healthful to begin with, then culturing it in a lab will do nothing to amend that problem, since it's going to have exactly the same nutritional composition as farmed meat. And there are also questions about what growth medium will be used, and therefore about the ultimate environmental impact of the product. As far as I'm concerned, the jury's still out on this one.

CHICKEN

In general, chicken has less saturated fat than red meats such as beef, pork, and lamb. As a result, many people believe that birds make for a healthier option than cows or pigs. And they have a point. Chicken meat is an abundant source of protein, niacin, selenium, and vitamin B_{12}, without the levels of saturated fat found in red meats.

But chicken brings its own set of dangers.

Part of the problem comes from how it's cooked. Grilled chicken often carries the chemical PhIP, which may contribute to breast and prostate cancer.[8] And when chicken is fried, additional problems emerge. Compounds known as heterocyclic amines, or HCAs, are produced in the frying process and found in all fried chicken—and they have been linked to an increased risk of many forms of cancer.[9]

Another problem stems from what chickens are fed. A common industry practice involves feeding chickens arsenic to make them grow faster.[10] The trouble is, arsenic is poisonous to humans. It can cause cancer, dementia, neurological problems, and other ailments. The industry responds by assuring us that arsenic residues in commercial chicken tend to be low.

Call me a Chicken Little if you like, but personally, I prefer my food arsenic-free.

And there are enormous sanitation and food safety concerns in the modern industrialized chicken industry. A *Consumer Reports* analysis found that 97 percent of broiler chickens purchased across the United States had high levels of campylobacter, salmonella, or other dangerous bacteria that cause food poisoning.[11] According to *Consumer Reports*, more than 48 million people become sick each year as a result of contaminated food, and chicken is the number one source of food-based contamination in the world.

FISH

Unlike the animals raised in factory farms, many fish still swim wild and free in the oceans. Fish meat can contain an abundance of protein and healthy fats, and is the most abundant source of omega-3 fatty acids available directly from foods. But wild fish also swim in polluted waters and exist at the top of very long food chains. As a result, many wild fish today are contaminated with dangerous levels of mercury, polychlorinated biphenyls (PCBs), and other toxins. And industrialized fishing operations are practically strip-mining the oceans, leaving fishery stocks depleted and threatening the viability of the commercial fishing industry for future generations.

The industry is changing fast, as more and more fish is being produced in fish farms. Already, over half the world's fish harvest comes from aquaculture. Unfortunately, this isn't great for the oceans, either. Most fish farms depend on stocks of wild fish to feed their amphibious residents, and it can take up to five pounds of wild fish to produce a single pound of farmed salmon.[12] Many fish farms provide an intensely unnatural environment, and in a spectacle remarkably similar to factory farming of cows and pigs, fish are given routine doses of antibiotics simply to keep them alive under miserable conditions.

If you choose to eat fish, the best options are likely to include wild salmon, sardines, anchovies, and herring—which are all uniquely high in omega-3 fatty acids and tend to be low in mercury. Some fish farms are developing more sustainable methods, but the industry is highly unregulated—and many fish farms are environmental disasters. What's more, genetically engineered salmon is now on the market, and in many places, including all of North America, it's unlabeled. As of this writing, it's only being produced in Canada. But if you want to avoid it, steering clear of any Canadian-sourced farmed salmon may be a wise move.

GOT MILK? YOU NEED TO SEE THIS . . .

In my family, we know a bit about the unhealthy side of dairy. At one time, my grandfather had manufactured and sold more ice cream than any human being who had ever lived. Ice cream consists mainly of two things: dairy fat and sugar. Naturally, no one is about to make a case for ice cream being a health food (unless they happen to work for Baskin-Robbins).

What about other dairy products?

The dairy industry has spent millions of dollars touting milk as "nature's most perfect food." And it is—for a baby calf. But what about humans?

We are the only species on earth that drinks milk after infancy, and we're also the only one that would think to drink the milk of another species. So while cow milk consumption does go back through thousands of years of human history, in the grand scheme of things, it's actually a bit of an acquired habit.

In order for cows to keep producing milk, they have to be repeatedly impregnated. To secure the milk for humans, the baby calves are typically taken away from their mothers in their first day of life—often, if they're males, to be turned into veal calves.

Dairy contains all the nutrition that's needed to nurture a growing calf. It provides an abundant source of calcium, vitamin D, vitamin B_2, vitamin B_{12}, potassium, and phosphorus. But since modern milk always comes from recently pregnant cows, it also contains hormones that don't do a human body any good.

Many studies have explored the correlation between dairy products and heart disease. Perhaps the largest of them, conducted by Harvard T.H. Chan School of Public Health researchers and published in the *American Journal of Clinical Nutrition* in 2016, reported on research done with 43,000 men and 187,000 women. When calories from full-fat dairy products were replaced with carbohydrates from whole grains, risk of heart disease dropped by 28 percent.[13] Replacing dairy products with red meat, on the other hand, led to a 6 percent *increase* in heart disease risk.

Dairy is known to stimulate the release of insulin and IGF-1 (insulin-like growth factor 1). This is thought to be the reason that dairy consumption is linked to increased rates of acne.[14] These hormones are also believed to increase the risk of certain cancers—especially prostate cancer.[15]

Another widespread problem with dairy consumption is lactose intolerance. When we are infants, our bodies produce a digestive enzyme called lactase, which breaks down lactose from mother's milk. But as we grow up, many of us lose the ability to do that.[16]

By adulthood, about three-quarters of the world's population is unable to break down lactose, and there's a strong racial dimension to lactose intolerance.[17] Caucasians are the only ethnic group on the planet that can usually digest lactose in adulthood. Most people of African, Asian, Jewish, Arab, and indigenous ancestry cannot.[18] As Caucasian-centric entertainment, food companies, and government policies have promoted dairy product consumption around the world, they've unintentionally subjected billions of people to significant digestive problems. Lactose intolerance can cause nausea, vomiting, and diarrhea.

If you do choose to eat dairy products, here are two pointers to keep in mind.

1. *Cows should eat grass.* Cows raised in pastures and fed grass have more omega-3 fatty acids and up to 500 percent more conjugated linoleic acid in their milk.[19] Their milk is also much higher in fat-soluble vitamins, especially vitamin K_2—a nutrient important for regulating calcium metabolism and with major benefits for heart and bone health.[20]

2. *You might want to skip the "low-fat" option.* In a long-term study published in 2016 in the *American Journal of Clinical Nutrition*, 18,438 middle-aged women were found to be less likely to be overweight if they consumed full-fat dairy than if they consumed low-fat dairy.[21] Other studies have indicated that compared to full-fat dairy products, low-fat versions don't confer benefits, and may even be harmful, when it comes to risk of heart disease or of type 2 diabetes.[22]

SHOULD YOU GO VEGAN?

Compared to the modern industrialized meat-centered diet, an eating pattern low in animal products and high in whole plant foods is correlated, for most people, with a healthier heart and brain, reduced inflammation, and higher quality and quantity of life.

But how low in animal products is it best to go? Should you go all the way, and become 100 percent vegan? Increasing numbers of people are. According to a report by research firm GlobalData, between 2014 and 2017 there was a 600 percent increase in the number of Americans who identified as vegan.[23] And the trend is spreading around the globe.

For many people, this can be a wonderful choice. Some people thrive on a vegan diet for long and vibrant lives. But that doesn't necessarily make it optimal for everyone at every phase. I've known a number of long-term vegans who found that their health improved with the addition of a modest amount of wild fish or grass-fed and pasture-raised meat in their diets.

Personally, I've been mostly vegan for my whole life. But I now choose from time to time to include low-mercury wild fish (mainly salmon, sardines, and herring) and pasture-raised eggs. That's not to say this is what's best for everyone. Nor that it will be what is best for me in the years to come. Our needs tend to change over the course of our lives.

My wife, Phoenix, was, like me, predominantly vegan for many years. Now she sources a small but, to her, important slice of her calories from wild fish and pasture-raised animal products. She likes to interview farmers personally to assess their ethical and sustainability practices before she buys their products.

As someone who wants to build a healthier and more compassionate world, I don't take the killing of animals lightly. However, I think each of us must include ourselves as well as all of life in our circle of compassion. This means listening honestly to see what our bodies need in order to optimally thrive.

A vegan diet is technically defined by what it omits (meat, dairy, eggs, and other animal products), and not by what it includes. "Junk food vegans" can expect to suffer from many of the standard American diseases. Whole foods–based vegans, who enjoy a rich abundance of fruits, vegetables, legumes, whole grains, nuts, and seeds will generally have a major advantage. And there are some nutrients to which all of us, and especially strict vegans, need to pay special attention.

Nearly everyone in the modern world, whether vegan or not, should probably consider supplementing a healthy diet with vitamins D_3 and B_{12}. Unless you eat fatty fish with some regularity, supplementing with the omega-3 fatty acids DHA and EPA (both of which are available from algal as well as from fish sources) is likely to be wise. And some plant-based eaters may also benefit from supplementation of zinc and vitamin K_2. For more on these nutrients, as well as iron, visit 31dayfood revolution.com/nutrients.

People living in the Blue Zone of Loma Linda, California, tend to be vegetarian, and many are vegan. They are the most thoroughly studied long-term vegans and vegetarians in world medical history. The extraordinary Adventist Health Studies (most of the people living in this Blue Zone are Seventh-day Adventists) investigated the long-term health outcomes for 96,000 vegans, lacto-ovo-vegetarians, pescatarians (who eat fish), semivegetarians, and nonvegetarians.[24] Among these groups, vegans were found to have the lowest rates of obesity, hypertension (high blood pressure), diabetes, and cancer, and the second-longest life spans. (Pescatarians came in second to vegans on most metrics, and first on life span.)

People living in the world's other Blue Zones—Ikaria, Greece; Okinawa, Japan; Ogliastra Province, Sardinia; and Nicoya Peninsula, Costa Rica—tend to get between 5 and 10 percent of their calories from unprocessed, pasture-raised, or wild animal products.

I think it's wise to be informed by what others have experienced and found to work, and by credible research, and then to apply best practices in order to discover what works best for you. You're the world's number one expert on your own experience.

ACTION:

Option 1: Replace luncheon meats or hot dogs with avocado, strips of baked tofu, a veggie burger, or roasted vegetables. For breakfast, instead of bacon, try some tempeh or a tofu scramble. (If you'd like some ideas and guidance, check out the recipes starting on page 277 or the five-day meal plan on page 319.)

Option 2: If you want to ditch the dairy, substitutes can be made for virtually every dairy product. In many stores, you'll find cultured cheeses made from a base of almonds or cashews; milks and yogurts made from pea, soy, almond, rice, oat, hemp, or coconut; butters thickened with coconut or palm oil; and even cultured kefirs from nondairy sources.

Option 3: Try swapping out meat and adding more legumes (including organic soy products), whole grains, nuts, and seeds to your diet. Many people enjoy tofu, tempeh, seitan, or even jackfruit as meat substitutes that provide a pleasant "meat-like" texture and become delicious when marinated or otherwise seasoned to soak up intense flavors. If you're going to eat meat, I suggest you think of it as a garnish, or "condi-meat," not the main ingredient—and that you get it from pasture-raised sources. Pasture-raised meat is pretty expensive, sometimes exceeding $30 a pound. For many people, this is a significant obstacle. But if you do choose to eat meat, the price of pasture-raised can be a good impetus to use it in modest quantities.

PART THREE

GATHER

Modern science confirms what many of us learned in kindergarten: Having friends is good for you, and not having them can be hazardous to your health.

Researchers at Brigham Young University concluded that a lack of good friends and connections to others is as damaging to your health as being obese, or as smoking 15 cigarettes per day.[1]

Loneliness kills just as surely as cigarettes. And by the same token, bonding and social connection are statistically correlated with higher life expectancy and long-term wellness, and with prevention of heart disease and even breast cancer.[2]

Gathering around a table to share food can be a beautiful way to forge bonds. But food can also be a source of division. Many families and relationships suffer when kitchens turn into zones of conflict. And I know a lot of people who compromise their food choices because they don't want to alienate people who are close to them.

Perhaps this is a concern for you, too. You might fear that if you live your food values, they could lead you to feeling lonely. You may worry about not being able to share a meal with a loved one at a restaurant, missing out on a weekend barbecue, having to decline a friend's invitation to dinner, or being unable to eat in the cafeteria at work.

In a toxic food culture, it can feel isolating to do something different.

When people are bonding around a beer or a burger, you may feel some disconnection if you choose not to participate.

That's why it's so important to navigate social dynamics around food as skillfully as possible, and to build new networks and friendships that will support your eating goals.

For all the diet books and programs available, this is one area where most of them come up short. They fail to recognize that humans are not lone wolves. Without the social network in place to help you sustain your path, chances are you'll slide back into old patterns.

But when you have a strong community behind you, it becomes easier and easier to do the right thing. You'll be pulled as if by gravity toward habits that serve your well-being. You'll find that your Food Revolution can be a doorway to new and deeper connections, beneficial not just for your health but also for your social life.

In the chapters to come, I'll share how you can go to a restaurant and know what to order on (or off) the menu, how to get back on track if you slip up over the holidays, how to navigate complex social dynamics so you can maintain your integrity without coming off as a killjoy, and how to be a positive influence. Few things are more rewarding than being a positive influence on friends and family—helping them to lose weight, heal from illness, or achieve their goals.

There doesn't need to be anything drab, dreary, or lonely about healthy food. So get ready to share some delicious and nutritious meals with old—and new—friends.

Take the Quiz: How Strong Is Your Healthy Food Community?

I share a meal with other people:

0. Twice a week or less.
1. Three to six times per week.
2. Pretty much every day.

In general, the people I share the most time with:

0. Tend to eat sugar, processed foods, and/or conventionally raised meat frequently.
1. Try to eat healthfully but don't always succeed.
2. Are strong healthy-eating role models.

The food at my family's holiday gatherings tends to have:

0. Lots of sugar, processed foods, and conventionally raised meat.
1. Both healthy and not-so-healthy options.
2. Pretty healthy and consciously chosen options.

Most of the restaurants I go out to:

0. Probably don't even know what kale is.
1. Offer reasonably healthy options if I order carefully.
2. Offer foods I feel great about eating.

I usually start a meal:

0. By diving right in, if I even notice that I'm eating.
1. With a quick moment of gratitude, when I or the people around me think of it.
2. With some way of expressing gratitude or appreciation, either in silence or in community with others.

I share healthy recipes or food ideas with other people:

0. Rarely, if ever.
1. Once in a while.
2. Frequently and happily.

If a friend or coworker is on a healthy eating path, I express my appreciation and support:

0. Rarely, if ever.
1. Once in a while.
2. Frequently and happily.

Add up your points to score from 0 to 14. The higher the better! Go to 31day foodrevolution.com/quiz3 to take the quiz online, connect with new like-minded friends, and participate in the 31-Day Food Revolution with others.

If you scored low, that's actually good news—because things are about to get a whole lot better. If you scored high, congratulations! You have cause for gratitude. Now, let's build on what's working and take it even further.

CHAPTER 18

Bring Friends and Family Along

Do you ever worry about the health of the people you love—and wish they ate healthier food? If you've tried to help others move in a positive direction, has it ever felt as if you were banging your head on a brick wall?

When I was a child, before my grandpa Irv (the cofounder of Baskin-Robbins) read my dad's bestselling books and turned his health around, we had our fair share of food conflict in the family. When my mom, dad, and I would visit my dad's parents, we sometimes stayed in a rented condo because sharing meals could become such a point of friction. My grandma famously declared, "You will NOT cook tofu in my kitchen." She was clear who was in charge, stating: "When you're in my house, you will eat what I serve."

Since my grandma wasn't exactly a black-belt champion in flexibility, we prepared most of our meals separately. We weren't about to let differences over food keep us from being a family. But we struggled with the separation they caused.

Eventually, of course, my grandpa's health crisis led him to change his diet radically—and things became infinitely more amicable. In time we came to agree that in the long run, blood is thicker, even, than ice cream. But that change was a long time coming.

As you find out how powerful food is in shaping the destiny of your physical and mental health, how can you be a positive influence without coming off like a nag or alienating people?

Some of us discover what *doesn't* work the hard way. Take me, for example.

I spent my formative years as an only child on a remote island. With our nearest neighbors living almost a mile away, I didn't develop social skills in any great abundance.

Add to that the fact that I'd been raised as a vegetarian, and prior to attending school, I hadn't often been around people, other than my grandparents, who ate meat. When we moved to a suburb of Victoria, Canada, so I could attend a school, lunchtimes were, at first, traumatic. I found the whole notion of eating animals to be barbaric.

Midway through grade school, I decided to speak my mind.

When lunchtime rolled around, I took it upon myself to inspect the lunches of the other kids. I would inform my classmates that their *Star Wars* or Cabbage Patch Kids lunch boxes were coffins.

I was passionate, and I was also strident. One day I told one of my best friends, Damien, that his beef sandwich was the product of a murder. We got into a fistfight, and before long, Damien's sandwich was in the garbage, and I was in the principal's office.

There I was, preaching compassion. But I was getting into fights with my friends over the contents of their lunch boxes.

MY BITE OF STEAK

My dad, who'd raised me as a vegetarian and who always encouraged me to respect animals and to cherish their right to life, was increasingly concerned about my fanaticism.

One day, he told me that he had a request—and he knew it might be hard for me.

I had no idea what was coming next. I imagined that maybe my dad wanted me to join in his daily yoga practice, starting at the crack of dawn.

But it was worse. A lot worse.

He wanted to take me out to dinner at one of the fanciest steakhouses in town. It sat on top of an 18-story building. The waiters dressed in suits, and the ambience was elegant. My dad planned to order me a grass-fed filet mignon.

He explained that he wanted to give me a better sense of connection to the masses of humanity for whom meat was a part of life. And since he'd raised me as a vegetarian, he also felt it was important for me to be the author of my own choices rather than blindly following in his footsteps.

I felt horrified. I think I might have been happier if my dad had asked me to sleep on a bed of nails.

Now, keep in mind that my dad was someone who would become one of the world's leading spokespeople for a more humane world. He was a passionate vegetarian. What he was requesting of me had to be incredibly hard for him. But it was also born of a deep conviction that this would help me develop in important ways—while perhaps salvaging what was left of my social life.

When the fateful night came, and my order of steak arrived, I looked at it with disgust. "Meat is murder," I fumed.

My dad smiled patiently. "It's true," he said, "that every piece of meat is the flesh of an animal that once drew breath from the same source as we do. I'm glad you recognize that, and I hope that you never forget it. But if you want to connect with people, you need to understand their viewpoint. And most people, when they look at meat, see food—and a highly desirable one, at that. All I ask is that you take a single bite. If you take one bite, I'll be satisfied, and won't ever ask you to do this again."

So I did. And as repulsed as I was to be eating the flesh of a sentient animal, I had to admit that the taste was pretty...interesting.

I didn't finish that steak. I didn't even take another bite. My dad asked the server to bring me some pasta. But something had changed in my life.

I had challenged my belief system in which there were sharp lines of right and wrong, good and bad, dark and light. And after that moment, slowly but surely, my judgment and sense of moral superiority faded away. I kept my deep conviction about respect for all life, which has persisted to this day. But I'd discovered that there's a world of difference between dedication and dogmatism.

Years later, I would hear and begin to understand the words of Dr. Martin Luther King Jr., who told us, "You have no moral authority with those who can feel your underlying contempt."

The fact is, when we judge people, and when we pathologize them, we lose our moral standing. Shoving ideology down people's throats isn't just obnoxious. It's also highly ineffective.

I hope you're more tactful than I was in elementary school. But many of us still ask: How do we influence our loved ones on a healthy eating path?

- **Make healthy and delicious food for your loved ones.** It's amazing how powerful a tasty meal can be to win people over. Sometimes the mouth is the fastest doorway to the heart. A pot of spicy chili served with homemade pan corn bread, or a slice of warm chocolate banana bread, can put a smile on anyone's face, even if it's much healthier than what they're used to eating.

- **Look for openings.** A lot of people are motivated to change when confronted by their mortality or a scary diagnosis. They might be moved by the illness or death of a loved one. Some people will be galvanized by caring about animals or the environment. When you see an opening in someone's consciousness, that's the perfect time to share what you know. Watering a seed at the right time can lead to the birth of a tree. But at the wrong time, it might just flood the soil.

- **Ask questions.** When you get to know what someone cares about and what their struggles are, then you might be able to help them. Most people don't like being told what to do. But a lot of people want support from their friends.

- **Always love them.** If yours is a family where there's a lot of hostility, defensiveness, and misunderstanding, it might be as hard to get traction when it comes to food differences as it is with everything else. Where there's love, communication, and mutual respect, the pathway is infinitely easier. When you bring kindness and clarity to your relationships, it can open the doorway to the highest level of rapport.

- **Lead by example.** Your example is the best teacher of all. When you're lit up, when you're vibrant and it shows, people will naturally gravitate toward you. Enthusiasm is contagious. People will be asking how you lost weight, or why you're looking so great.

Shannon Briggs of Covington, Washington, is a good example of this. In 2016, Shannon was diagnosed with cancer. She believes that eating a rainbow of organic vegetables complemented her treatment and helped her to overcome her cancer. Today Shannon is overjoyed to be alive. Recently, she received a surprise letter from a coworker who credited her with inspiring him and his whole family to improve their food choices. The letter brought Shannon to tears.

- **Take advantage of the experts.** You don't have to memorize all the facts or recite a litany of medical studies in order to influence people. That's what TED talks, books, films, and events like the Food Revolution Summits are for. Tens of millions of people have had their lives changed by the resources I've listed in the back of this book. The fact is, conversations about food can easily turn into power struggles. You might find it easier to share a film, book, article, or event.

HOW TO GET STARTED

Think about some people you'd like to influence. Based on all you know—what they value, what they struggle with, what stage of life they're in—what could be your best opening for being a positive influence? Are they concerned about their health or their weight? About increasing athletic performance? About preventing Alzheimer's or other aging-related ailments? Are they concerned with ethical, environmental, or social issues? Do they love fresh and tasty food?

Many people have to hit bottom with a health crisis before they'll shift course. But sometimes the vision of a long life, more energy, and a clearer mind is a catalyst. And a surprising number of people, if they'll admit it to you, want more fulfilling sex lives. (You probably don't need me to remind you to tread lightly on this topic!)

You might give them a copy of a helpful book (you'll find a massive boost in engagement if you insert a Post-it note revealing a teaser like "this page made me think of you"), or make them a meal, or share an article, or start up a conversation. Test the waters and see where things lead. Worst case: You back off and try another approach another time. You detach with love and let life unfold the way it will. Best case: You change their lives and gain more allies. Most cases will be somewhere in between. Pay attention to what they're telling you with their words but also to what their actions are saying. Express your consideration and respect.

Here are three ways to start a conversation about healthy eating:

1. *I want to eat more vegetables because they're good for my health. Do you have any favorites, or favorite ways to prepare them?*
2. *Would it be all right with you if I tell you about something that's making me really happy?* (If they say yes, then share something exciting about weight loss, energy level, a health condition disappearing, or whatever benefit you've experienced.)
3. *I just watched what's probably my favorite food and health movie [or read my favorite food and health book] ever. May I tell you about it?*

Remember, too, that even if people don't personally wish to match your healthy journey with their own, you can still ask them to respect and support yours. You might say, for example:

I've decided to make some big changes in my diet, because I'm not getting any younger, and frankly, I'm not ready to die. You might think my new way of eating is a bit weird, or extreme, but I'd really like your support. You don't need to join me, but I'd like you to respect me.

What would help me is if you would think about my food needs when we share a meal, so I don't feel alone. I'd also love to ask if you could hold off on any wisecracks, even if you think they're funny. Please don't tease me for not eating certain things, or tell me what I'm missing out on. It's not easy for me to make these changes, and I'd love it if you could do your best to treat me with respect. How does that sound?

You'll find your own words, of course. What matters is that you speak from the heart, and that you engage your loved ones in meaningful ways that create the conditions for a healthier life and family environment. You are a participant and a cocreator of your family and community.

None of us can control what anyone else will do. But we do get to decide how we respond, and how we can make the best out of what comes into our lives.

Sometimes you'll find that when you're true to your integrity, it sends out ripples to others. Ginny Trierweiler from Colorado recently lost 65 pounds after giving up sugar, flour, and alcohol. But she didn't always receive support from her colleagues. At one point, she was working with a nurse who was battling weight issues by drinking meal-replacement shakes. The nurse asked about Ginny's approach, and would often try to tempt her with whatever sweet treat was available on the unit for staff. One day, there was a beautiful box of chocolates and she offered Ginny one. Ginny said no thank you, and her colleague replied, in a scolding, don't-be-ridiculous voice, "Not even one?!" Ginny held up her fingers in a zero sign and said, "I will have zero!" The nurse replied, "Wow, so that's why you're losing weight!"

Ginny later overheard the nurse, impressed by Ginny's determination, telling the story to other people. You never know the lives you may be touching when you choose to be true to your own values.

ACTION:

Option 1: *Choose one person to share your journey with. Send them an article or a link, buy them a book, or invite them over for a film night.*

Option 2: Ask a friend or loved one if you can make them a whole-foods, plant-powered meal using one of the recipes from this book—and share it together. You might want to open the mealtime with a gratitude go-around.

Option 3: Invite a group of friends over for a movie night to watch an educational film about food. Lead a discussion afterward. If possible, have a go-around so that no one voice dominates and everyone gets a chance to engage.

CHAPTER 19

Find a Healthy Eating Ally

A study in the *New England Journal of Medicine* in 2007 looked at the health outcomes and social ties of 5,124 adults over the course of 32 years.[1] Researchers

> At times our own light goes out and is rekindled by a spark from another person. Each of us has cause to think with deep gratitude of those who have lighted the flame within us.
> —*Albert Schweitzer*

found that if one sibling became obese during the study, the chance that another sibling would become obese increased by 40 percent.

Of course, this could just be genetics in action. But then the researchers noticed that the same pattern occurred in marriages. If a spouse became obese, the odds of a partner doing the same shot up dramatically. Could this be simply because spouses share meals and lifestyle habits? Well, maybe. But apparently there's more to it. The study also found that if a participant had a close friend who became obese, the odds of the participant herself becoming obese rose by a stunning 57 percent.

We're all susceptible to social influences. When we don't know how to leverage this, it can pull us toward ill health. But by the same token, we can leverage peer support to help us achieve our goals.

Some people just prefer to do things on their own. And if that sounds like you, then more power to you! You can always apply the most effective principles as a soloist. But if you're like many folks, it helps to have someone who will root for you. Someone who will stand by you and stand up for you. Someone you can confide in when things get tough, and who will celebrate your victories.

Accountability can make your actions visible, and give you a reference point for success.

Decide what you'd like someone to help you accomplish. Do you want to lose weight, give up sugar, or go organic? Would you like to eat greens at least once every day, go vegetarian or vegan, or do more home cooking?

Choose one goal, and then pick a good ally. It could be a spouse, a sibling, a coworker, or a friend. Your ally will probably be most supportive if she has the same personal goals. Even if she doesn't, she can help if she fundamentally loves and supports you.

When you make a request of someone, you might want to communicate your "why." Do you want to prevent cancer, heart disease, dementia, or diabetes? Do you want to shed excess pounds? Do you want more energy, better digestion, or a stronger immune system? Do you want to walk more lightly on the earth or contribute to a more compassionate world? Let your friend know what you intend to accomplish, especially if you have specific aims.

Once you have your allies established, create an accountability system. Maybe you'll check in every day, every week, or every month—or they'll check in with you. The harder the change you want to make, and the stronger the temptation to slack off, the more consistently a check-in will be beneficial. Your allies can be a resource to troubleshoot obstacles or to celebrate victories. And for big changes that involve shifting deeply entrenched habits, they should be willing to field calls or requests for support any time temptation strikes.

Create built-in rewards, too. Depending on the relationship with your ally, she might agree to help you create a celebration if you reach a goal. If you want to lose 20 pounds, then reaching that goal might mean that your ally joins you for a spa day, ski trip, or hike. Perhaps she'll buy you a gift card for a massage, or come over and wash all your dishes.

Avoid celebrations that involve junk food! I had a friend who celebrated losing 15 pounds by going out for cake and ice cream. You won't be terribly surprised to hear that her 15 pounds came back (and then some) within a matter of weeks.

In 2016, Sarah Medlicott from Santa Cruz, California, decided to take on a series of health goals that included kicking sugar to the curb. She asked a friend of hers, Jenny Brewer, to be her ally. Jenny and Sarah started taking a regular Monday hike to check in, catch up, and support each other. These hikes became something of a touchstone for

Sarah—giving her support and accountability and helping her to stay on her path.

When Sarah was feeling especially critical of herself and impatient that she wasn't seeing faster progress, Jenny was there to remind her of the distance she'd come, and of the ways that her mind was tricking her to slide into old habits. Even when they're in different towns, they still do a "walk 'n' talk" phone call to stay connected and supported.

Many people struggle to jog, go to the gym, take exercise classes, or follow through on exercise routines on their own. If you decide to share a consistent exercise activity, it could solidify your bond while contributing to your health.

My dad and I have been working out together at a local gym for nearly 20 years. We typically go twice each week, and we like to egg each other on. We know each other's records and averages, so we can hold each other accountable. It's amazing what being watched and encouraged can do to catalyze an extra burst of effort. When I work out on my own (and to be honest, when I don't have my dad's companionship, I rarely make the effort!), I don't push myself nearly as hard. Something about being watched and tracked brings out my urge to excel. And by making it a routine that we share, I have strong encouragement to stay in a regular groove.

ACTION:

Option 1: Tell someone you love about what motivates you to pursue healthy eating, and mention a tangible goal. Ask if they'd be willing to support you, and then find a mutually agreeable way of connecting and creating accountability.

Option 2: Form a healthy partnership with somebody you trust and create individual goals. Develop agreements about what each of you intends to accomplish, how frequently you'll connect, how you'll measure success, and what you'll do to celebrate.

Option 3: Bring it to work! Invite colleagues to join in a fitness competition. Some people have used contests involving planks or push-ups, and others have used hiking, jogging, or team sports. Create a shared method of tracking or scoring, and provide daily updates on a leaderboard. Of course, different people start with different levels of fitness. Whoever improves the most in a week could be the winner.

CHAPTER 20

Start a Healthy Meal Swap Team

Do you ever feel lonely? As if something in you, deep down, longs for a stronger sense of community or belonging? If you do, then you've got a lot of company. A 2016 Harris Poll found that loneliness is something that most people—72 percent of Americans, in fact—report feeling.[1]

For all the technological connectivity of the modern world, it seems as if something important has been lost. We can "friend" people on Facebook and "love" their tweets. But we all know that friendship and love take more than clicks of a button.

One of my favorite antidotes to loneliness is sharing food. I enjoy cooking. But I probably enjoy preparing food 10 times more when the food will be feeding other people.

Preparing healthy food for people who don't eat the same way you do can be a challenge. But it can offer its own special reward.

Gina Bonanno-Lemos of Orange County, California, grew up in an Italian family—one that owned an Italian deli and sold authentic home-made Italian food. She was known for her culinary skills. Her parties were popular and well attended. But when Gina adopted a plant-based diet, her friends and family became skeptical and scoffed at the idea that her new food could possibly taste good. That all changed when Gina attended a Fourth of July party at her brother's house.

Gina prepared a large pot of her now-famous three-bean vegan chili and set it out for everyone to enjoy. And enjoy it they did. Many family members remarked about the amazing taste—with no idea who'd made it or that it was meat-free. When her mother announced that it was in fact Gina's homemade chili, the room of 50-plus people grew silent. An uncle said, "I thought you didn't eat meat?" To which Gina explained that it wasn't meat that they were eating. Knowing that her meat-loving family would want something to bite into, Gina had added her secret weapon—Beyond Meat Beefy Crumble.

Gina's family was blown away that what they were eating was 100 percent plant-based and filled with the muscle-building power of pea protein. They vowed never to doubt Gina's kitchen prowess again, and they now reach out to her for advice and recipes.

Not everyone has a big family that likes to converge around food. Many people live alone or with people who don't eat as they do. And even if you're lucky enough to share food consistently with family members, the routines of cooking and cleaning can get a little old.

This is where forming a healthy meal swap team can truly shine.

The basic concept is simple: Find another person, or a team of people, who want to eat healthfully like you do, and agree to create and share meals with one another.

This can start as simply as making some extra quinoa with coconut curry sauce and asking the neighbors if they'd like you to drop some off for their next night's dinner. If their response is positive, you could ask if they might like to consider a routine of sharing extras back and forth.

If you're setting up swaps with colleagues from work, you might decide to rotate who makes lunch for the bunch. If five people are in on the deal, a different one might feed the clan each day of the week. But you can also start small and just make lunch for a few colleagues on Monday and build from there. A big batch of chickpea salad served with all the fixin's—sliced tomato, pickles, lettuce, sliced avocado—can make a fabulous, easy-to-transport, crowd-pleasing lunch.

Bringing healthy lunches to school can sometimes feel isolating for a kid whose friends are chowing down bologna sandwiches and candy bars. Try inviting a few other parents to band together in creating healthy school lunches. A rotating host or family can provide for the troupe of kids on designated days. Or better yet, join together to improve school lunches for everyone (more on that in chapter 24).

You can even get a meal going with people you hardly know.

With family spread out around the world, little time off from work, and their duties as new parents absorbing most of their free time, Aryana and Aaran Solh of Austin, Texas, were feeling isolated as Thanksgiving rolled around. Instead of spending it feeling lonesome at home, they rented out a local community event space and invited everyone they knew, as well as the greater Austin community, to join in a vegan Thanksgiving potluck and dance party.

The Solhs had been thriving on a plant-based lifestyle for more than 10 years. Most of their friends didn't eat the same way, but the Solhs wanted everyone to feel wholeheartedly welcome. Aaran made vegan latkes, and Aryana made a rainbow mandala salad with tahini dressing and a raw vegan chocolate cheesecake. Their guests commented that they had never tasted such delicious food. Over the course of the evening, over 100 visitors stopped by to dance and eat. They also used the occasion to invite donations for Amala Foundation, a local nonprofit that supports refugee youth. Aryana reflects that to this day, it was one of the most joyful and meaningful evenings she's ever been a part of. It showed what can happen when we intentionally create gatherings that have a greater purpose than ourselves.

You might find interested people by hanging a flyer at your gym, natural-foods store, community center, senior center, library, college campus, yoga studio, or church; by asking friends, family, or neighbors; by emailing colleagues at work; or even by posting an invitation on Facebook or Meetup.

Here's an example of what you might say:

WANT TO JOIN A HEALTHY MEAL SWAP TEAM?

Do you ever get tired of cooking the same foods over and over? Want to share your favorite healthy dishes with others—and to have healthy meals made for you? Contact me to join our Healthy Eaters' Meal Team! When you cook, you can make enough to share. Then take a few days off while other people cook for you! Let's build community, lighten our cooking load, and support healthy eating—all at the same time! Contact me to find out more and join in!

If you have specific dietary desires or commitments, be sure to include that information in your outreach. For example, if you want to organize your healthy-eating team around foods that are sugar-free, or vegan, or low-carb, or high-carb, it's best to say that up front. You might also suggest incorporating rules. (For example, every meal has to include a leafy green vegetable.)

It's possible the other swap team members won't share all your food values or priorities, in which case you might have to do a little negotiation and decide what are your deal breakers and where you're willing to be a little flexible.

By cooking in quantity, you'll save time. By sharing meals, you'll build social connections and discover new flavors and experiences. And by organizing your meal-swap team around healthy food, you'll support nutritious eating for everyone.

AND YES, THERE'S AN APP FOR THAT

Did you know that there are also meal-sharing apps? They function something like an Airbnb for home-cooked meals. You can volunteer to host, setting the price and stating what kind of food you're offering to prepare—and then takers will book meal slots and can pay to join you for dinner. Or you can be a guest and search for hosts, taking them up on their offer of home-cooked meals. Meal-sharing apps such as Eatwith and Meal Sharing connect eaters with home-cooked meals provided by local people. Customer reviews, dietary preferences, and clear pricing help to ensure that it's all aboveboard and that you get what you want, whether it's as a host or as a guest.

ACTION:

Option 1: Make a healthy meal or dish for a friend, neighbor, colleague, or family member. Lead with generosity, and see where it takes you!

Option 2: Check out Eatwith.com, mealsharing.com, or another online meal-sharing app, and either offer to host a meal for guests or sign up to attend someone else's meal as their guest.

Option 3: Create a flyer, email, or post and share it publicly or with at least 10 friends, inviting them to join a swap team. Follow up with everyone until you have a solid group set to make plans.

CHAPTER 21

Eat Well When You Eat Out

Phoenix and I have a date night almost every week, and it usually starts with dinner at a restaurant. We leave our kitchen chores behind and let someone else plan, prepare, and clean up.

It's not necessarily the healthiest way to go. And it can get pricey. But restaurants provide a lovely ambience along with a chance to experience new flavors and cuisines.

It's good to choose with care, however, because not all restaurants are necessarily safe places to eat.

DANGEROUS INGREDIENTS

Unless you've been hiding in a cave for the last 40 years, or you work in the McDonald's PR department, you probably know that fast food is often a nutritional disaster. Nearly everything is loaded with sugar, salt, chemicals, factory-farmed meat, and processed carbs.

But did you know that even many upscale and gourmet restaurants use ingredients you'd never intentionally bring into your kitchen— including some that should probably come with warning labels?

Even the fanciest restaurants are heavily influenced by the need to cut costs and increase sales. And since most of them don't have to reveal the ingredients they use, they're often driven by market pressures to sneak in cheap fillers and taste boosters.

Many use highly processed oils and foods laced with artificial flavorings, added sugars, and preservatives. Unless they explicitly tell you otherwise, restaurant salad dressings could contain chemicals like disodium guanylate and monosodium glutamate (MSG). And almost all restaurant meats are sourced from factory farms.

Even when salmon is advertised as "wild," that may not be a guarantee that it actually is. In 2015, the nonprofit ocean conservation group Oceana used DNA analysis to study samples of salmon from upscale and takeout restaurants in New York; Washington, DC; Chicago; and Virginia. They found that two-thirds of the "wild" salmon on restaurant menus was incorrectly labeled. It was farmed.[1]

Many countries have rules and regulations to ensure that the food restaurants serve is sanitary. But you can never be totally sure of the ingredients being used, or how the food has been stored, prepared, or cooked. To some extent, eating out requires a leap of faith.

HOW TO FIND THE GOOD ONES

There are some great tools to help you appraise restaurant options. I thought I knew all the restaurants worth knowing in my town. But recently I loaded up Google and Yelp, using search terms like "organic," "natural," "sustainable," and "vegetarian." Lo and behold, I found a whole string of new establishments that I hadn't known about, complete with price information and customer reviews.

One of the restaurants I discovered was a local organic Sri Lankan restaurant that my wife and I went to on a date night. During our meal, the owner, who is also the head chef, came out to say hello to all the patrons. She asked me for feedback on the spices she'd used in the vegetable curry I was eating and shared some of the thinking that had gone into her choice of ingredients. She cared about her guests. Offering nourishing food that delighted people was more than a job—it was a passion.

It's always possible there's a jewel hidden in your neighborhood or nearby.

There's also a growing trend toward healthier "fast food" options. For example, Chipotle now has more than 2,000 locations worldwide, and despite some challenges with safety in its supply chain, the restaurant has led the way by going non-GMO and offering vegan options and meat from grass-fed animals. Amy's Kitchen has opened an organic drive-through restaurant in California and has plans for franchise-based expansion. And there's a growing body of health-minded chains opening up, with names like Veggie Grill, Native Foods Café, Lyfe Kitchen, and Sweetgreen.

HOW TO ORDER SMARTLY

Before visiting a restaurant that's new to you, check to see if its website has an online menu. When you arrive, don't be afraid to tell your waitperson your preferences or needs and ask for recommendations. And if you don't see anything on the menu that feels like a good fit, you can often order "off the menu," requesting combinations or options that make use of ingredients the restaurant has—assembled in a way that works for you.

For example, recently I was staying in a hotel and decided to try my luck at its restaurant. I didn't see anything on the menu that I felt comfortable eating, but I didn't let that stop me. I ordered steamed vegetables with lemon wedges and a baked potato topped with olive oil, Tabasco sauce, salt, chopped parsley, and curry. I also ordered a salad, and instead of the house dressing, I requested olive oil, lemon juice, salt, and an Italian seasoning mix the restaurant had on hand.

It certainly wasn't the high point of my culinary life. But by the time I added the seasonings, I had a reasonably tasty (and unique!) meal and felt glad that I hadn't compromised my values or taste buds.

When I'm eating breakfast at a restaurant, I opt for porridge instead of bagels, pastries, or sugary boxed cereals. For lunch or dinner, I try to incorporate steamed vegetables and salads along with quinoa, rice, potatoes, or sweet potatoes and some tasty curries. A lot of restaurants can accommodate these kinds of options. Selections at many eateries can be bountiful if you're creative and willing to ask for substitutions. Notice a veggie-packed stir-fry with chicken on the menu? If you like, you can politely ask that the chicken be left out and replaced with extra veggies, sautéed mushrooms, or tofu.

The way I look at it, you shouldn't feel guilty about requesting a little extra attention. Restaurants are in business to serve their customers. By telling them what you need, you're helping them do their job. And besides, if they get "out of the box" requests often enough, they just might decide to change the box. How else would they know there was customer-based demand for healthier food?

Stephanie Prima of Friday Harbor, Washington, is a vegan whose top food goal is to eat a lot of vegetables. In restaurants where chefs are cooking with the seasons, she'll order a collection of vegetable side dishes. On occasion the chef will beautifully plate all the sides on one platter for her, complete with garnishes and sauces—giving her a variety of colors, textures, cooking techniques, and temperatures.

Stephanie has enjoyed such delicacies as grilled polenta cake with marinara; sweet pea purée; sautéed greens with garlic; roasted asparagus with balsamic glaze; seasonal herbed vegetable medley; rosemary roasted red potatoes; and roasted brussels sprouts with mushrooms. When chefs prepare dishes especially for her, Stephanie feels like a VIP. She's grateful for the special care, and happy that she made her wishes known toward honoring her health priorities.

Personally, I have slightly different (and more lax) standards when I'm eating out or traveling than I do at home. I eat out about once a week, and I figure that if the occasional meal is at a slightly lower standard, my overall health shouldn't suffer too much. I do want to be able to move through the world, and to have a social life, without too much trouble.

And remember—once you decide to eat something, there's no benefit in carrying guilt. Enjoy it. Take pleasure in it. And if you're with friends or loved ones, enjoy their company, too. Using your five senses while eating enhances your mealtime experience tenfold. Relishing the crunch of freshly picked fruits and veggies, seeing the vibrant array of colors across your plate, hearing the sizzle of a pan, smelling the intoxicating aroma of sautéing garlic and onions, tasting a fiery-hot spiced curry, and taking in the smile of a friend or loved one—these make for a sublime culinary experience.

AND A WORD ABOUT KINDNESS

Behind most restaurants is an owner, of course. But there are also chefs, servers, dishwashers, janitors, and other staff who work hard to bring us our meals. Many of them aren't paid a whole lot. Some of them face hostile working conditions. Did you know that 40 percent of female fast-food workers are subjected to sexual harassment on the job?[2]

When you go to a restaurant, even if you find the food or the service disappointing, remember that the workers are probably under a lot of stress. Smiling, saying "thank you," tipping generously, and being friendly can brighten everyone's day—including your own.

HEALTHFUL EATING "ON THE GO"

I hope to live in a world someday in which every convenience store and fast-food restaurant has healthy food. But we're not there yet. And until we get there, it can be wise to plan ahead so you don't get stuck choosing between Skittles and fried pork rinds.

When I need to find food in a new town, I use Google or Yelp to see if there's a Chipotle or, if it's a big enough city, to check for a natural-foods store such as a co-op or a Whole Foods Market.

There are also more specialized apps and tools. Bookatable.com is a popular online restaurant scouting, review, and reservation service based in Europe. Vegetarians and vegans find wonderful options and reviews all over the world on happycow.net. Another fun tool designed for the road is Food Tripping, a GPS-based app that's especially helpful if you want to find local, sustainable food at convenient spots while you're traveling. Food Tripping has a growing database of healthy food markets, farmer's markets, quick eateries, organic coffee shops, and juice bars.

As nice as it is to find options in new communities, many people prefer to leave home with supplies. I nearly always head out on long drives or flights with some food packed. Try sandwiches with avocado or with pesto and bean spreads; chickpea salad wraps; Mediterranean mezze platters, olives, flatbread, roasted peppers, and tabbouleh; chia puddings; nut "cheeze" and crackers; homemade energy bars or energy balls; trail mix; dried fruit; sturdy veggies (such as broccoli, cauliflower, or celery) with hummus; vegetable sushi rolls; or cold bean-and-pasta salads with tangy herb vinaigrette and veggies. Fruit travels well, too. Apples, oranges, pears, and bananas can be ready to go, no refrigeration necessary. (Do be careful with bananas, though. I can tell you from personal experience that squished bananas and laptop computers don't get along!)

Some people use a dehydrator to make their own kale and vegetable chips or flax crackers. Season your homemade chips and crackers with nutritional yeast, smoked paprika, and garlic powder, or rosemary and oregano for an Italian twist. Make your trail mix more interesting by adding coconut flakes, chocolate chips, goji berries, or a simple dusting of cinnamon. (If you like any of these ideas and want to find recipes to help you put them into action, try searching online for the concepts, or go to allrecipes.com and enter "kale chips," "flax crackers," "homemade energy balls," or the preferred recipe of your choice into the search bar and see what you come up with.)

If you're going camping, you might want to bring porridge and dried fruit, cold cereal and nondairy milk in nonperishable packaging, rice or quinoa, canned beans, and spice mixes. Nut butter and jelly sandwiches work well, too. You might also be able to steam some cabbage, carrots, onions, or courgette, which store reasonably well, especially if you're "car camping" and can bring a cooler.

SHARING HEALTHY FOOD AT PARTIES

Most people don't exactly think of parties as optimal venues to showcase healthy foods. They're more often associated with alcohol and processed snacks than with chia seeds and organic kale. But who says that having fun and eating well can't go together? Even if most of the foods at a social event are packed with hyperprocessed and chemical-laden products, that doesn't mean you can't bring something nourishing. Serving a bowl of warm marinated olives, rosemary roasted cashews, or homemade roasted red pepper hummus is sure to attract the attention (and appetites!) of the guests, without sacrificing flavor or good nutrition. In fact, the less healthful other party foods might be, the more of a difference your contribution will make.

You might be surprised at how people respond.

A STORY OF CAKE AND BERRIES

Judith and her boyfriend, Jon, were invited to a potluck. They were running late and decided to stop at a Whole Foods Market on the way to pick up something to bring.

Judith decided to bring a fancy decorated cake. But Jon was more of a healthy eater and insisted they bring a tray of fresh blueberries, raspberries, blackberries, and strawberries. Unfortunately, they were both adamant and got into an argument.

When neither of them was willing to budge, they ended up bringing both offerings. When they arrived, Judith placed her cake at the center of the dessert area. There weren't a lot of spots left, so Jon put his berry tray at the end of the table, where people would see it only after making their way past all the other desserts—if they saw it at all.

Since they were both highly competitive, they decided to bet on which would be more popular. Judith was confident about her cake, and Jon acknowledges now that he thought she was probably right, but he was too stubborn to admit it at the time.

At the end of the evening, Judith and Jon were shocked that the cake had barely been touched, and the berries were all gone. What made matters worse, from Judith's point of view, was that somebody left a note next to the berry tray that said, "Thank you for bringing these! Glad to find them instead of the usual pastries."

Sometimes people will default to bringing unhealthy items because they think that's what everyone wants. But as increasing numbers of people want better food, it's becoming more and more cool to offer healthier options.

BRINGING SOMETHING THAT WORKS FOR YOU

If you're attending a gathering hosted by someone else who isn't likely to be amenable to making foods that work for you, you might ask if it's okay if you bring something to share. That will at least ensure you'll have something nutritious. And this gives you the opportunity to spread the love and to shift the food culture in a positive direction.

Anne Swan from Owosso, Michigan, brings healthy food to parties because it gives other partygoers an opportunity to try out plant-powered foods.

At Anne's instigation, family gatherings have turned into potlucks. A number of family members are, like Anne, plant-based eaters, and they bring plenty not only for themselves but for the "traditional crowd," who end up appreciating the variety. Anne loves creating a food culture that works for her while exposing everyone else to wholesome options.

WHAT TO BRING

Wondering what to serve at a party? The foods that work best fit on small plates and are easy to eat while people stand and chat. Some people love

to include veggies or wholesome crackers served with hummus, gua-
camole, or salsa; sushi rolls; slices of apple, pear, orange, or other fruit;
mixed nuts or trail mix; crispy potatoes with a nacho "cheeze" sauce;
baked courgette chips; popcorn; and mini courgette pizzas. (You'll find
recipes for many of these scrumptious delights in the Recipes for Health
section of this book.)

If you're going to a public event, see if you can request healthy options
in advance. Sometimes event organizers get so busy that they take the
path of least resistance and serve food that isn't well thought out. Your
inquiry could inspire them to rethink the menu.

The same Stephanie Prima who loves to order thoughtfully at restaurants also serves as the volunteer and event coordinator for an annual
TEDx event on San Juan Island in Washington. For years, the organizers hired a caterer to provide deli sandwiches on white bread, with a
plain green salad. But to Stephanie it felt odd that an event focused on
new innovations and ideas would serve food that might contribute to
brain fog.

In 2017, Stephanie volunteered to coordinate a different menu. She
was nervous about how it would be received, since the event attracted
all kinds of eaters, some of whom might prefer sandwiches and pizza to
a kale salad. But she found a caterer who could provide a delicious meal
made from whole foods that were nourishing, colorful, and plant-based.
The menu, sourced mostly from local growers, included a mixed green
salad with house-made vinaigrette, seeds, veggies, and seasonal fruit;
kale-and-chickpea salad with lemon, sumac, and pepitas; East Indian
lentil soup; cauliflower, sweet potato, and black bean chili; non-GMO
corn cakes with seasonal fruit; and gluten-free naan. For dishware, her
caterer provided compostable bamboo plates and utensils.

The caterer received abundant compliments, as attendees exclaimed
how great it was to have "REAL FOOD!" Stephanie felt happy that her
efforts were so warmly received. To her delight, several attendees asked
the caterer if he could provide healthy meals for events that they were
hosting.

Stephanie could have easily settled for the status quo. But she took a
risk. She did the research to find a talented caterer. And not only were

her efforts warmly received, they sent out waves that directly affected future gatherings.

You never know whose life you might touch when you bring healthy food into a new place. But step by step, one dish at a time, you're contributing to healthier lives and ultimately to a healthier food culture.

GETTING BACK ON TRACK

At the first Thanksgiving in the United States, the pilgrims worried about having enough food to survive the winter. But these days, we worry about how to survive Thanksgiving without feeling more stuffed than a 20-pound turkey. Holidays have become a tour-de-force of overindulgence. I know many people who eat healthfully most of the time, but around the holidays, they slip faster than Santa could ever slide down a chimney on Christmas Eve.

A 2016 study in the *New England Journal of Medicine* found that Germans gain an average of 1.7 pounds during the Christmas and New Year's season, and Americans gain 1.3 pounds.[3] People in Japan gain an average of 1.1 pounds during their Golden Week (a week that features four national holidays). And most of this weight gain is never lost—thus contributing to an ever-expanding obesity epidemic.

If you find yourself falling off the wagon over the holidays, don't panic. Just pick up where you left off and get back on the path.

Many people go on diets in the new year to get rid of holiday-fueled spare tires. But sudden deprivation is often a prelude to episodes of slippage or, worse, bingeing. This is an important time to treat yourself with compassion, and to get lovingly back on track. In the long run, what matters most isn't what you eat 2 percent of the time. It's what you eat the other 98 percent.

And perhaps it's time we remembered what holidays are really for. Christmas can be about a lot more than maxing out your credit cards and stuffing your belly. It can also be a time of generosity, love, family connection, and spiritual reflection. Thanksgiving can bring us so much more than just a "turkey day." Giving thanks can actually be a profound opportunity to bring loved ones together. And, as you'll see in the next chapter, they can be very good for your health, as well.

ACTION:

Option 1: *Decide on a tasty, nutritious offering to bring to a party or family gathering. Mark it in your calendar, along with a note about the recipe or a link to it.*

Option 2: *Use Google, Yelp, or a smartphone app to find one new restaurant that markets to a health-conscious audience, and give it a try.*

Option 3: *Invite loved ones to join you at your favorite healthy restaurant. Francine Regan-Pollock from Vancouver, British Columbia, invited six friends to join her and her husband at their favorite plant-based comfort-food restaurant. Some of their friends eat healthfully, and others don't. But all of them were willing to give it a go. They dined on tofu "buffalo wings" and cauliflower bites, and they taste-tested every plant-based burger on the menu. The troupe had a blast. Two of Francine's guests tell her they have since moved their diets in a healthier direction.*

CHAPTER 22

The Stunning Neuroscience of Gratitude

Have you ever had someone say sweet things to you, but you were so distracted that you hardly noticed? On the other hand, have you ever listened to someone sharing appreciation and felt it reach deep into your heart?

It could have been the same person, saying the same thing, in each instance—but you had a completely different experience because of your level of receptivity.

Food can be a little like that. When you're present for the interaction, your salivary glands, your digestive process, and your cells can be in a more meaningful relationship with food.

People say "You are what you eat," and that's a half-truth. It might be more accurate to say "You are what you digest."

THE BEGINNING OF DIGESTION

Have you ever gotten an upset stomach just from thinking about a certain food? Or felt your gut relax as you sat down to a cup of warm tea?

From the moment you first interact with food, which can include thought, sight, or smell, your mouth may begin to form salivary enzymes, and your belly may start to secrete gastric juices. This preparation is important. Saliva, combined with chewing, helps to break down food, enabling your body to absorb critical nutrients.

What's even more remarkable is that in response to anticipation, smell, and taste, your stomach goes to work preparing the way with the gastric juices needed to digest the specific food that's about to enter. If you're thinking about an apple, your body prepares to meet the apple. By the time it reaches your tummy, that apple is greeted by the perfect acidity level and the optimal enzymes for exquisite digestion. It's an extraordinary interactive process that can make the difference between nutrition being absorbed, or going in one end and out the other.

When you savor your food—by smelling, chewing, and letting saliva develop—you're shifting the course of your digestive process and setting yourself up to more efficiently absorb what you're eating.

It's been well documented that when your nervous system is in a state of ease and relaxation, your digestion improves, your metabolism stabilizes, and a myriad of benefits ensue.[1]

Your relationship with food is intimate. When you bring consciousness and care to any relationship, it becomes richer and more meaningful. Slowing down and paying attention doesn't just change how you eat. It might also change what kinds of foods you're drawn to. Your body has tremendous wisdom, and sometimes, if you slow down a bit, you become better able to hear it.

GRACE AND GRATITUDE

In most of the world's major religious traditions, it's a common practice to pray, give thanks, or say grace before a meal.

And today, science is discovering that gratitude can have profound benefits to your quality and even *quantity* of life. It doesn't just make things *feel* better. It actually also makes them *get* better. According to recent research, gratitude is good for your physical, emotional, and mental health.[2] People who express more gratitude have fewer aches and pains, better sleep, and expanded mental clarity.[3]

When I heard all this, I was skeptical. What if people who are fortunate or particularly healthy already just feel more grateful? Does gratitude really cause good fortune, or is it more of a by-product?

The answer surprised me.

In a study led by Robert A. Emmons, PhD, at the University of California at Davis, randomly assigned participants were given one of two tasks.[4] Each week, participants kept a short journal. One group was asked to briefly describe five things they were grateful for that occurred during the week, while the second group recorded daily hassles that displeased them. Keep in mind that these groups were randomly assigned. Nothing about their lives was inherently different, other than the journaling required of them.

The people in the grateful group listed things like "sunset through the clouds," "the chance to be alive," and "the generosity of friends." And in the hassles group, people listed familiar things: "taxes," "hard to find parking," and "burned my dinner."

After 10 weeks, participants in the gratitude group reported feeling better about their lives as a whole. They ended up being a full 25 percent happier than the hassled group. They reported fewer health complaints, and they were exercising an average of 1.5 hours more per week than the hassled group.

Studies have shown that the expression of gratitude leads to measurable effects on multiple body and brain systems, including mood neurotransmitters (serotonin and norepinephrine), social bonding hormones (oxytocin), cognitive and pleasure-related neurotransmitters (dopamine), inflammatory and immune systems (cytokines), stress hormones (cortisol), blood pressure, and blood sugar.[5]

Apparently, positive vibes aren't just for flower children. They can be good for everyone. So how can you put gratitude to work for you and the people you love?

THE ART OF SAYING GRACE

In our home, before dinner we often go around the table, with each of us sharing something we're grateful for. Sometimes we talk about simple things, like that the sun came out today, or that a friend had a birthday. Other times, we might express gratitude for a family member.

When he was 16, my son River told me that he was grateful to me for my work for Food Revolution. He said that he missed me when I was working long hours or traveling, but he wanted me to know that he was proud of me. I don't know if words can express how deeply his comment touched me.

Rick Hamlin, editor of *Guideposts*, appreciates how "saying grace" can help families cross partisan divides, commenting: "My Republican brother-in-law always holds hands when we say grace. My Democrat brother-in-law gives these thoughtful, heartfelt graces that make me cry. I love them both. They are people of deep, abiding, probing faith. We can disagree about many things but we can always agree about this: We are blessed."[6]

Saying grace can also be a moment to give thanks for the many people and forces that make our meal possible. Lauren F. Winner, associate professor at Duke Divinity School, likes to say grace at restaurants because she finds it so easy, when she goes out to eat, to take for granted the low-paid folks who set the table, wash the dishes, and generally make her night on the town possible. "To pray before my meal," she reflects, "even if it's awkward, reminds me how privileged I am, how much I owe."[7]

Here's a "grace" poem I shared at a family dinner recently. Please feel free to use it or adapt it any way you like.

> *I give thanks for the farmers and the farmworkers who grew our food. I give thanks for the people who dug the wells that irrigated the soil, and the truck drivers who brought the vegetables to the market. I give thanks for the many hands and hearts that worked so hard to bring us every single ingredient we are now blessed to enjoy.*
>
> *I recognize that some people who labored to bring us our food are struggling to feed their own families. I hope and I pray that we may be fed by this nourishment and use it to build a world where everyone has healthy food and the opportunity to live with dignity.*
>
> *I give thanks that we are together, and that we are blessed to share this meal with one another.*

You can write your own gratitude and share it (as well as reading gratitude prayers from others) at 31dayfoodrevolution.com/gratitude.

Gratitude reminds us that we are not alone—and that there are, in fact, a great many people and forces that play critical roles in bringing us the food we eat.

When we're aware of them, we're less likely to take them for granted. And we're more likely to become conscious of the real impact of our food choices, not only on our own lives or on the health of our loved ones, but also on farmers, animals, and the whole world.

Food, we quickly see, is not just a commodity, but also a community. Food is a web of relationships that's intertwined with who we are, and with how we live.

I'm grateful for the opportunity to be nourished by real, healthy food. And I'm also happy that, with our food choices, we have immense power to contribute to building a healthier world.

To me, that's cause for gratitude.

ACTION:

Option 1: Before your next meal, take a deep breath and pause for a moment to smell and savor your food.

Option 2: Convene friends, family, or colleagues around a moment of thanksgiving. Ask them to share one thing they are thankful for. I've even known companies that start business meetings with a moment of thanksgiving.

Option 3: Create a daily gratitude routine. If you're with friends or family for regular meals, you could suggest that every dinner begin with a thanksgiving go-around. Or record in a journal five things you're grateful for at the end of every day. Stay with it. Gratitude is one of the healthiest habits in the world.

CHAPTER 23

Feed Our Children Well

Whether you're a parent or grandparent, an aunt or uncle, a brother or sister, a teacher, a caregiver, or simply a friend, chances are you have kids in your life.

> There can be no keener revelation of a society's soul than the way in which it treats its children.
>
> —*Nelson Mandela*

It isn't easy to raise a youngster in the modern world.

American children see an average of more than 300 food ads per week.[1] And most of these ads aren't for broccoli or organic flaxseed. They're for hyperprocessed, sugar-laden junk foods.

The junk food industry isn't spending billions of dollars marketing to kids as a public service. They're doing it to make money. And in the process, they're hooking our kids on products that lay the foundations for a future of disease.

They employ highly paid, highly trained multidisciplinary teams of scientists and spend enormous sums of money with the explicit goal that large numbers of people will be unable to stop eating their products—regardless of devastating health consequences. "Bet you can't eat just one" is more than an advertising slogan for a brand of potato chips. It's also throwing down the gauntlet with a sobering threat to public health.

While many food industry advertisers try to brand their products as fun, we all know that there's not a whole lot of fun in being obese, or in suffering from diabetes, heart disease, or cancer.

Our toxic food culture may be hitting kids the hardest of all. Millions of children are growing up overweight, mentally and physically lethargic, and suffering from preventable type 2 diabetes.

I once saw a child wearing a T-shirt that said, "If you love me, don't feed me junk food." The fact is, children depend on us to protect them from harm. And we all have a stake in their well-being. You don't need to be a health nut or a food activist to want kids to be healthy.

Dietary changes can even impact academic performance. A study in Canada published in the *Journal of School Health* found that students who ate a diet rich in fruits, vegetables, protein, and fiber did better on their literacy tests than those eating foods high in salt and saturated fat.[2]

But children face negative peer influences and are surrounded by junk food that's normalized and even celebrated. And as unhealthy as they are, there's no argument that sugary and processed foods can taste good—and be highly addictive.

HELPING KIDS TO LOVE HEALTHY FOOD

River and Bodhi, our teenage twins, love vegetables.

They've been known to scarf down an entire head of steamed savoy cabbage before they even start eating the rest of their dinner—and then ask for more. But it wasn't always this way. When they were little, they were extremely picky eaters. Sometimes it seemed like the only way to get them to eat at all was to serve an abundance of bread. And as I've mentioned, we had our fair share of fights over potato chips.

When our kids were about nine years old, I realized that for all my talk about healthy eating, our family wasn't really living it. Phoenix and I had to make changes.

The first thing we noticed was that our kids would get hungry while we were making dinner. They would scrounge the cupboards and fridge and would typically score the most processed, salty food around. When dinner arrived, they were no longer hungry.

We realized that our kids loved eating with their hands, and this was one reason they were drawn to bread, chips, cookies, and packaged snacks. So we came up with the idea that we could wash or steam vegetables and make a dip or sauce. It took some time to find which vegetables and sauces worked best. A family favorite is the Terrific Tahini Dressing that you'll find on page 302.

We developed a routine. About half an hour before dinner, we'd put a sauce or dip in a bowl and set out some lightly steamed broccoli, kale, cabbage, carrots, collards, and/or cauliflower. Sometimes our twins would even skip the sauce and just have at it with the vegetables.

To this day, putting vegetables in the middle of the table is a family tradition. Even after dinner, we often leave vegetables out for late-night snacking. Sometimes, when River is feeling rebellious, he'll grab some steamed cabbage even after brushing his teeth.

His dentist might not think it's the best idea, but it sure beats late-night doughnuts.

If you want to share healthier food options with children, here are a few of my favorite tips.

To-Go Packs

We make organic trail mixes and put them in ready-to-go packets. Ours have ingredients like walnuts, cashews, dried apple, almonds, and raisins. Other healthy snacks include bags of popcorn, vegetable chips, fruit and nut bars, or seasoned mixed nuts. The key is to have things available on demand that can fit into an active life.

Share Meals

Eating together as a family encourages healthy food habits. In 2012, researchers studied 2,000 elementary school children in London, and found that those who shared in family meals as little as once or twice a week consumed an average of 3.4 ounces (1.2 portions) more fruits and vegetables per day than those whose families never ate together.[3] Other studies have found that families who eat dinner together tend to eat fewer fried foods and to drink less soda.[4] Sharing meals has many other benefits, too—like positive social connection and family bonding.

Don't Bring Unhealthy Foods into the House

Create a healthy environment at home. Clean out those cupboards and replace junk food with fruit or cut-up veggies that are convenient to grab when hunger strikes. (You can clean and cut up fruits or veggies in the evening and then have them around to munch for the next day or two.) Don't bring junk foods, such as chips or packaged cookies, into the house. Make rules and, if kids are old enough, get everyone on board. For example, we never have sugary sodas in our home. Period. Teaching self-control and clear boundaries can be important not only with food but in all areas of life.

Talk About Food Honestly

Growing up as part of the Baskin-Robbins empire, my dad gained an insider's perspective on the way that sugar and chemicals drive addiction. He also discovered from firsthand experience how the junk food industry tries to turn kids into lifelong consumers before they can even talk.

So by the time I was five, my dad was already trying to prepare me to defend myself from these dangers, offering his critiques of the processed food industries—and helping me to see beyond advertising jingles to understand the dark side of unhealthy products.

It might sound odd to think of telling a five-year-old how sweets can spike blood sugar, or about the danger of sodium nitrate in processed meats. But the reality is that in a toxic food culture, kids need to begin developing the equivalent of a food immune system at a very early age. Junk food addiction is, in many ways, a kind of socially communicable pathogen. If you don't have an immune system, then exposure can and often does lead to disease.

I'm glad my dad started preparing me to resist these dangers early on. I've done the same with my kids. I learned that it's important, when initiating a conversation about food with a child, to tie it to things that matter to them. Many kids are more motivated by concerns about things like animals, the environment, and social equity than they are about their personal health.

Once they understand the "why," many kids can actually become leaders in helping a whole family to implement healthier choices. And beware: They may hold you accountable for your own decisions and slip-ups, too!

I remember an occasion when I took seven-year-old Bodhi shopping in a natural foods store. He was getting fussy, and I had a big shopping list to get through. To calm him down, I reached frantically for something he could munch on, so that he would stop bugging me long enough that I could finish the shopping. I settled on a cookie, which I pulled out of the bulk bin (making a mental note to pay for it upon checkout).

The cookie was organic and vegan. I decided that under the circumstances, that was good enough. One cookie wasn't about to kill my son.

But Bodhi looked at it, noticing its red and blue sprinkles. "Is this cookie coated in candy?" he asked. I sheepishly acknowledged that it was.

He handed it back with disgust, exclaiming, "Don't you *ever* feed me junk food again!"

I found myself feeling both startled and proud. Sometimes when you talk the talk, it's your kids who remind you that you also need to walk the walk.

STRATEGIES TO STOP PICKY EATING

Some families make tofu and vegetables for the parents and buy chicken nuggets and fries for the kids. In other families, the parents drink sodas while forbidding their children to have any. "Do as I say, not as I do," they admonish. Neither of these approaches creates a healthy family ecosystem.

So what to do? Not all toddlers are ready for kale salads, but many meals can be adapted even for little ones. Some kids can be persuaded to try just a small taste, which can be a bite-sized way to open their minds and taste buds.

You can also tell them that it takes time to adjust to new foods, and that foods can taste different depending on how they're cooked, what they're served with, and how we feel that day. So they may need to try something a few times before deciding if they like it or not.

Get Kids Involved

Kids tend to love to eat foods they grow, or prepare, themselves. Gardens, including school gardens, have been correlated with higher levels of life satisfaction and vegetable consumption. And finding healthy, simple recipes can be an empowering experience for children. Getting kids involved in recipe planning and cooking can be a great way for them to develop important life skills and experience the self-confidence that can come from being able to feed themselves and to make a contribution to others.

If you've been raising kids on a modern industrialized diet and are making the switch late in the game, don't worry—it can be done! It may seem challenging to "deprive" kids if their favorite foods are things like pop, chips, and candy. But having family meetings about the subject can help. And you can find healthier alternatives to family favorites. For example, instead of chicken nuggets, you can make homemade baked chickpea nuggets (you'll find a recipe on page 288). You can also keep some frozen berries or frozen fruit on hand, and let kids dig in when they want a snack or a dessert.

Instead of heating up packaged frozen french fries, make homemade oven-baked sweet potato fries, sprinkled with sea salt and freshly ground black pepper. And even if you're vegan and gluten-free, your family can still enjoy pizza if you make it on a corn tortilla or gluten-free pitta bread, smothered in oregano-flecked marinara and piled high with sautéed garlic, onions, spinach, and mushrooms (or your veggies of choice!) and, if you like, a sprinkling of nondairy "cheeze."

Be Patient and Persistent

It takes time to build new habits—even for kids. It can take 8 to 15 tastes of a new food to develop an affinity for it. If kids are used to burgers and fries, and you're switching to burritos and coleslaw, it may take a few tries for them to adjust. Be positive, patient, and persistent. Present foods in new and different ways. And keep it playful. Especially for kids, laughter is one of the best doorways to a new way of eating.

ACTION:

Option 1: Next time you serve kids a meal, put veggies and a sauce on the table before the meal and invite everyone to nibble.

Option 2: Engage a child in preparing a healthy meal or snack. Depending on their age and level of interest, they may be able to choose a recipe, and to harvest, wash, chop, measure, or stir. Even a little bit of active engagement can change a child's relationship with food.

Option 3: Pick a youngster you'd like to nurture toward a lifetime of healthier eating. You could read them a book (there are lots of great children's books that will help—check out Gregory, the Terrible Eater; Eating the Alphabet; The Adventures of Alex the Vegetarian Coyote; and Yummy Plants ABC). If they're older, have a conversation, give them an educational or inspirational book, or show them a film. The bottom line: 1) Pick a person; 2) pick a strategy; and 3) put it into action.

CHAPTER 24

What About School Lunches?

In 1966, Martin Luther King Jr. broke down in tears as he described watching a teacher in Marks, Mississippi, cut an apple into slices to feed her desperately hungry students.[1] And still today, many of the United States' 15 million kids growing up in poverty depend on school meals for their survival, while more than 30 million kids eat lunch at school every day.[2]

School meals provide important sustenance to kids around the globe. Teachers in the United Kingdom describe malnourished pupils "filling their pockets" with food from school so they can have something to eat when they get home.[3]

What goes into school meals has a tremendous impact on the next generation and the future of a nation. Well-balanced school meals have been linked to fewer sick days, improved concentration in class, and better educational outcomes.[4] But unfortunately, healthy school meals are all too often a rarity, as they get lost in a sea of sugar, white flour, and fried chicken.

A series of studies in the 1980s removed chemical additives and processed food, and reduced levels of sugar, in the diets of juvenile offenders.[5] Over 8,000 young people in 12 juvenile correctional facilities were involved. *The result was that problem behaviors fell 47 percent.*

In Virginia, 300 juvenile offenders at a detention facility housing particularly hardened adolescents were put on a similar diet, with no chemical additives and little sugar, for two years. During that time, the incidence of theft dropped 77 percent, insubordination dropped 55 percent, and hyperactivity dropped 65 percent.[6]

In Los Angeles County probation detention halls, 1,400 youths were put on a diet that eliminated processed foods and chemical additives and greatly reduced sugar levels. Again, the results were excellent. There was a 44 percent reduction in problem behavior and suicide attempts.[7]

These and other studies suggest that when troubled youngsters are put on a healthy diet based on nutrient-dense foods such as vegetables, fruits, seeds, legumes, and whole grains, and that avoids sugar, preservatives, and artificial colors and flavors, the results are predictably outstanding.

There are two things I want to point out here, and they're both significant. The first is that these studies are stunning, and they clearly show criminality and antisocial behavior being dramatically reduced with nutritional improvements. The second is that these studies took place decades ago, and nothing has been done to seriously follow up on them, or to implement their discoveries on a vast scale.

When I think about all the parents and grandparents who stay up late worrying about their kids' future, and about how many children and teens are struggling with hyperactivity and feelings of confusion and hostility, I start to wonder when we'll decide it's time to act on what we know—*now*.

WHAT'S WRONG WITH AMERICA'S SCHOOL LUNCHES?

In recent years, important efforts have been made to make school meals healthier in the U.S. and other countries, but many nutritional experts still find them woefully inadequate. And our kids are paying the price.

A 2010 study conducted by the University of Michigan found that in Michigan, 38 percent of students who routinely ate school lunch were overweight or obese, compared to only 24 percent of children who brought their own meals.[8] The study found that 91 percent of the children who brought lunch from home consumed fruits or vegetables on a regular basis, as compared to only 16 percent of children whose diets were dependent on the food provided by the school.

For parents who can afford it, having kids bring healthy options to school is a great way to go. But as long as tens of millions of families depend on school meals for a fundamental part of daily nutrition, we all have a stake in making them healthier.

In the U.S., many school food service directors want to serve healthful food but face an uphill battle. They must confront challenges with staffing, budgets, and making many groups happy (including students, parents, administrators, and their state's education department, which administers the USDA school meal program). Public school food programs must be financially self-sufficient, too. While public schools have budgets that district residents vote on, and that are paid for primarily through property taxes, those budgets typically don't include funding for school meals. Public school food programs depend instead on income from students who pay for food, coupled with reimbursements from the federal and state governments that subsidize meals for students from low-income families.

Another longstanding challenge is the USDA's Foods in Schools Program. This is a program through which the USDA purchases hundreds of millions of dollars' worth of agricultural products and gives them to schools free of charge. The U.S. government devised this to stabilize prices and ensure abundant demand for some of the nation's agricultural goods. However, the net effect is to tilt the marketplace toward the foods that the USDA chooses to purchase, which unfairly supports the farmers who grow them while creating a competitive disadvantage to farmers who do not. This also floods schools with the donated products— something that budget-strapped food service directors feel unable to turn down.

So what is most of the USDA Foods Program money going toward? If you're thinking cabbage, lentils, and blueberries, guess again.

In 2015, the USDA allocated 64 percent of food program procurement expenditures to meat, dairy, and egg products, virtually all of which came from factory farms.[9] As long as these systems are in place, farmers will have an unfair incentive to produce factory-farmed animal products, and schools will have an unhealthy incentive to serve them.

Considering that more than 60 percent of Americans eat more saturated fat than is recommended by the nation's official dietary guidelines, while less than 15 percent of Americans eat the recommended amount of vegetables, this subsidy system tilts the playing field in the wrong direction.[10]

Economic forces place many school food service personnel in a bind. They have limited budgets. The options most affordable to them, in part because of taxpayer subsidies, are centered on animal products. And the most convenient choices are often heavily processed.

Despite rising food costs and unhealthy government subsidies, however, many school districts are working hard to move their menus in the right direction. School gardens are on the rise, and increasing numbers of schools are seeking to rely less on animal products and processed foods, and to serve more whole foods, fruits, and vegetables. Since 2012, by law, all public schools in the U.S. have been required to provide minimum levels of fruits and vegetables. The levels are far lower than would be optimal, but they're a good step in the right direction.

Many countries in Europe have policies to help schools provide nutritionally balanced meals that also reflect the general culture of each nation.[11] In England, certain foods are restricted (deep-fried foods are limited to no more than two portions per week), while others are promoted (students must receive at least one portion of fruits and one portion of vegetables every day). In France, by law, at least 50 percent of school meals must include vegetables. As a result, French school lunches include salads featuring foods like carrots, tomatoes, onions, lettuce, and coriander, as well as vegetable dishes featuring green beans, broccoli, parsley, and other nutritious greens.[12]

In 2017, the European Union announced plans to invest €150 million per year in a new program to help cover the cost of school lunches—and to subsidize inclusion of fruits and vegetables.[13]

Also in 2017, the environmental organization Friends of the Earth announced the results of a partnership with the Oakland Unified School District in California.[14] Motivated by environmental concerns and a desire to support student health, over the course of two years, the district reduced the amount of animal products served in its schools by 30 percent. And much of the meat it served (in reduced quantities) was purchased from carefully chosen sources including Mindful Meats, a company that sources beef from organically raised retired dairy cows.

The results were extraordinary. Students reported increased satisfaction with the healthy, regionally sourced meals. And we'll look at the impact industrialized meat production has on our water, soil, and climate in chapter 28, but suffice it to say that there's a big one. In fact, according to Friends of the Earth's report, the changes enabled the district to save

42 million gallons of water—enough to fill 63 Olympic-sized swimming pools—and to reduce net carbon emissions by 600,000 kilograms—the equivalent carbon savings of installing 87 solar panels, which would cost approximately $2.1 million dollars. However, this carbon-saving strategy did not cost the district any money. In fact, the food shifts actually *saved* the district $42,000.

If changes like this were implemented in schools across the United States, they would lead to saving 700 million kilograms of carbon emissions—equivalent to planting 17 million trees. And over time, the health implications of making these kinds of changes would be profound.

In Los Angeles, the county's Department of Public Health has undertaken a major campaign to lower rates of childhood obesity.[15] Through education, shifting policy, and a "meat-free Monday" in the Los Angeles Unified School District (which serves 1.5 million meals per year), the region is having some success. Since 2009, kids have been eating more vegetables and drinking less sugary soda. During that time, the rate of early childhood obesity in the county has fallen by 10 percent.[16]

Some people worry about the financial impact of changing food policy. But when it comes to moving toward more plant-food-centered meal plans, *savings* are more likely. In 2010, Johns Hopkins School of Public Health released a study, which found four hospitals in the San Francisco Bay Area were saving $400,000 in meat costs each year by incorporating more vegetarian dishes into their menus.[17] And by introducing Meatless Mondays, New Jersey's Valley Hospital saved nearly $50,000 in a year.[18]

In November of 2017, Marianne Bradley-Kopec accepted the position as cook at a new school in downtown Salt Lake City. When Marianne started the new job, she was given a sample menu that featured foods like hamburgers, chicken nuggets, and meatloaf. For the first week, Marianne stuck with the suggested menu. But she saw that the students came from varied cultures and religious backgrounds, so she quickly replaced the meals on the menu with new offerings that featured plant-based cuisine from around the world. With the money saved by not buying meat, Marianne was able to purchase organic produce. She received wonderful feedback from the students, staff, and parents. And she reports something truly extraordinary: Some parents are coming to school specifically so they can eat lunch with their children.

In the largest plant-based eating initiative in school lunch history, the Brazilian cities of Serrinha, Barroca, Teofilândia, and Biritinga announced a commitment in 2018 to making all their school meals 100 percent plant-based.[19] The plan was designed to help stem Brazil's obesity epidemic while making the nation more environmentally sustainable. It impacts more than 23 million meals annually.

SO WHAT CAN YOU DO?

Things like government food subsidies and school district meal plans can feel overwhelming to everyday folks. As a result, even people who care a lot about how we feed our kids tend not to get involved.

But because hardly anyone engages, when you do speak out, even in a simple way, you can have a tremendous impact.

Amie Hamlin is executive director of the New York Coalition for Healthy School Food. The organization works directly with dozens of schools in the state of New York, and worldwide, helping them implement healthier options. They've developed a Wellness Wakeup Call program that provides schools and classrooms with daily healthy eating tips that can be read in classrooms and over PA systems. Amie gave me this example: *"Good morning! This is your Wellness Wakeup Call. Try to find foods that don't have ingredients like high fructose corn syrup, partially hydrogenated fats, artificial colors, and artificial flavors. Enjoy your day, the healthy way!"*

These daily tips are now being used by hundreds of schools, and the coalition has also shared whole-foods, plant-based recipes with more than 25,000 schools worldwide.

Some people fear that kids won't eat healthy foods because their taste buds have been too jaded by junk foods. And some schools have, indeed, offered healthier options and found that students didn't eat them. The key is often to combine healthier lunches with education and to bring creativity and care to the recipes, so that nutritious food is tasty and looks good. Some schools offer a variety of meal options and let the students vote on their favorites. Over time, they develop a steady rotation of meals known to be popular. And student taste buds and habits evolve.

If you care about what kids are eating, and about how taxpayer money is being spent in your community, you have a right to speak up and an opportunity to make a difference. I worked with Amie Hamlin to create a simple action kit for healthier school meals, and you can download it at 31dayfoodrevolution.com/schoollunches.

ACTION:

Option 1: *Use your favorite Internet search engine to find out how many schools are in your local district (type in "what's my school district" and then "how many schools are in [name] school district?") and then get the name of the food service director (type in "who is the food service director in [name of district]"). Just having this information will give you a sense of empowerment. Decide if you want to contact the food service director to put in a word of encouragement toward healthy foods.*

Option 2: *Reach out to your local school district's food service director to ask if they've considered participating in meat-free Mondays or offering plant-based meat-alternate options. You can also ask if the schools have a salad bar, how many fresh fruits and vegetables (as opposed to canned) are offered, and if they participate in farm-to-school programs. Let them know you care.*

Option 3: *Set up a meeting with your local school district's food service director or your school superintendent to find out what's already being done to support or encourage healthy school lunches in your community—and see how you can help.*

PART FOUR

TRANSFORM

Your food choices are a kind of vote. With every bite, you vote for the health you want and also for the world you want.

There's a huge and growing demand for food that's organic, sustainable, fair trade, non-GMO, ethical, healthful, and delicious. In cities worldwide, we're seeing ever-expanding farmer's markets and community-supported agriculture programs. More young people are getting into farming. Grocery stores (even big international chains) are displaying local, natural, and organic foods with pride. The movements for healthy food are growing fast and starting to become a political force.

From rural farms to urban dinner plates, from grocery store shelves to state ballot boxes, millions of people are rising up and taking action. We're reclaiming our food systems and our menus. And we're taking responsibility for our health.

Do you want to support an end to child slavery in chocolate production? Do you want animals to be treated with respect, free from cruelty? Would you like the people who grow our food to have the capacity to feed their own families? How about wanting honest labels, and healthy food for our kids?

Some people worry that the problems we face are too big and overwhelming. Many of us struggle just to make ends meet and survive another day—without having to try to save the world on top of that.

But the truth is, you and I have immense power. We have the power to choose what we take into our bodies. We have the power to invest in the kind of food system we want. And we have the power to contribute—in a tangible, meaningful way—to building a more healthy, ethical, and sustainable future for ourselves, our loved ones, and our planet.

Take the Quiz: Are You a Food Revolutionary?

The impact that different foods have on the world's climate impacts my choices:
    0. Never.   **1.** A little.   **2.** A lot.

I eat animal products that come from factory farms:
    0. Frequently.   **1.** From time to time.   **2.** Never.

I've signed food-policy related petitions or letters:
    0. Never.   **1.** From time to time.   **2.** Frequently.

My relationship to eating GMOs is:
    0. What's a GMO?
    1. I avoid them if I can.
    2. I know what foods they're in and steer clear.

I share books, films, and/or online summits or classes on food policies with other people:
    0. Never.   **1.** From time to time.   **2.** Frequently.

Food-policy issues affect how I vote, lobby, or engage in political dynamics:
    0. Never.   **1.** Somewhat.   **2.** A lot.

I have asked to speak with a restaurant manager, in person or on the phone, to share my appreciation or concern about the health or ethical impact of foods they serve:

   0. Never.   **1.** Once or twice.   **2.** At least a few times.

Add up your points to get a score from 0 to 14. The higher your score the better! Go to 31dayfoodrevolution.com/quiz4 to take the quiz online and see how you compare to other quiz takers, and to participate in the 31-Day Food Revolution with others.

CHAPTER 25

GMOs and the Food Giants

Sixty-four nations, including Japan, China, Russia, and all of the European Union, require mandatory labeling of GMOs. In 2013, with national polls showing that 93 percent of the American public wanted GMOs labeled in the United States, too, voters in Washington State put GMO labeling on the state ballot.[1] The resulting initiative was called I-522.

Monsanto and the junk food industry teamed up to shatter Washington's all-time ballot measure spending record. They dumped more than $22 million into fighting I-522, burying the state under a barrage of misleading ads designed to make consumers think that the addition of labels would cost consumers enormously and cause significant harm to the agricultural industry.[2] (Consumers Union, publisher of *Consumer Reports*, found both of these allegations to be completely false.)

While the "yes" side, the side that wanted GMOs to be labeled, had many thousands of volunteers and in-state donors (as well as some help from concerned citizens in many other places, including our family), the "no" side was entirely corporate-funded. In fact, only a paltry $550 of the "no" campaign's $22 million came from sources within Washington State.

The "no" side prevailed by 38,000 votes, or about 2 percent. But after the election, controversy raged. It turned out that the largest single donor to the "no" campaign, the Grocery Manufacturers Association (GMA), was guilty of laundering money. The state attorney general sued the GMA for channeling more than $11 million into the "no" effort and then trying to hide their actual donors from the public. The GMA was forced to reveal that companies like Coke and Pepsi had been pouring millions into the "no" campaign—but had apparently been trying to hide their lobbying efforts behind the GMA. It seemed that these corporations didn't want to face a consumer backlash, so they tried to use the GMA as a cover.

In 2016, Thurston County Superior Court Judge Anne Hirsch slammed the GMA for "intentional" violations of state law and fined them $18 million—quite likely the largest campaign-finance penalty ever issued in the United States.

But the damage had been done. The GMA and its misleading ad campaign had won. GMO labeling had, for the time being, been blocked. After pouring years of effort into advocating for the consumer's "right to know," I felt dispirited. I knew there could be other ballot initiatives in other states, but I hated to think that corporate interests could buy their way to keeping the public in the dark.

That's when one of my twin sons, River, showed me the doorway to a new strategy.

It all started innocently enough. I was in the grocery story with him. I was hot and tired, my blood sugar was low, and I reached for a bottle of Mango Tango–flavored Odwalla smoothie. River, then a preteen, was not pleased. "Odwalla is owned by Coke!" he implored. "Do you want to give your money to Coke?!"

I stopped, looked at River with a mixture of guilt and parental pride, and put the bottle back on the shelf.

Little did I know that my son was tipping me off to what could become a breakthrough strategy in the struggle for GMO labeling.

River was right. I knew that Coca-Cola had made a million-dollar contribution to the GMA's campaign to oppose GMO labeling in the state of Washington. The fact that the company was obscuring its efforts by routing contributions through the GMA implied to me that executives were nervous about the potential for consumer reaction.

Natural-food lovers like our family don't buy much Coke. But we do tend to buy products like Odwalla, Honest Tea, Zico Coconut Water, Dasani, and Simply Orange, which are all natural brands owned by Coke. If we were going to put our money where our mouths were, then River had nailed it: Until the company changed its ways, it was time to stop giving our money to Coca-Cola.

So Food Revolution Network joined with the Center for Food

Safety, launching a campaign calling on Coca-Cola to stop funding the fight against GMO labeling. We invited our members to boycott not just Coca-Cola, but also the natural brands it owned.

That's when I got wind of data showing that sales of Honest Tea and the other natural brands Coca-Cola owned were growing fast, while sales of Coke itself were on a multiyear decline. The company's future, I realized, was going to be in part shaped by the views of the increasingly vocal and engaged natural-foods consumer.

Within a matter of months, more than 300,000 people had signed on to our efforts, and our members were contacting Honest Tea and Coca-Cola regularly—making calls, sending letters, and posting on their public Facebook pages, demanding that they stop fighting GMO labeling.

Coca-Cola began to take notice. By 2014, we had entered into regular dialogue. Together, we ended up convening a series of meetings. Coca-Cola brought executives from the company, along with leaders from Nestlé, Mars, Unilever, and the American Beverage Association. On our side, we brought in leadership from the Center for Food Safety, Just Label It, and Consumers Union, along with our Food Revolution Network.

The goal of these meetings was to see if the food movement and the food industry could arrive at a consensus about GMO labeling. Food industry leaders readily acknowledged that they hated spending money fighting against transparency and against consumer empowerment. They were afraid that GMO ingredient disclosure would harm sales, but they were eager to find a way out of what was increasingly feeling like a PR black hole.

In essence, our campaign was working. Natural-foods consumers might be a relatively small share of the overall food marketplace, but our voices were getting through, and it was clear to me that the largest food companies in the world were getting nervous.

I was asked to facilitate this series of meetings, which took place over the course of 2014, 2015, and 2016.

I found myself collaborating with senior executives from companies that had policies that disturbed me. Companies that were making billions of dollars selling junk food to kids, selling chocolate that may have had origins in child slavery in the Ivory Coast, and promoting a way of manufacturing and serving food that was fueling obesity, heart disease, and cancer for millions.

But as I sat with these corporate executives, with the stated intention of creating a safe space and seeking common ground, I saw the humanity of everyone assembled. None of the leaders in that room wanted to exploit kids or to make anyone sick. Many of them felt trapped in a system that they knew was, at times, ethically dubious. As a Nestlé executive told me privately, "We know that most of our products aren't exactly healthy. And to be honest with you, we'd like to do better."

As a lifelong food activist, I've dispensed plenty of judgment about corporate policies wreaking havoc on humans, animals, and the future of our planet. But as a human being, sitting in that room, I felt compassion and, in an odd way, even partnership with the food industry executives gathered with me.

We all wanted to find a way to grow, manufacture, and label food that was accountable to the consumer. And because of economic realities, we wanted to do so in a way that could be viable for the future of these companies. If any company that does the right thing goes out of business, that sends a terrible message to the rest of its industry.

I realized that as consumers, we have enormous power to influence corporate policy. By withholding our purchases, and speaking out, yes—but also by investing in the brands and practices that we want to support.

I suggested to the companies that had convened that they stop identifying with Monsanto's interests and recognize that their ultimate accountability was to the consumer. If, as they feared, a "contains GMOs" label would be negative in the minds of consumers, perhaps that was a reason to consider going non-GMO. Around that time, as if to prove my point, Whole Foods reported a sales bump of 15 to 30 percent when products were certified non-GMO.[3]

Our dialogues were passionate, and at times heated. But with respect, and focus on our shared outcomes, we arrived at a good deal of common ground. By early 2016, our little assemblage had jointly chosen attorneys who could team up to flesh out a plan that we hoped to pitch to the U.S. Congress.

While confidentiality agreements prevent me from sharing the details of the bill we were discussing, I can say that it would have been a game changer. It would have had the backing of both food industry and food movement leadership. If we had pulled it off, we'd have brought to Congress one of the most unlikely alliances in history. It's not every day that Food Revolution leaders join with corporate food industry executives to advocate for a national solution that they can both get behind.

That's almost what we achieved.

Almost.

In July of 2016, the U.S. Congress beat us to the punch—narrowly passing legislation that gave lip service to GMO labeling while nullifying state-level initiatives and giving companies the option to, essentially, keep consumers in the dark. Companies could label GMOs on the package, but they could also simply post information on websites, linked to QR codes on packages. When S. 764 became law, the dream bill that our unlikely alliance had been cooking up became, suddenly, irrelevant.

But the relationships we'd built live on. And the dialogue we shared continues to send out waves.

Although S. 764 rendered the nature of GMO labeling essentially voluntary, some companies nevertheless decided to label. Mars, for example, concluded that the dangers of appearing to have something to hide were greater than the dangers of disclosure. In 2016, the company announced that when selling food products that contained GMOs in the United States, it would disclose that fact on its packages.

Writing to me about this decision, a Mars vice president said: "It has been an unnecessarily long journey to get to where we all could have gotten to more than a year ago, but we ended up in the right place. I value the work we all did together and hope we can continue to find new ways to continue it."

Mars wasn't the only one. In that same year, four other major companies—General Mills, Conagra, Kellogg's, and Campbell Soup Company—also announced plans to voluntarily label GMOs on their packages.[4] And many large-scale companies began to come out with certified non-GMO products and product lines. In fact, between 2012 and 2017, certified non-GMO products went from nothing to over $22 billion in sales in the United States alone.[5]

By 2018, companies began leaving the GMA in droves. Campbell's

Soup Company, Nestlé, Dean Foods, Mars, Tyson Foods, Unilever, the Hershey Company, Cargill, the Kraft Heinz Company, and DowDu-Pont all cut ties with the association. While the companies didn't say much about their rationale publicly, some executives privately explained that the public outcry over the GMA's policies on GMOs, sugar, food labeling, and other controversial topics were driving their choice to disengage.[6]

Consumer pressure was changing the food industry—making companies more transparent and more accountable. And something in me was changing, too.

I've always felt a certain righteous indignation about the corporate food industry. It seems to me that anyone who places profits ahead of the health of our kids should be held accountable. But at the same time, I think it's important to remember something my dad taught me when he asked me to consider that my "meat is murder" attitude wasn't helping anyone. If we want to have real impact on someone, we need to see how things look from their point of view.

Pretty much everyone who has kids wants them to be healthy. But a lot of people want to make money. And so long as it's more profitable to peddle sugary, pesticide-contaminated food than to offer food that's real and organically grown, and so long as it pays to use GMOs without labeling, there will be companies standing firmly on what I believe to be the wrong side of history.

That's why it's becoming more important than ever before for each of us to get informed about what we're eating, and to recognize the power of the consumer choices we make to shape policies, practices, and profits all around the globe.

ARE GMOS REALLY A PROBLEM?

You might be asking why this GMO issue matters so much. Aren't GMOs just a new and more scientific way of developing seeds that will grow under more difficult conditions, reduce pesticide and water use, and help to feed a hungry world? Might they not, in time, even bring us foods that are tastier and more nutritious?

That's what Monsanto/Bayer, and its allies have claimed. And if they were right, I might be an enthusiastic fan. But the facts tell a very different story.

The vast majority of corn, soybeans, canola, cotton, and sugar beets grown in the U.S., and many grown around the globe, are genetically modified. These GMO crops have not been engineered to increase flavor, nutrition, or crop yield. They haven't been engineered to require less water or fewer pesticides. Instead, they've been engineered with one or both of two traits: pesticide *production*, and herbicide *resistance*.

Pesticide Production

Bt corn, for example, has been developed so that it contains the pesticide bacillus thuringiensis (Bt) in every cell of the plant. When certain bugs eat it, their intestines explode, and they die. The pesticide is "built in."

There are many natural pesticides that have been approved for use in organic agriculture, and Bt is one of them. Just because they've been approved doesn't necessarily make these pesticides entirely nontoxic. But we do know that Bt has been used in food production for many decades, and that it's generally thought to be safe for humans, at least at modest levels of exposure. Now, however, Bt crops have fundamentally changed the equation. Historically, Bt was sprayed on the outside of plants, and could even be washed off. But with GMO crops, it's found in literally every cell of the plant. Human beings are eating it in utterly unprecedented quantities.

What's the long-term impact of eating these Bt-infused GMO crops? Nobody truly knows, because no long-term studies have been conducted. But many people are concerned about the potential risks. Scientific studies have linked GMOs to toxic and allergic reactions in people; to sickness, sterility, and fatalities in livestock; and to damage to virtually every organ studied in lab animals.[7]

The United Nations/World Health Organization's food standards group and the American Medical Association have each called for mandatory safety testing of genetically engineered foods.[8] But in the U.S., the FDA has so far failed to require or conduct any long-term testing at all.

And the reality is, with GMOs, we don't just have to worry about what's *in* the crops. We also have to worry about what's *on* them. Because the second major trait that's been engineered into GMO seeds is . . .

Herbicide Resistance

In 2016 Bayer bought Monsanto for $57 billion.[9] One of Monsanto's most prized assets was Roundup—the most popular herbicide in the world. The company had come up with a fairly ingenious business model in which it genetically engineered seeds that were resistant to its famed herbicide. This meant that farmers growing Roundup-resistant crops could spray their fields with this chemical and the weeds would die—but the crops would not.

Before the invention of genetically engineered Roundup Ready seeds, no one ever sprayed herbicides on food crops, because to do so would have killed the plants. But now, thanks to genetic engineering, Roundup was being sprayed directly on food crops destined for human consumption. This created a historically unprecedented reality: The vast majority of us began eating weed killer on a daily basis.

In 1987, only 11 million pounds of Roundup were used in the United States, but today nearly 300 million pounds of Roundup are applied each year.[10] This chemical is now being sprayed on 89 percent of the U.S. corn crop and on 94 percent of the soybeans.[11]

Worldwide, 9.4 million tons of Roundup have been used on fields growing our food.[12] That's more than two pounds for every single human being on Earth.

So how does Roundup impact human health? In 2015, the World Health Organization classified glyphosate (the primary active ingredient in Roundup) as a probable human carcinogen.[13] The state of California has listed Roundup as being carcinogenic, seeking to require warning labels on Roundup and other glyphosate-containing products, on the basis of this recognized cancer risk.[14]

Research has also shown that glyphosate is an endocrine disruptor, meaning that it interferes with the proper functioning and production of hormones in human cell lines.[15] And as we discussed in chapter 9, many scientists now fear that glyphosate, which was patented by Monsanto as an antibiotic, might have damaging effects on your microbiome (the bacteria in your digestive tract).[16]

HOW TO AVOID GMOS AND GLYPHOSATE

Foods that are grown organically are, by definition, non-GMO and glyphosate-free. So if you want to avoid GMOs and glyphosate, choosing organic is more important than ever.

But not everyone can afford to go organic. If that's the case for you, it may be comforting to know that most fruits and vegetable are still not being genetically engineered or sprayed with glyphosate. And it can also help to know which nonorganic foods are likely to contain them.

The major crops that are genetically modified are:

- *corn*, much of which is fed to livestock and used for ethanol for our cars, but some of which is used in many refined foods
- *soy*, also often turned into animal feed, though much of it is processed into refined foods eaten by people
- *sugar beets*, which supply about half the sugar in the U.S., and almost all of which are genetically modified (though cane sugar is not genetically modified)
- *canola*, mostly used for canola oil
- *alfalfa*, most of which is fed to animals
- *cotton*, mostly used for clothing as well as for cottonseed oil.

But keep in mind that corn and soy, in particular, are used as the raw ingredients for all sorts of food additives, including aspartame, sodium ascorbate, vitamin C, citric acid, sodium citrate, ethanol, natural flavorings, artificial flavorings, high-fructose corn syrup, hydrolyzed vegetable protein, lactic acid, maltodextrin, monosodium glutamate, sucralose, textured vegetable protein (also known as TVP), and xanthan gum.

GMOs can sneak their way into a broad range of food additives and enhancers. If a product isn't certified organic or certified non-GMO, and if it has more than a few ingredients, there's a pretty good chance that it does, in fact, contain GMOs.

And now, some new GMO crops are beginning to be grown more widely, including Hawaiian papayas. Some Canadian farmed salmon is itself genetically engineered, though this is still a relatively small portion of the overall salmon for sale. (GMO salmon presents a unique set of health and safety concerns, including the danger that it could escape pens, cross-breed with wild salmon, and obliterate native salmon species within a matter of years.) And across North America we have increasing amounts of genetically engineered courgette, summer squash, apples, and potatoes coming on the market—and (so far mainly in South Africa) wheat.

For a more complete listing of some of the foods and hidden ingredients that can be genetically modified, as well as more information on the risks of GMOs and how to avoid them, download my special report on this topic at 31dayfoodrevolution.com/gmo.

To keep it simple, my non-GMO advice is:

1. Go organic.
2. If organic isn't available or affordable, go certified non-GMO.
3. Read labels so you can avoid corn, soy, canola, and sugar if they aren't either organic or non-GMO.
4. Avoid processed foods—which is a good idea anyway.

ACTION:

Option 1: If there's a GMO food in your life, switch to an organic or non-GMO alternative.

Option 2: Review any consistent exposures to GMOs in your diet (such as corn, soy, sugar, or canola that are neither organic nor certified non-GMO) and eliminate them. Move toward a non-GMO kitchen.

Option 3: Call a local restaurant with a reputation for relatively healthy food during "off hours" (not during the 6 to 9 p.m. dinner rush). Ask to speak with an owner or manager.

You might say something like this:

"I'm a huge fan of your restaurant. And I wanted to let you know something that would help me be a more enthusiastic patron. I think there are a lot more people like me. Would you like to hear it, and if so, would now be a good time?"

[If yes]

"I'm sure you're aware how many products in stores now are certified non-GMO or organically grown. Non-GMO certified is a $22 billion industry. So I wanted to give you the feedback that eating non-GMO is important to me and to my family, and we'd be a lot more excited to eat at your restaurant if you were able to be non-GMO or organic, or to offer some non-GMO or organic items. I know it's hard for a restaurant because you have so many ingredients to consider. But I thought you might appreciate the feedback, because it also might get you some new, enthusiastic customers."

Worst case: They'll be annoyed, but at least you will have shown them that consumers care. Best case: They'll make a change and help usher in a new era in your community.

CHAPTER 26

Is Organic Worth the Cost?

I love organically grown food. But I don't love its price tag. At my local natural-foods store, I can buy organic onions for $1.29 a pound. But a conventional supermarket, down the road, carries commercially grown onions for $0.69 per pound. While neither price is especially high for a pound of nourishing food, the cumulative impact of opting for a higher price can be overwhelming for many families struggling to make ends meet.

In 2012, *New York Times* columnist Roger Cohen went so far as to declare that the "organic ideology is an elitist, pseudoscientific indulgence."[1]

I think you'd have a hard time convincing migrant farmworkers that choosing organic food is elitist. It's no big mystery that many of them have tough lives—often working brutally long hours with no insurance, substandard housing, and unreliable compensation. Add to the mix that many of them are being literally poisoned on the job.

Pesticide exposure causes farmworkers to suffer more chemical-related injuries and illnesses than any other part of the workforce. The pesticides used to grow nonorganic food are a primary reason the average life span of a migrant farmworker in the U.S. has been reported to be as low as 49 years.[2]

You'd also have a tough time convincing Teri McCall of Cambria, California, that organic food is elitist. Teri lost her husband of 40 years, Anthony "Jack" McCall, to terminal cancer in 2015.[3] For nearly 30 years on his 20-acre fruit and vegetable farm, Jack had used the herbicide Roundup.

In 2016, Teri cited a rapidly growing body of evidence linking Roundup to cancer and filed a wrongful death lawsuit against Monsanto (now Bayer). She alleged that the company had known for years that exposure to glyphosate—the main ingredient in the agribusiness giant's flagship weed killer—could cause cancer and other serious illnesses or injuries. And she blamed the company for her husband's death. (As of this writing, the lawsuit is ongoing.)

Roundup, like hundreds of other widely used synthetic herbicides and insecticides, is banned in organic agriculture.

BUT WHAT ABOUT YIELD?

Organic crops have historically had a per-acre yield found to be about 10 to 20 percent lower than large-scale industrialized monocultures.[4] But before we jump into hysterics about the need for pesticides and petro-chemical fertilizers in order to feed humanity, let's put this in perspective. Nearly half of the world's crop calories are not eaten by humans, but rather used as feed for poultry, pork, cattle, and even farmed fish.[5] As we'll discuss in chapter 28, it can take between 4 and 12 pounds of feed to produce 1 pound of meat, eggs, or dairy products. The vast majority of the calories animals consume are turned into hoof, hide, bone, or manure and expended as energy that the animals use to live. The majority of animal feed is, in a caloric sense, wasted.

In *The Global Benefits of Eating Less Meat*, Mark Gold and Jonathon Porritt write that after factoring in all inputs, the world's cattle alone consume a quantity of calories equal to the caloric needs of 8.7 billion people—more than the entire human population on Earth.[6]

If we're serious about feeding humanity, shouldn't we consider eating less meat, so we could turn less of our cropland into livestock feed, freeing up more of it to grow food sustainably for humans?

HOW ORGANIC CAN WORK

When it's practiced well, organic agriculture can lead to crops more resistant to droughts and floods (which climate change is making increasingly common). It can also enable a more diverse agricultural output, which means that you might get less of one monocrop, but more diversity and, in many cases, more net food value per acre. If your metric is health per acre, small-scale organic farming often wins by a large margin.

In 2013, the UN Conference on Trade and Development issued a landmark report titled *Trade and Environment Review 2013: Wake Up Before It's Too Late.*[7] The report concluded that small-scale organic farming is the only way to sustainably feed the world for future generations. It called for "a rapid and significant shift from conventional, monoculture-based and high-external-input-dependent industrial production toward mosaics of sustainable, regenerative production systems that also considerably improve the productivity of small-scale farmers."

But so far, many governments and research institutions are pushing in the opposite direction. Over the course of the last century, billions of dollars have been spent researching and promoting chemical-intensive, pesticide-laden forms of agriculture. With only a tiny fraction of those resources, organic agricultural researchers are continually finding breakthroughs and developing methods that are increasing yield, sequestering carbon out of the atmosphere, and creating more nutritious and resilient crops.

CAN YOU TRUST ORGANIC?

Each country has its own form of organic certification. The United States uses the USDA Organic label, which indicates that the food or other agricultural product has been produced through methods that integrate practices that foster cycling of resources, promote ecological balance, and conserve biodiversity. Sewage sludge, irradiation, genetic engineering, and most synthetic pesticides and fertilizers may not be used.

European products certified organic by Ecocert carry a very similar set of requirements. While enforcement could always be stronger, both the USDA Organic and the Ecocert labels provide a significant measure of confidence to the consumer.

Maintaining the integrity of organic certification takes vigilance. Organizations like Organic Consumers Association point out that large-scale corporate agribusiness has chosen to invest heavily in organic food production. Now that transnational corporations are out to make money off the organic brand, many of them push to drive down standards. As consumers, we have to be attentive to make sure that the real meaning of organic foods doesn't get diluted.

WHY DOES ORGANIC FOOD COST SO MUCH?

Part of the answer is that organic certification is expensive. It can cost farmers many thousands of dollars to certify their farm, and the cost and regulatory burden of certification can be especially hard on smaller farms.[8] In effect, organic farmers are being penalized for growing food in a way that protects the fertility of the soil and spares farmworkers and the entire web of life, including us, from poisons.

Imagine what would happen if this were reversed. What if all the farms that used pesticides and chemical fertilizers had to pay a fee for their environmental contamination and were subject to inspections? What if the organic farmers had a lower, instead of a higher, regulatory burden? The economics of organic food would change in an instant.

If we had more sane food policies, organic food would cost less than it does now. But until that time, the frustrating reality is that it can still be difficult to afford for a great many people.

PESTICIDES

Pesticides have been linked to a wide range of human health hazards, ranging from short-term problems such as headaches and nausea to chronic impacts like reproductive harm and endocrine disruption. Pesticides have been linked to many types of cancer, including non-Hodgkin's lymphoma, as well as brain, breast, ovarian, prostate, stomach, testicular, and liver cancers.[9]

In 2010 scientists at the University of Montreal and at Harvard University released a study that found that exposure to pesticide residues on food may double a child's risk of ADHD.[10] Another study conducted by researchers at the Public Health Institute, the California Department of Health Services, and the UC Berkeley School of Public Health found a sixfold increase in risk factors for autism spectrum disorders for children of women who were exposed to organochlorine pesticides in their environment during pregnancy.[11]

In response to worries about eating foods sprayed with neurotoxic poisons, as well as concerns about the social and environmental implications of pesticides, more and more consumers are buying organically grown foods.

Does consuming organic food really reduce your body's burden of toxic chemicals? Seeking to answer that question, Liza Oates, PhD, and a team at RMIT University in Australia randomly selected 13 adults. The research team fed some an organic diet and others a nonorganic diet. The study found that a mostly organic diet for only one week led to a 90 percent reduction in pesticide levels detected in urine.[12]

Which Foods Carry the Most Pesticides?

Fortunately, not all conventionally grown foods carry large amounts of pesticides. The Environmental Working Group (EWG) analyzed pesticide residue testing data from the U.S. Department of Agriculture and the Food and Drug Administration to come up with rankings for 48 popular fresh produce items in the United States.[13] These are listed below, in order from most contaminated to least. Lower-number rankings indicate more pesticide contamination. The first 12 are what EWG refers to as the "dirty dozen," the most pesticide-contaminated foods, and the last 15 are what they refer to as the "clean 15," the least pesticide-contaminated foods. While these rankings are based on data taken in the United States, it's probable, given the global nature of food distribution systems, that numbers are similar in many other countries. But we don't know with certainty.

The Dirty Dozen (highest pesticide contamination— buy organic if at all possible)

1. Strawberries
2. Spinach
3. Nectarines
4. Apples
5. Grapes
6. Peaches
7. Cherries
8. Pears
9. Tomatoes
10. Celery
11. Potatoes
12. Sweet peppers

The Middle 21 (medium pesticide contamination— moderately important to buy organic)

13. Cucumbers
14. Cherry tomatoes
15. Lettuce
16. Snap peas
17. Blueberries
18. Hot peppers
19. Kale / collard greens
20. Green beans
21. Plums
22. Tangerines
23. Raspberries
24. Carrots
25. Winter squash
26. Oranges
27. Summer squash*
28. Bananas
29. Green onions
30. Watermelon
31. Mushrooms
32. Sweet potatoes
33. Grapefruit

The Clean 15 (lower pesticide contamination— least important to buy organic)

34. Broccoli
35. Cauliflower
36. Cantaloupes
37. Kiwis
38. Honeydew melons
39. Aubergines
40. Mangoes
41. Asparagus
42. Papayas*
43. Sweet peas (frozen)
44. Onions
45. Cabbages
46. Pineapples
47. Sweet corn*
48. Avocadoes

* Some genetically modified summer squash, papayas, and sweet corn are now under commercial cultivation. If you want to avoid GMOs, choose organic options for these items.

I'm often asked whether people who can't afford organic foods should steer clear of conventionally grown fruits and vegetables. The answer is an unequivocal *no*. Hundreds of medical studies have illustrated the huge health benefits of eating fruits and vegetables. Most of the fruits and vegetables eaten in the studies that have found these tremendous benefits were grown conventionally—with pesticides.

If you can afford organic, I encourage it. And if you can't, then I hope you won't let that stop you from eating and enjoying a vast array of fruits and vegetables. Let's not make the perfect the enemy of the good.

Researchers have found that pesticide residues can persist on many fruits and vegetables. So especially if it's not grown organically, you may want to wash produce. Plain water appears to be just as effective as (and a lot less costly than) using commercial produce cleaners.[14] If you want to go a step further, you can create a bicarbonate of soda solution, folding in 1 ounce of bicarbonate of soda for every 100 ounces of water. Studies have demonstrated that when you soak produce in this solution for 15 minutes, most pesticide residues will be removed. If you like, you can spin produce in a salad spinner afterward to dry it out.[15]

ACTION:

Option 1: Find at least one item in the "dirty dozen" that you consume regularly and commit to buying it organically grown.

Option 2: Go organic with as many foods as possible, including all the foods in the "dirty dozen."

Option 3: Ask to speak to the produce buyer at your local supermarket or grocery store. Find out how many organic foods they sell, if this portion has changed in the last year, and in what direction it's headed. Encourage, congratulate, support, or nudge.

CHAPTER 27

The Simple Act of Growing Food

I was raised with parents who grew most of their own food. They almost named me Kale, after all. And although I didn't much care for putting my hands in the dirt as a kid, I usually did my part, and I'm glad that I grew up feeling connected to the seasons, to the sun and the rain.

Today our twin teenage sons take leadership roles in growing our family garden. They love to plan what to plant. They love to harvest. And they love to comb through recipe books to find fun things we can make with our bounty.

There's nothing quite like creating a salad packed with tons of flavor (and medicine) in minutes: lettuce, spinach, rocket, sorrel, celery, chives, radish, dill, parsley, and even mint can all be harvested, and in a mere five minutes, offer an explosion of nourishing appeal.

FOOD FOR HUMANS

When people, and especially children, spend time growing food in a garden, they eat more fruits and vegetables.

A few years back, master gardening teacher Stacey Murphy was leading a gardening class at the High School for Public Service in Brooklyn, New York. The students had planted a mix of different types of lettuce seeds, and a month later, it was harvest day. Each student harvested a leaf of each kind of lettuce so they could share in a group taste test. Many had never seen these types of greens in their lives. They marveled at the variety of colors and shapes, and wondered aloud what the leaves were going to taste like.

Stacey instructed the students to try the first bite all together, on the count of three. Amid all the different reactions to the flavor, she noticed one girl just staring as she held an untasted piece of lettuce in her hand. Stacey asked the girl why she hadn't tried it, and the girl replied, "Because it was just on the ground." When Stacey asked where her lettuce usually came from, the girl replied, "In a bag."

While Stacey was wondering what question to ask next, the girl's classmates started daring her to try her lettuce, telling her how tasty it was. After washing her handful of lettuce samples thoroughly, the girl tried many of the different leaves and discovered that she loved sorrel.

The next day, Stacey noticed this same girl, at a moment when she thought nobody was watching, sneaking into the garden to pick and eat sorrel.

Not everybody loves gardening, of course. Some people feel too overwhelmed caring for themselves or their family to want to feel responsible, as well, for a bunch of plants. It's not for everyone.

But in an unpredictable world, there's something empowering about knowing you can grow food. And gardening can be good for your spirit as well as for your health. It can increase your time outdoors, relieve stress, induce greater relaxation, and even boost your immune system.

On a global level, gardening also reduces your carbon footprint. Not only does it keep food from traveling potentially thousands of miles to get to your dinner plate, but a healthy garden and composting system can also contribute to the process by which plants absorb carbon dioxide and then sequester it into the soil.

And let's not forget what's perhaps the best and most basic contribution of gardens—they feed people.

David Young knows a bit about that. He's an urban farmer in the lower Ninth Ward of New Orleans. Since 2009, he's started gardens on 30 abandoned lots left over from Hurricane Katrina. People in the lower Ninth Ward don't have access to a lot of good food. In fact, the nearest grocery story is three and a half miles away. But David helps to fill the gap, providing produce for free or at low cost to people most in need in the community. He's created a small orchard's worth of fruit trees, and the community is welcome to pick the fruit freely. David also rescues bees that would be killed by exterminators, and he maintains more than 60 hives throughout the lower Ninth Ward.

In 2015, he gave out over 2,500 pounds of food in the community. His programs are funded partly by honey sales, and he works entirely as a volunteer. David may not be paid in dollars, but he loves what he does and feels blessed to grow food that truly serves his community.

WHAT IF YOU'RE A TOTAL BEGINNER? HOW DO YOU GET STARTED?

You don't have to spend your whole life growing food, like David does, in order to plant a few vegetables and reap a satisfying harvest.

I asked Stacey Murphy what steps new gardeners can take to start growing some food, and she and I created a simple guide to beginning a garden. You can get it at 31dayfoodrevolution.com/startgardening.

WHAT IF YOU DON'T HAVE MUCH ROOM?

Liz Hodge lived in an apartment in Brooklyn, New York, that had no yard. But she wasn't about to let that stop her from growing food, so she created a grow closet with potted plants and full-spectrum light bulbs.

One day Liz's five-year-old son asked what she was doing. She said she was pollinating the peppers. Her son asked why, and she explained that there were no bees inside, and bees typically pollinate pepper flowers so they can grow into peppers. After watching his mom for a minute, he insisted on helping because, he explained, she was "doing it wrong."

Liz showed her son how she used a Q-tip to spread the pollen. Her son tried it, too, but then added the missing touch. He buzzed like a bee as he pollinated the flowers—giggling all the while.

Sometimes, even in small spaces, gardening can be fun.

Many people who don't have dirt use containers that they place on a tiny outdoor patio, a rooftop, a fire escape, or even a windowsill.

GROWING FOOD AND GROWING HOPE

In 2016, before taking her later stint as the innovative cook for a Salt Lake City school, Marianne Bradley-Kopec served as a cook and kitchen manager for her local Meals on Wheels program, which fed local elderly and housebound individuals in her community of Hamilton, Montana. When Marianne began cooking for the program, she was disappointed to see the quality of the vegetables she was expected to send out with every meal. Everything was canned and most of it was packaged in China. Marianne knew there had to be a way to improve the quality of the meals she was delivering, but the budget wouldn't allow it. So she researched organic farms in her area and found one, Homestead Organics Farm, that was literally down the street—and she came up with a rather ingenious plan.

Marianne recruited local high school students to come work on the farm as a community service project. Laura Garber and Henry Wuensche, the owners of Homestead Organics Farm, dedicated an entire plot to the project, and the students spent their summer planting, cultivating, and harvesting thousands of pounds of produce, which was in turn donated to Meals on Wheels.

A local bank helped sponsor the project, which came to be known as Cultivating Connections—donating enough money for each student to earn $1,000 by the end of the summer. Laura and Henry taught the students about growing organic food, composting, recycling, and sustainability, and they also brought in guest speakers to teach the students life skills like team building, checkbook balancing, and budgeting.

As the summer came to a close, Marianne fixed a huge lunch featuring vegetables from the farm. After lunch the students went with the volunteer drivers to meet the people who they'd been growing food for all season. It was emotional to see the bond that the elderly clients immediately had with the students. There were many tears shed, and there was much hugging and hand holding in those homes that day.

Some of the students ended up staying connected to the Meals on Wheels program by becoming volunteer delivery drivers, while others continued to work at the farm as paid employees. The Cultivating Connections program is ongoing today and has actually expanded, thanks to the dedication and generosity of Homestead Organics Farm. Marianne states, "In my wildest dreams, I couldn't have asked for a better outcome. I merely planted the seed of an idea that grew into something amazing thanks to a lot of wonderful, loving people."

Growing food is powerful. It can bring people together, and sometimes it can even help to knit the fabric of a community.

But if we were to grow a lot more food, we'd need more land. Where would that land come from? There's one excellent source that many people have right in their backyard. Literally.

FOOD, NOT LAWNS

In the United States alone, there are more than 32 million acres of land dedicated to growing lawns.[1] Meanwhile, there are about 16 million acres of land being used to grow all our fruits and vegetables. This means that if half the lawns in the nation were converted to organic gardens, fruit and vegetable production could double. That would be a great thing for our environment, too, considering that every year U.S. lawns are sprayed with 90 million pounds of pesticides.

The typical American lawn uses 10,000 gallons of supplemental water (not including rainwater) annually.[2] Of course, edible gardens need to be watered, too. But researchers estimate that gardens use only about one-third as much water as lawns.[3] And organic gardens use even less water.

HOW TO TURN A LAWN INTO A GARDEN

First, if you're interested in converting a lawn to a garden, clarify whether the lawn has been sprayed with any herbicides that might inhibit vegetable growth. Herbicides will eventually wash away, but if they've been used, it's best to wait for at least a few inches of rain to cleanse the area.

If your terrain is steep, you may need to do additional preparation (such as terracing) or consult with a landscape specialist.

If you're herbicide-free and have a reasonable slope, your next step will be to clear out the grass. The easiest method is to cover it with cardboard or plastic and wait for the sod to die and its root structure to loosen. Plastic is typically faster and can be effective in as little as a week, but it may take up to three weeks for grass to die off. (If you have Bermuda grass, it's a lot tougher. Talk with a landscape specialist for advice on that one.)

Next, flip the top four inches of sod over in place in squares that are approximately six inches by six. With the grass upside down, it can no longer photosynthesize and any remnants will die. By turning it over, you'll also create a looser soil structure that your future vegetable plants will love. Wait until soil clumps easily break apart in your hands, indicating that the grass root structures have dried up.

Next, add two inches of compost (which can be homemade or purchased from a landscaping or garden supply store) and gently rake it flat. Break up the sod clumps as you go.

Your planting bed is now ready for seeds or seedlings.

Note: If you have very dense clay soil, or if you're impatient, an alternative is to simply cover the grass until it dies off, and then to add four inches of soil on top of the dead grass, two inches of compost on top of that, and start planting.

THE GROWING FOOD REVOLUTION

Some people grow food in abandoned lots, on rooftops, or in backyards. Some grow it in containers on windowsills or on median parkways. Others are converting lawns into gardens.

You don't have to grow everything you eat, or even 10 percent of it. Raising even a single tomato, courgette, or parsley plant can be liberating. The simple act of nurturing or harvesting living things, on any scale, can permanently change your relationship to food. You'll save money. You'll be reducing your carbon footprint. And you can enjoy healthy, fresh food that's free of pesticides, herbicides, and chemical fertilizers.

ACTION:

Option 1: Sprout a batch of nuts, seeds, or legumes (such as almond, radish, pea, chickpea, mung bean, alfalfa, sunflower, lentil, broccoli, or soy) by soaking for 12 hours, and then rinsing and draining twice daily for at least two days. When you see "tails" beginning to form, you'll know that your food is, literally, alive! You don't have to plant it in the ground to participate in the cycles of life (and to add bonus bioavailability to the nutrients in your food). Remember that legume seeds should be cooked well before eating them.

Option 2: Fill a container with potting mix to ¾" from the top, and set it in a place that either gets at least six hours per day of sun in the summertime or has access to a grow light. *As soon as the seasons allow, plant at least one edible seedling, then water it regularly until harvest.*

Option 3: Turn a lawn, patio, rooftop, fire escape, or yard into a vegetable garden or a community garden. Enjoy growing fabulous food and helping to make the world a more fertile and beautiful place.

CHAPTER 28

Eat for a Healthy World

What we eat impacts our health and the health of our children. But its impact is much bigger than that. It also affects the entire planet.

> You cannot get through a single day without having an impact on the world around you. What you do makes a difference, and you have to decide what kind of difference you want to make.
>
> —*Jane Goodall, PhD*

FOOD AND OUR CLIMATE

The facts are sobering.

Carbon dioxide (CO_2), methane, nitrous oxide, and other gases are building up and surrounding our planet like a blanket, trapping heat and destabilizing our climate.

Rising global temperatures are causing the polar ice caps to melt and the oceans to rise, threatening the homes and livelihoods of hundreds of millions of people. Climate change is bringing desertification and droughts to some areas and floods to others, making it increasingly difficult to reliably grow the food upon which our lives depend.

While some people debate what's causing climate change, and how important human activities are in driving it, one thing is clear: It's happening. And if we can do anything to ameliorate this growing crisis, then future generations have every right to expect us to do it.

If you're like me, you may feel overwhelmed by the scope of the problem. Sometimes I feel less like a drop in the bucket and more like a drop in the sea.

How can any one of us measure the impact of our own choices against those wrought by the totality of humanity?

Many companies and political leaders have resisted facing the enormity of the dangers that climate change presents, or acknowledging the role that human activities are playing, because they fear that serious action to reduce greenhouse gas emissions could have a devastating impact on the global economy. And there are some reasons to be concerned.

THE COST OF CHANGE

In 2008, the International Energy Agency issued a report entitled *Energy Technology Perspectives*.[1] This meta-analysis explored the economic impact of stabilizing global CO_2 levels at 450 parts per million—a level that many scientists say is needed to help prevent devastating droughts and flooding induced by rising sea levels. The report concluded that this could be accomplished through massive investment in new systems of transportation, energy production, and energy efficiency—at a long-term cost of up to $45 trillion.

I don't know about you, but that sounds like an awful lot of money to me. Sure, it would all feed into the economy, and it would create a lot of jobs. But the cost sounds more than a little daunting.

But what if we could slow or even reverse climate change without it costing a cent? What if there were ways we could take action, individually as well as collectively, that might actually save money while improving health and quality of life for humanity?

It turns out, there just might be.

In 2009, researchers from the Netherlands Environmental Assessment Agency offered a ray of hope. They published a study in *Climatic Change* in which they weighed the costs of large-scale CO_2 reduction through changes in energy infrastructure and compared them to what could be accomplished through changes in agriculture.[2] The researchers concluded that if the average human shifted to a low-meat diet (which they defined as a maximum of 70 grams, or one small serving, of beef and 325 grams, or three servings, of chicken and eggs per week), there would be a tremendous savings in greenhouse gas emissions. This shift would free up approximately 15 million square kilometers of farmland, which could in turn be planted with vegetation that would mop up carbon dioxide.

The bottom line? According to this study, scaling back on foods like beef burgers and bacon could over the course of decades wipe $20 trillion off the ultimate cost of fighting climate change—effectively cutting it in half.

The researchers also referenced how substituting beans for burgers could lead to dramatic reductions in rates of heart disease, cancer, diabetes, obesity, Alzheimer's, and other chronic, diet-caused illnesses. And this, in turn, could lead to profound economic savings. Right now, the world spends more than $60 trillion on health care every decade.[3] Much of this goes to treatment of chronic and preventable disease. If global dietary patterns shifted, we could not only take a massive bite out of climate change, but we could also save untold lives while reaping immense economic benefit.

HOW YOUR FOOD AFFECTS YOUR CLIMATE

Why does modern animal agriculture have such an enormous effect on greenhouse gas emissions? It's not as if cows are driving around all day in air-conditioned Hummers or forgetting to turn the lights off when they leave the room.

Remember that most of the world's meat, eggs, and dairy are produced in factory farms—what the livestock industry calls concentrated animal feeding operations (CAFOs). In these establishments, large numbers of cows, pigs, chickens, and other livestock are packed together in extremely close quarters. Instead of eating grass, leaves, bugs, roots, or anything resembling their natural diet, the animals are fed a diet based heavily on corn and soybeans. Instead of their manure fertilizing grasslands, it piles up in massive lagoons that pollute nearby air, rivers, and groundwater. Most of the pigs and chickens eaten by humans spend their entire lives in CAFOs. Many cows start on pasture but are "finished" by being fed corn and soy in feedlots, where they gain much of their weight.

After cows come into the feedlot, they gain enough weight to produce about 1 new pound of beef for every 12 pounds of feed input.[4] Pigs produce about a pound of flesh for every 7 pounds of feed, while for chickens, it's about a pound of flesh for every 4 pounds of feed.[5] In all of these cases, the majority of the feed is being, essentially, wasted. (Most industry publications compare feed to animal weight gain, noting that cattle in feedlots typically gain about a pound of total weight for every six pounds of feed.[6] But keep in mind that less than half of the animal's weight is edible meat—which is why it actually takes about twelve pounds of feed to produce a pound of beef.[7])

According to Richard Oppenlander in his 2012 book, *Comfortably Unaware*, 80 percent of the world's soy crop, and 70 percent of the grain grown in the United States, goes to feed livestock raised for human consumption.

Cycling calories from plants through livestock is inherently wasteful. And it takes a lot of land to do it. In total, livestock systems (including pasture, animal farms, and land growing food for animals) occupy 45 percent of the total land area of the planet.[8] Worldwide, we use about eight times as much land to grow food for animals as we do to grow food directly for humans.[9]

One of the primary sources of CO_2 emissions in the world today is deforestation. Huge areas of forest, including vast swaths of tropical rain forest, have been cut down or burned in order to create land on which to graze cattle or to grow cattle feed. Forests that previously absorbed carbon from the atmosphere are now emitting it as vegetation is degraded or incinerated.

And as significant as CO_2 emissions are to our global climate, there are a couple of other gases that also play a major part. In fact, methane is actually up to 100 times more potent at trapping energy than carbon dioxide, and nitrous oxide is 310 times more potent.[10] Two of the main sources of methane emissions are cow manure and the eructations (belching and flatulence) from cows. And one of the primary sources of nitrous oxide emissions is the fertilizer that's used to grow livestock feed.[11]

WHAT THIS MEANS

Put it all together, and startling truths emerge. When the Food and Agriculture Organization of the United Nations set out to study the impact of industrialized agriculture on global climate, it concluded that livestock production, and especially industrialized beef production, is responsible for 18 percent of global greenhouse gas emissions.[12] This means that production of meat causes more net climate impact than the entire transportation sector—all of the world's cars, trucks, ships, planes, and trains—combined.

In 2014, researchers at Oxford University surveyed the diets of 60,000 people and analyzed their net impact on greenhouse gas emissions. According to this study, published in the journal *Climatic Change* in 2014, the average meat-eater in the U.S. is responsible for almost twice as much global warming as the average vegetarian, and close to three times that of the average vegan.[13]

Of course, you don't have to go vegetarian, or vegan, to support a stable climate. Whether or not you want to go veg, you can eat less meat and move away from industrialized animal agriculture—and make a very real impact. Every bite counts.

WATER IS LIFE

Water covers 70 percent of our planet. But despite the fact that we live on "the water planet," the reality is that fresh water—the stuff we bathe in, drink, and irrigate our farms with—is remarkably scarce. It makes up only about 3 percent of the world's total water supply. And I'm not just concerned because my name is Ocean.

As human populations, and our consumption of water, have grown, more and more water has been pumped out of the ground at increasingly unsustainable rates. The world's largest current underground water reserves in Eurasia, Africa, and the Americas are under stress.[14]

According to a report from *National Geographic*, two billion people rely on groundwater that is considered finite and threatened.

Some of our water comes from rivers, streams, and lakes. But can you imagine what would happen to humanity if our wells ran dry? Billions of people would starve.

Where is our groundwater going? Did you know that more than two-thirds of it is used to irrigate agriculture?

I live in California, a state of 40 million people. And California, like many parts of the world, faces a water shortfall. Up to 65 percent of the state's water comes from groundwater, which is not being replenished as quickly as it's being consumed.[15] The water we pump out of the ground has been stored up over countless millennia, and in most years, we just don't capture enough rain and snow to keep pace with the amount that we're using.

In response to this growing crisis, many state residents are taking steps to conserve. We're installing low-flow showerheads and taking shorter showers, and we're replacing lawns with shrubs and rock gardens.

These steps help. But to truly solve the water puzzle, we have to look at where the most water is going. Agriculture is at the center of it all. California's livestock industry alone uses more water than all the homes and businesses in the state combined.[16] And even with all that water, California still imports most of the meat consumed in the state. (The United States produces roughly the same amount of beef that it consumes. The state of California produces about 9 percent of the nation's total, but with 12 percent of the population, it consumes more than it produces.)[17]

One thing California exports is alfalfa.[18] And alfalfa is a thirsty crop. California, it turns out, exports more than 100 billion gallons of water per year in the form of alfalfa to countries like China, which use it for livestock feed. How much sense does it make, in a state facing a potentially devastating water crisis, to in effect ship away more than three times enough water to meet the needs of every household in the city of San Francisco, so China can eat more beef?

And it's not just California. In his book *Six Arguments for a Greener Diet*, Center for Science in the Public Interest founder Michael Jacobson, PhD, writes that crops grown for livestock feed consume 56 percent of the water used in the United States.[19] *National Geographic* reports that it takes 1,799 gallons of water to produce a single pound of grain-fed beef.[20]

If you want to save water, reducing industrialized beef consumption could be the most powerful single step you can take.

THE GROUND BENEATH US

Many people go organic because they want to steer clear of eating food that may be contaminated with polluting and neurotoxic pesticides. Others don't want to eat animals pumped full of antibiotics and hormones.

But now, add a new reason to the mix: dirt.

While many of us think of it as dead, the reality is that healthy soil is teeming with life. An acre of healthy topsoil can contain 2,400 pounds of fungi, 1,500 pounds of bacteria, 900 pounds of earthworms, 890 pounds of arthropods and algae, and 133 pounds of protozoa.[21]

It takes nature a thousand years to generate three centimeters of precious topsoil. But today we're losing our topsoil at an alarming rate. The average rate of soil erosion on U.S. cropland is seven tons per acre per year.[22] According to Maria-Helena Semedo, the United Nations Food and Agriculture Organization's deputy director general of natural resources, unless new approaches are adopted, the global amount of arable and productive land per person in 2050 will be only a quarter of the level that we had in 1960.[23]

If current rates of degradation continue, all the world's topsoil could be gone within 60 years.

Where is all this topsoil going? Most of it is being washed away with rains and irrigation, as unsustainable farming practices destabilize the soil and fail to replenish it with an adequate supply of new organic matter.

The sobering reality is that if we don't change course, then climate change, aquifer depletion, and topsoil erosion will mean that the next generation may be on course to witness mass starvation on a level utterly unprecedented in human history.

For an example of where none of us wants to be headed, take a look at the Sahara Desert, which covers large parts of Algeria, Egypt, Tunisia, Chad, Morocco, Eritrea, Niger, Mauritania, Mali, and the Sudan. Did you know that this was once a rich agricultural region? It grew abundant millet and other grains, and prehistoric cave drawings depict the region as rich in flora and fauna.

But not anymore. Today this desert gets average rainfall of 25 millimeters (less than one inch) per year, making it inhospitable to most forms of life. And it's huge. The Sahara Desert now covers more than 8 percent of Earth's total land mass—an area larger than the continental United States.[24] And it's growing. Unsustainable farming practices are combining with climate change to cause the mighty Sahara to expand steadily. In fact, it's grown by more than 3.5 million square miles in the last 60 years, and its rate of growth appears to be accelerating.[25]

But the good news is, we can address these problems—starting with a change to how we grow our food.

Ronnie Cummins, international director of Regeneration International, tells us: "The solution to global warming and the climate crisis (as well as poverty and deteriorating public health) lies right under our feet, and at the end of our knives and forks."[26]

The key to regenerative agriculture is that it not only does no harm to the land, but actually improves it. It incorporates technologies that lead to healthy soil that becomes capable of producing high-quality, nutrient-dense food while simultaneously improving, rather than degrading, land. Ultimately, regenerative agriculture leads to productive farms and healthy communities and economies. It's dynamic and holistic, incorporating organic farming practices such as composting, conservation tillage, cover crops, crop rotation, mobile animal shelters, and pasture cropping to increase food production, farmers' income, and especially, topsoil.

Healthy soil can sequester carbon. Plants breathe in carbon dioxide, and when farming is well managed this carbon can be taken out of the air and captured in the dirt.

Cam and Roxane McKellar run Inveraray Downs, a 1,250-hectare farm in New South Wales, Australia. They grow many crops, including wheat, sorghum, corn, sunflower, barley, chickpeas, mung beans, and soybeans.[27] In the year 2000, after decades of conventional cultivation, pesticides, and inorganic fertilizer, the quality and productivity of the soil had been harmed. Pest infestations were on the rise, and the crops the McKellars were growing needed increasing amounts of pesticides and inorganic fertilizers just to keep yields steady. At the same time, the costs of fertilizers, fuel, insecticides, and herbicides were becoming prohibitive. Cam recalls, "We were going broke. Everyone but me was making money out of the farm!"

The McKellars investigated alternatives, and started to practice organic composting, crop rotation, high-intensity rotational grazing, and adding abundant recycled green manure. They slowly reduced their reliance on nonorganic fertilizers, swapping them for options such as kelp, fish emulsions, and composts.

Over time, the McKellars restored the soil structure. Their soil now holds more water, making it less susceptible to drought and flood and requiring less irrigation.

Today, as a result of all these changes, Inveraray Downs' production costs have decreased, crop yields and quality have improved, and the structure, fertility, and resilience of soils are all being restored. All of this is good for the consumer, good for the planet—and also good for profits.

Cam reflects, "Fundamentally we need to work with nature, not against her.... I should have moved to a more natural system of farming a lot earlier in my life. It is not hard. Start small, experiment, then expand."

PUTTING IT INTO ACTION

If we are to have a stable climate for future generations, as well as water and soil for our grandchildren to grow food, there are a few things that we know we must do. We need to leave fossil fuels in the ground, to move as rapidly as possible toward renewable energy, to implement regenerative agricultural principles that sequester carbon, to eat mostly plants, and to remember that our actions *always* have an impact.

When you support organic agriculture, you're contributing to healthier soil and healthier food production systems. But organic alone may not be enough. Increasingly, organic food is grown on large-scale megafarms that may be an improvement over chemical-intensive industrialized agriculture, but which are still far from truly sustainable, much less regenerative.

When you have the opportunity, supporting small-scale, local, and organic farmers can be a potent way to contribute to healthy food for your family, a healthier local economy, and a healthier future for our world.

ACTION:

Option 1: Commit to a week of doing your part for the climate change solution by cutting down on (or eliminating) your industrialized beef consumption.

Option 2: Commit to a week of doing your part for the climate change solution by cutting down on (or eliminating) all your meat consumption.

Option 3: Interview a farmer (perhaps at a farmer's market) or a produce manager at a store. Find out if they've ever thought about carbon sequestration, and how they do (or don't) think about the health of soil. If they've never thought about it before, perhaps you'll get their wheels turning. If they have, perhaps you'll learn something new. Either way, you'll be advancing one of the most important conversations of our time: How can we sequester carbon and enhance soil health while sustainably growing abundant and nourishing food for the future of humanity?

CHAPTER 29

Make Your Food Cruelty-Free

Even people who eat meat—in fact, perhaps, especially people who eat meat—have a stake in wanting the animals raised for food to live in a good way and to be treated humanely.

And people from all walks of life are appalled when they learn about the conditions in today's concentrated animal feeding operations (CAFOs)—also known as factory farms.

Warning: The next few pages contain some truths that can be a little hard to stomach. But I think we're all more capable of conscious choices when they're informed by reality.

In the United States, as in much of the developed world, egg farms cram more than 90 percent of the nation's 280 million egg-laying hens into barren cages so small the birds can't even spread their wings.[1] Each bird spends her entire life given barely more space than a sheet of paper.

In these terribly cramped quarters, with no outlet for their normal foraging, dust-bathing, and exploratory activities, and unable to establish their natural pecking order or to have any personal space whatsoever, many hens are driven so crazy that they try to peck each other to death. The industry's response? Instead of giving these poor birds more breathing room, or access to the outdoors, the industry chops off their beaks.[2] Debeaked birds suffer acute and chronic pain in their beaks, heads, and faces. The procedure doesn't stop them from pecking each other, but it does mean that their efforts to cause harm will be largely futile.

Like chickens, pigs in industrialized farming operations are kept indoors in intensely crowded conditions for their entire lives. And, like chickens, many pigs are driven crazy by the stress. In this environment, many of them will attack one another's tails and rears, even becoming cannibalistic. The industry's response is to cut off the pigs' tails.[3] The process, known as "tail docking," is typically performed in the pig's first day of life. It is intensely painful, and yet it is usually conducted without anesthesia. The baby pigs squeal in agony as their sensitive tails are literally dismembered.

Meanwhile, in a reality that does not please fans of Wilbur or Babe, 60 to 70 percent of the more than five million breeding pigs in the United States are kept in crates too small for them to walk, turn around, or socialize.[4] Pigs are considered to be as intelligent as dogs, but they're raised like they're parked cars, side by side, cage next to cage in a filthy, stinky warehouse.

And it's not just chickens and pigs that are suffering. Cows are mammals, with a strong urge to bond with their young. Yet in industrialized animal agriculture, their babies are typically taken from them in the first day of life so that all the mother's milk can be available for humans. Mothers will cry helplessly, for days on end, with no hope of ever seeing their little ones again. Many of the baby males are sent off to veal barns, where they're confined in crates, some of which are just two feet wide.[5] Here they may be chained by the neck to restrict all activity, making it impossible for them to turn around, stretch, or even lie down comfortably. This severe confinement is created intentionally, with the goal of keeping the calves' meat "tender" because muscles cannot develop.

Some veal connoisseurs refer to the "soft, unresisting flesh that melts in your mouth"—apparently unaware that this flesh is the product of an animal that was never allowed free movement in its life.[6]

When I think about the conditions in which billions of animals are raised today, I feel deeply sad. I believe that if we as humans are going to raise animals, we have a responsibility to treat them as the sentient beings that they are. They belong in farms and fields—not in factories and feedlots. I don't know anybody who wants to see animals raised in torturous conditions.

And many farmers hate it, too. They didn't set out to raise animals because they wanted to be cruel. But they have to keep costs down, and in order to be competitive in an industry that often runs on very low margins, they must resort to practices that are heartbreaking.

THE CHICKEN FARMER WHO SPOKE OUT

In 1992 Craig Watts of Fairmont, North Carolina, put up four chicken barns on land that had been in his family for nearly 200 years and signed on as a contractor with Perdue Farms. Perdue brought him baby chicks and chicken feed, provided a guaranteed market, and gave Craig specific instructions for profitably raising the birds. He earned five cents for every pound of chicken—never enough to escape a cycle of farm debt.

Driven by economic pressure, Craig did what Perdue instructed him to do—even when it meant treating chickens terribly. He spent decades presiding over barns jammed with tens of thousands of miserable birds. They'd been bred to grow massive breasts at the utmost speed, and their legs were unable to support morbidly obese bodies. *Poultry Science* journal has calculated that if humans grew at the same rate as today's chickens, a human would weigh 660 pounds by the age of eight weeks.[7]

Instead of clucking around in the dirt digging for worms, as chickens are meant to do, these birds spent their lives sitting in their own excrement as their bellies grew red, sore, and bare of feathers.

Craig's contract with Perdue explicitly forbade him from ever giving his birds sunshine or fresh air. The stimulation, Perdue told him, would make the birds move—thus expending caloric energy and decreasing profits.

Craig didn't like it, but felt he had no choice. Perdue, meanwhile, inspected his farm weekly, and gave him nothing but glowing reviews—naming him "top producer" numerous times.

One day in 2014, Craig saw an ad on television in which Jim Perdue, the company's chairperson and third-generation leader, walked through a clean, uncrowded chicken barn with full-grown birds while talking about "doing the right thing" and "raising chickens cage free." Then, as now, the company's packages even carried a seal from the U.S. Department of Agriculture with verification that the birds were raised "cage free." According to Craig, that's when his BS alarm sounded. It was one thing to be forced by economics to keep chickens in abject misery. But it was quite another to be complicit in lying about it.

Craig invited Leah Garces, the U.S. director of Compassion in World Farming, to visit his broiler barns—and to bring a camera. Leah documented the conditions in which Craig's chickens were forced to live and wound up releasing a video that rocked the chicken-farming world. This wasn't an undercover investigator revealing a worst-case scenario. This was a farmer showing the world what's actually done as standard practice in a USDA-certified operation.

The resulting video doesn't show Craig tucking the chickens in and reading them bedtime stories. Craig showed suffering birds unable to stand, lying in heaps of excrement, as he said, "I can't speak for a chicken. All I can say is what I observe. And no, they're not happy. And they're definitely not healthy."

The video went viral and was seen by millions of people.

Craig continued his operation for another year and then could take it no longer. He canceled his contract with Perdue, rented his land out to a crop farmer, and jumped in full-time with Socially Responsible Agriculture Project—an organization working for an end to the factory-farming system. Craig's job now is to spread the word about the madness of factory farms, and to help farmers transition to more humane and sustainable operations.

The factory-farming system, Craig told me, has gone completely off the rails. The companies that drive it have massive political influence, and they force farmers into a form of indentured servitude. Animals are suffering, and the environment is deteriorating. And he, for one, has made it his mission to expose the truth and work for change.

THE NORMALIZATION OF CRUELTY

In many countries around the world, there are laws against cruelty to animals. But in the United States, each of the states specifically exempts animals destined for human consumption from protective laws.[8] The result is that the animal agriculture industry routinely does things to animals that, if you did them to a dog or a cat, would get you put in jail.

Gene Baur, president of Farm Sanctuary, told me: "Most of the anti-cruelty laws exempt farm animals as long as the practices are considered to be normal by the agriculture industry. What has happened is that bad has become normal, and no matter how cruel it is, normal is legal."

A poll conducted by Lake Research Partners found that 94 percent of Americans believe that animals raised for food deserve to be free from abuse and cruelty, and that 71 percent of Americans support undercover investigative efforts by animal welfare organizations to expose animal abuse on industrial farms.[9]

TRYING TO HIDE THE TRUTH

Worried that consumers are starting to find out the truth and will demand changes to the treatment of modern farm animals, industry leaders have pushed for "ag gag" laws to hide factory farming and slaughterhouse abuses from public scrutiny.[10] Six U.S. states now have these laws on the books, threatening jail time for anyone who takes pictures or videos of farms without permission.

One of those states is Kansas. On June 28, 2013, George Steinmetz, a photographer working for *National Geographic*, was arrested and briefly jailed after taking aerial pictures of a feedlot for a series on food issues. George has taken award-winning photos in many dangerous situations, including war zones. But it was his photographs of U.S. feedlots, taken from a paraglider in an area with hundreds of thousands of cattle, that put him behind bars. The Kansas law makes it illegal to "enter an animal facility to take pictures by photograph, video camera, or by any other means." Apparently, the feedlot executives considered paragliding to be a form of illegal entry.[11]

"It was quite a surprise to me," Steinmetz commented. "I've been detained in Iran and Yemen, and questioned about spying, but never arrested. And then I get thrown in jail in America."

What is it that these farm owners don't want us to see? I'll tell you one thing: They didn't put these laws in place because they were scared that we would take pictures of broccoli farms.

WHAT HAPPENS WHEN CRUELTY IS DISCOVERED

The job of meat inspectors for the USDA is to monitor animal treatment and food safety. They're responsible for ensuring that the laws against excessive cruelty to animals, however weak these laws may be, are enforced.

Unfortunately, thanks to the weight of agribusiness interests, USDA meat inspectors are often given overwhelming volumes of animals to review—with animals flying by at rates as fast as 140 per minute.[12]

And when these inspectors do find problems, they aren't always thanked.

After 29 years as a USDA meat inspector, Jim Schrier was stationed at a Tyson Foods slaughter facility in Iowa in 2013.[13] Under federal law in the United States, pigs are required to be completely unconscious and unable to feel pain prior to shackling. At the Tyson Foods plant, Jim witnessed that pigs being shackled for slaughter were kicking and thrashing violently—a direct violation of federal regulations.

Jim did exactly what he was supposed to do. He reported the clear humane-handling violations to his superior in the chain of command. But when he presented his concerns, the supervisor reportedly became very angry, and a week later Jim was directed to work at another facility 120 miles away. Then the USDA reassigned Jim permanently to a plant in another state.

In what looks an awful lot like a form of whistleblower retaliation, after nearly three decades of service, Jim Schrier was forced to choose between his job and his family.

When Jim's wife, Tammy, launched a petition on Change.org exposing this story and calling for Jim to get his old job back, some of the first signers were other employees who had worked at the same plant and corroborated his findings.[14] Instead of being punished, they said, he should be rewarded and the whole plant should be inspected.

By the end of 2013, more than 200,000 people had signed the petition. Feeling the heat, the USDA offered Jim a job much closer to home, and the plant where Jim had worked, in Columbus Junction, Iowa, was forced to take corrective action. The campaign was declared a victory.

Most of the time, it's only when the truth comes out that change becomes possible.

In 2012, undercover investigations led to a $497 million judgment against Chino, California's, now defunct Hallmark Meat Packing Company, and to the temporary shutdown of Central Valley Meat Company over what federal investigators termed "egregious, inhumane handling and treatment of livestock."[15] In response to widespread public outcry, California and Michigan passed laws that phased in a ban on battery cages for hens, and nine U.S. states have joined Canada and the entire European Union in heading toward a ban on confining pigs in gestation crates.

We still have a long, long way to go before we make human treatment of food animals anything like humane. But we are beginning to make some progress.

THE ANTIBIOTIC CONNECTION

To keep animals alive under miserable conditions, and as a means of making them gain weight more quickly, the industrialized meat industry has taken to routinely mixing antibiotics into the feed of factory-farmed animals.

Most of the antibiotics used today (80 percent of the antibiotics used in the United States, and 66 percent in Europe) are not given to humans who are sick, but are rather fed routinely to animals in CAFOs.[16]

This practice has led to the rapid development of antibiotic-resistant bacteria, sometimes called "superbugs," that are no longer treatable by any known antibiotic.

In 2011, an Environmental Working Group study found these antibiotic-resistant superbugs on 81 percent of the ground turkey and 55 percent of the ground beef in America's supermarkets.[17]

Superbugs now threaten to make common infections once again lethal. Many public health authorities fear that we could be on the verge of entering into a "post-antibiotic world" that threatens to kill millions of people annually by 2050.[18]

With antibiotic-resistant bacteria already costing more than $55 billion in medical treatment and hospitalizations, and now killing tens of thousands of people each year in the United States alone, you could say that today's factory farms have become a kind of biological weapons factory.[19] They are breeding bacteria that are killing more people than all forms of terrorism in the world combined.[20]

WHAT YOU CAN DO

If you, like me, are appalled by the way that industrialized animal agriculture is treating animals, and if you want to preserve the viability of antibiotics for future generations, I have good news.

There's a lot you can do.

You can opt for a mostly or entirely plant-based diet. Every factory-farmed burger or chicken wing you don't eat is going to take a bite out of an inhumane system—and do a good deed for our water, topsoil, and climate, as well as your health, to boot.

And if you do choose to eat animal products, you can do so in a way that encourages the operations that do the right thing.

There's no reason you should ever spend your hard-earned money supporting industries that profit from torture.

If you want to eat meat, dairy, or eggs, it's important to know what the labels and certifications mean. Some of them represent serious commitment to ethical behavior. Others are little more than image management designed by PR companies.

For example, in the United States, the term *natural* does not tell the consumer anything about what the animals were fed, what drugs they may have been given, or whether their living conditions were humane.[21] An animal could have been fed a totally unnatural and genetically modified diet, treated with unspeakable cruelty, and pumped full of hormones and antibiotics—but its meat could still be slapped with a "natural" label before it reaches the market. All that's required for a "natural" label on meat products is for the manufacturer to assert that the product doesn't contain any artificial additives or colors, and that it's been "minimally processed" after slaughter.

WHAT THE ANIMAL WELFARE LABELS MEAN

In the United States, the "USDA Organic" label on animal products tells you that the animals were fed organic feed, and are free from added hormones and antibiotics. Unfortunately, it tells you nothing about how they were treated. And there are many animal welfare claims on the market that are not third-party verified, and therefore may or may not mean anything.

Third-party-verified animal welfare labels that do mean something are "Certified Humane," "Animal Welfare Approved," "Certified Grassfed," and for fish, "Certified Sustainable Seafood."

When USDA Organic is combined with Certified Humane, Animal Welfare Approved, or Certified Grassfed, you can know that the animals were not only fed organically grown food, but also raised free from the most egregious forms of cruelty. And if you're going to eat animal products, there's nothing more authentic than visiting the farm to see how the animals actually live.

Buyer beware: With chicken and eggs, "cage free" and even "free range" often don't mean much. Cage-free birds typically must be given at least 1.5 square feet of space per bird, while for free range, they get at least a whopping 2 square feet. "Pasture-raised" birds, on the other hand, are supposed to get 108 square feet per bird. This leads to a significantly different quality of life for our feathered friends.

For a full directory of labels on food and what they mean, visit 31day foodrevolution.com/labels.

IS IT WRONG TO EAT MEAT?

Ethical vegetarians raise an important question. Why do we love pets and eat pigs?

I mean, seriously, why is it that we can take a dog or cat into our homes and our hearts, and consider them part of the family, but at the same time, we can take a cow or a pig that may be just as smart and sensitive as a dog or a cat and subject it to immense cruelty before killing it for our supper?

The way I see it, we each draw the line of ethical eating based in part on what feels close to us. Many people in the modern world would be horrified at the thought of eating chimpanzees, dogs, or cats, as we tend to see them as more akin to us. For some people, that sense of proximity extends to all mammals. For some it even extends to birds, fish, or even shellfish.

I have deep respect for each person's felt sense of moral integrity. And I also know that we live in the real world. Anyone who's ever grown a garden knows that even growing organic kale can involve the murder of aphids and slugs, as well as keeping out hungry rabbits, gophers, and deer, some of whom may starve. Simply to live in the world is to partake, in some way, in death as well as in life.

As a human being of conscience, I want to do the least harm, and the most good, that I reasonably can. And I want to help bring consciousness to the real impact of the choices we make, so that we can be as congruent as possible with the values that we hold not just for animals, but also for ourselves.

For this reason, I've made the personal choice to be mostly vegan (with some wild low-mercury fish and some pasture-raised eggs in the mix upon occasion). But that doesn't mean this would be the optimal choice for you. You don't have to be a vegetarian or an animal rights activist to care about animals and to want them to be treated with respect. You don't have to swear off animal products in order to eat less meat and to steer clear of factory farms.

We can all play a part in helping to end senseless cruelty to animals, and in helping to shape a more humane system of food production.

ACTION:

Option 1: Download the food labels guide available at 31dayfoodrevolution .com/labels. On your next shopping trip, go to the meat, dairy, and/or egg sections, and see which claims and labels are used. Review what they actually mean. If you learn something new, tell at least one other person.

Option 2: Inspect the labels on any animal products in your fridge, freezer, or local food stores—and say no to at least one product that doesn't meet your ethical standards.

Option 3: Next time you're in a restaurant that serves animal products, ask your server if they are antibiotic-free, and if the animals were pasture-raised or lived in factory farms. If they don't know, ask if they can check. If the answer is yes, thank them. If the answer is no, ask them to let their manager know that you'd appreciate if they make the switch to antibiotic-free. For bonus points, ask if you can share your concern with a manager directly. You don't have to eat meat to care and to raise awareness. Anyone can do it.

CHAPTER 30

Stand Up for Healthy Food for All

A few years ago, I walked into a 7-Eleven in Oakland, California. In the checkout line ahead of me was a woman, probably in her

> Anyone who has ever struggled with poverty knows how extremely expensive it is to be poor.
>
> —James A. Baldwin

forties, with two small children. She looked so weary. Her kids were tugging on her, and she seemed exhausted. She also looked to be about 50 pounds overweight.

My heart went out to her as I saw her fatigue. She was having a pretty hard day.

I don't usually make it a habit to look at the contents of other people's shopping baskets. Frankly, I think it's rude. But as I waited in line, I couldn't help but notice the sugary cereals and sodas, processed meats, chips, ice cream, and canned soups filling her grocery basket.

I started to feel a bit of judgment, thinking that this woman's weight, and her fatigue, were probably being fueled by her diet.

That's when I noticed that she was paying for her groceries with food stamps.

And then it hit me. The woman in front of me was probably struggling to feed her family at all. The last thing she needed was some snooty shopper behind her arrogantly critiquing her for the contents of her basket.

The family checked out and left for the parking lot. As they walked out, I felt humbled and sent a little prayer their way—a prayer for their health and happiness.

But I also knew it was going to take a lot more than prayers to help this family, and millions of families like them, to have access to the healthy food, and the healthy life, that they deserve.

In 2014, an estimated 795 million people worldwide, including more than 48 million Americans (one out of every seven people), 4 million Canadians (one out of eight) and 13.5 million Europeans (about 2 percent of the population) were hungry or living in households designated as "food insecure."[1] According to official definitions, "food insecure" means that a household doesn't have a ready availability of nutritionally adequate and safe foods.

And while many of us associate food insecurity with images of starving people in Ethiopia or India, the reality is that in the developed world, it is more often linked with obesity. A 2012 study of 66,553 adults found that those who were food insecure had 32 percent greater odds of being obese than those who were not.[2] The cheapest calories are often also the junkiest ones, thus fueling increased rates of obesity and other health problems. Food insecurity and poverty have been directly linked to increased incidence of cancer, heart disease, diabetes, and most of the other lifestyle-fueled chronic ailments of our times.[3]

In fact, children living in poverty are seven times more likely to suffer from poor health, compared to children living in high-income households.[4]

As I bought my batteries in that West Oakland 7-Eleven, I found myself thinking about that family and wondering…how did it get this way? Why is it that people who are already struggling just to pay rent and to feed their families at all are the most likely to be suffering from diet-fueled and life-threatening illnesses that they, of all people, can least afford?

FOLLOW THE MONEY

There are many factors that feed into poverty. And there are a multitude of reasons why many people of low income, especially in the developed world, also lack access to safe, affordable, and healthy food—and tend to depend on junk food even more than the general population.

One reason for this is being financed by taxpayers.

Since 1995, the U.S. Department of Agriculture has handed out more than $277 billion in subsidies—primarily to growers of "commodity" crops like corn, soy, rice, and wheat.[5] These crops, some of which are shipped around the world, mostly wind up as cattle feed or get refined and converted into processed foods and sweeteners like high-fructose corn syrup.

But between 1995 and 2012, less than 0.03 percent—that's less than 30 cents out of every $1,000—of total U.S. farm subsidies went to growers of apples or vegetables.[6] This same pattern plays out around the world, as governments essentially subsidize junk food at the expense of the foods we all know we should eat more of—creating a market distortion that pushes everybody, rich as well as poor, in the wrong direction.

Whether you're a free-market economist or a government-intervention-loving socialist, this system is just plain crazy.

In theory, farm subsidies could make some sense. Farmers work hard, and many of them take risks in the face of droughts, floods, and marketplace forces beyond their control. Personally, I kind of like the idea of a government protecting farmers while also bringing down the price of foods that poor people need to feed their families.

The trouble is, most of our subsidies are going to mega-agribusiness operations already making quite a bit of money without taxpayer help.[7] And the effect of this support is to create a marketplace distortion, unfairly bringing down the prices of the very foods that are making us sick.

Hostess Twinkies are cheaper than carrots, for example, in part because they contain 14 ingredients made with highly subsidized processed ingredients, including corn syrup, high-fructose corn syrup, cornflour, and vegetable shortening.[8]

When I met with Coca-Cola executives to discuss what it would take for their company to go non-GMO, they explained that their products are, in fact, non-GMO in Europe, where they sweeten their soda with sugar. But in the United States, the economics are different and push them to use high-fructose corn syrup instead. The reason? In the United States, corn is subsidized by the U.S. taxpayer. High-fructose corn syrup, which is made almost entirely from genetically engineered corn, is therefore also subsidized. This makes it cheaper than sugar, thus bringing down the price of the product.

The bottom line is that U.S. taxpayers are subsidizing companies like Coca-Cola, and incentivizing them to use genetically engineered high-fructose corn syrup in abundance. Consumption of this sweetener is starting to decline, but it's still used so widely that in the U.S. the average woman eats her own weight of it every two and a half years.[9]

THE LINK BETWEEN SUBSIDIES AND CONSUMER CHOICE

Okay, so these subsidies create an artificial effect on the price of foods. But do we know if they are really and truly affecting the health of low-income people? In a word: yes.

In a study published in *JAMA Internal Medicine* in 2016, researchers from the Centers for Disease Control and Prevention and other institutions looked at what 10,000 Americans reported eating.[10] They then calculated how much of their diets were made up of food that was subsidized by the government.

They found that more than half of Americans' calories came from subsidized foods, and that diets full of subsidized food were high in dairy, simple carbohydrates (like sugar and white flour products), and factory-farmed (grain- and soy-fed) meat. They found that the more subsidized foods that people ate, the lower their diets were likely to be in fruits, vegetables, nuts, seeds, and overall quality.

Poorer and less educated segments of the population were found to be eating vastly higher quantities of subsidized food. The old adage that "beggars can't be choosers" is playing out on a vast scale, fueled by subsidized industries that, in effect, leave the poorest segments of our population dependent on junk food to survive.

Compared to people who ate the least amount of subsidized food, those who ate the most had a 37 percent higher risk of being obese, a 34 percent higher risk of having signs of elevated inflammation, and a 14 percent higher risk of having abnormal blood cholesterol levels.

What all this means is that in the United States, taxpayers are spending hundreds of billions of dollars effectively making junk food cheaper—and creating a competitive disadvantage for real, healthy food.

Unfortunately, this phenomenon isn't limited to the United States.

Among the 30 member-countries in the Organisation for Economic Co-operation and Development, governments provide a series of subsidies known as "producer support."[11] These subsidies combine to an average of 31 percent of total revenue for the primary grain, oil, sugar, and livestock products.[12] Somehow fruits, vegetables, nuts, seeds, and legumes—the very foods we know we should be eating more of—are largely left out of the equation.

No one is being forced to eat junk food, of course. Whether certain crops are subsidized or not, we are all—each of us—ultimately responsible for the foods we put in our mouths and for what we feed our children. But wouldn't it make more sense if we as a society made it a little easier to do the right thing? Isn't subsidizing junk foods, and thereby making healthy food more expensive, a little like rewarding us for *not* wearing seat belts and fining us if we use them to stay safe?

What kind of a world would we have if instead of subsidizing junk food and grain-fed livestock, we made healthy foods more affordable for everyone?

As I uncovered the reality of agricultural subsidies, and as I thought about all the tens of millions of people suffering from diet-related disease that is being promoted with taxpayer money, I felt awful. But then I realized something important. This is not the way it has to be. There's nothing natural or free about a marketplace that's heavily manipulated to serve the interests of an agribusiness elite.

Anytime you learn about something that's wrong in the world, the good news is, you're also discovering something that could be better. Every problem is also a solution waiting to happen—an opportunity to make a difference.

And some people are finding and promoting solutions that work.

In the United States, Wholesome Wave has launched a program that matches the value of SNAP (food stamp) dollars when they're used to buy fruits and vegetables. Users shop with SNAP as they normally would—but they get their purchasing power doubled in the form of tokens or coupons called "nutrition incentives." The program has been found to be highly effective, reaching 500,000 people in the regions it serves and unlocking $10.6 million (and counting!) in fruits and vegetables annually. This not only helps the poor and the elderly to buy more fresh, locally grown, organic produce, but it also helps the farmers to sell more of their harvests. You can find out more at wholesomewave.org.

THE SURPRISING SOURCE OF MOST OF THE WORLD'S FOOD

A decade ago I was in Guatemala, on the shores of Lake Atitlán, in a community where I was told the villagers grew most of their food organically. They didn't have much money, but the food that they grew for themselves didn't cost them a cent. They saved their seeds, composted their food waste, and nourished the soil as if their lives depended on it—which they did.

The Guatemalan villagers I visited are not alone. Despite the corporate takeover of big agribusiness in much of the industrialized world, small farmers and backyard gardens are fundamental to the world's harvest. Worldwide, about 500 million family farmers grow 80 percent of the world's food.[13]

While many of us may think of farmers as male, the reality is often quite different. Women in rural areas grow at least half the world's food.[14] Around the planet, it's women who are the primary seed keepers and, often, the custodians of food biodiversity.

Not that women get the credit they deserve. In India, as in many places, the people classified by the government as "farmers" are the landowners. Fewer than 13 percent of the women who grow food own land titles. So women who grow food are usually classified as farmworkers, while men who may simply hold title to the land are likely to be classified as farmers. According to Oxfam International, women in India do 80 percent of the farm work.[15] The statistics are similar in Africa, where women are said to be responsible for 80 percent of the continent's food production.[16]

Why is this gender distinction important? Because women should be honored for the work they do. And for another reason, too: When women have access to more dignity and opportunity, the well-being of their whole family as well as their community tends to be uplifted. The U.N. Food and Agriculture Organization reports that in the developing world, a monthly increase of $10 to a woman's income achieves the same improvements in children's nutrition and health as a $110 monthly increase to a man's income.[17]

If we truly want to see an end to hunger in our lifetimes, we'll need to address the root causes of poverty. Contrary to popular misconception, world hunger is not, in fact, caused by a shortage of food. It's caused by a shortage of justice. We produce more than enough food to feed everyone alive. People go hungry because they are poor and don't have enough money to buy the food being produced.

Small-scale farmers, most of them women, are fundamental to the world's food security. In general, compared to industrialized operations, small-scale farmers grow more food per acre of land they cultivate, and require less water and chemicals. They grow more diverse, abundant, safe, sustainable, and healthy food—and produce less waste. And the money they earn is immediately reinvested locally.

According to a 2013 UN report, *Smallholders, Food Security, and the Environment*, investing in small-scale farmers can help lift more than 1 billion people out of poverty.[18]

Supporting the dignity and well-being of rural farmers may be one of the most potent steps the global community can take if we want to reduce hunger and increase food security on the planet.

AND IT'S NOT JUST RURAL COMMUNITIES

Areas without access to nutritious, high-quality, affordable food are known as food deserts.[19] According to official classifications, people who live in food deserts don't have a supermarket or grocery store within a mile of their home if they live in an urban area, or within 10 miles of their home if they live in a rural area.

South Los Angeles is a well-known food desert.

Ron Finley, who operates a large organic garden in the area, says that the drive-throughs are killing more people than the drive-by shootings. He adds that in his community, it's easier to get alcohol than it is to get a banana.

In 2011, Ron got sick and tired of having to travel 45 minutes to get real food. So he decided to grow some himself. He turned the 150-by-10-foot median strip parkway in front of his house into an edible garden, growing food that he freely shared with all passersby. This violated a city ordinance and led to a fine. When Ron refused to pay it, an arrest warrant was issued. Ron fought back, and ultimately won in court. And his fame as the "gangsta gardener" was born.

Today, Ron's TED talk about his journey has been seen by more than four million people. In 2016, when he was threatened with eviction from his rented home, a global GoFundMe campaign raised enough money for the nonprofit Ron Finley Project to buy it.

Now Ron's gardening has expanded far beyond the median in front of his home, providing a backyard garden shared by hundreds of family, friends, neighbors, and interested groups. In 2017, he was growing oranges, pears, pomegranates, papyrus, sugar cane, almonds, rosemary, artichokes, chard, flowering celery, Mexican marigolds, red Russian kale, mint, sweet potatoes, blackberries, fennel, plums, bananas, Christmas lima beans, sunflowers, volunteer Green Zebra tomatoes, apples, red dandelions, corn, nasturtiums, and apricots.

Ron still shares his harvest freely with the community. Sometimes neighbors stop by in the middle of the night for a snack. Ron feeds the hungry and brings real food to the people who need it most. But he's growing a lot more than vegetables. The way he sees it, he's helping to grow the very fabric of community itself.

And he's not the only one.

In central Detroit, Michigan, the Michigan Urban Farming Initiative has created an "agrihood" that provides free, fresh produce to 2,000 households within two square miles of the farm.[20] With financial sponsorship from BASF, General Motors, and other area businesses, it also supplies food to local markets, restaurants, and food pantries. This agrihood is one of many rays of hope springing up in Detroit. In the year 2000, there were an estimated 80 farms within Detroit's city limits.[21] By 2016, there were 1,400, with the city's urban farmers producing an estimated 400,000 pounds of fresh fruits and vegetables for city residents each year.[22]

THE SIMPLE POWER OF GROWING FOOD

When faced with the enormity of the problems in the world today, it's easy to hope for technological breakthroughs. And sometimes technology is truly dazzling. From iPhones to self-driving cars to drip irrigation, technology can add convenience, efficiency, connectivity, and knowledge to our lives.

But let's not forget that growing food is one of the most basic, and one of the most beautiful, things that a human being can do.

Endea Woods of Boardman, Oregon, is a mother of seven. When she was raising her family, they lived far from grocery stores, and money was tight. They lived in an environment that would, in her words, "make anyone starve." Her solution? Grow a garden! Cultivated with compost, the garden not only kept her family fed; it helped her whole clan to be robustly healthy. She remembers, though, that at times she was challenged to harvest enough veggies for cooking because her kids loved to eat straight from the garden!

When we grow food, we reclaim self-sufficiency. We connect ourselves with the living earth. We participate in something precious, and ancient, that has helped to define the human experience for millennia.

All over the world, from rural India to urban Detroit, people are growing fresh organic food to feed their families and communities. And wherever you live, whether in a tiny apartment or a sprawling ranch, you can join them, and you can celebrate them. You can support them at farmer's markets. You can raise money to assist their efforts. And you can cheer them on and tell their stories. I believe that every time a farmer or a gardener plants a seed to grow real, healthy food, they're also planting a seed of hope for our world.

ACTION:

Option 1: Contact a local food bank to find out how you can contribute something healthy.

Option 2: Make a donation or raise money to support an organization that's helping to lift communities out of poverty by investing in their long-term well-being. One of my personal favorites is Trees for the Future. For every copy of this book that's sold, I'm donating funds to enable them to plant an organic fruit or nut tree in a low-income community. Find out more and make a bonus contribution yourself at 31dayfoodrevolution.com/trees.

Option 3: Contact the elected officials representing your city, county, congressional district, state, or country to request a meeting. Or, if they host town halls, attend one. Ask what they're doing to contribute to greater nutrition and health for low-income community members. Let them know you care, and that you want them to take positive action. Many elected officials believe that every person who brings them an opinion could represent many thousands of others who feel the same way but didn't take the time to speak out. So make your voice heard!

CHAPTER 31

Seize the Day: A Time for Action

So... how's it going? You've reached the final chapter! Whether you've completed every single step in this book, or you've just skimmed around, I want to welcome you to this point and to thank you for being here.

Is your relationship with food, and your life, beginning to change?

Are you thinking about food differently in any way? Are you more aware of what's healthy and what's not? Are you taking any steps to get the support you need or to gather your community? Are you more aware of the ethical and global impacts of your relationship with food?

Do you feel a stronger congruency between your values and your actions?

Are there any more vegetables in your fridge, or in your plans?

Whatever your answers are, I hope you don't wait until you reach your goal to be proud of yourself. I hope you're proud of yourself every step of the way.

The truth is, you're part of the food revolution every time you choose real food over processed junk—every time you go for beans instead of burgers, or for crisp celery sticks instead of potato chips. You're part of the Food Revolution every time you support organic, local, fair-trade, humane, or non-GMO food. And every time you spread the word, sharing food or wisdom with friends, family, or your community.

Thank you for all the ways that you step outside the status quo and take a stand for the health and for the world that you want.

NOW FOR SOME SELF-ASSESSMENT

At the beginning of Parts One, Two, Three, and Four, I've given you a quiz. I'd like to invite you to take the quizzes again and see how you're doing.

If you like, you can take them online, compare your scores with others, and join a community of peers at 31dayfoodrevolution.com/quizzes.

If you're not exactly where you'd like to be, please don't feel any stress. Once you know where you stand, you can make conscious choices about where you'd like to go.

With your food choices, you literally have the power to shift the course of your destiny. You can eat the conventional diet, and in all likelihood, you'll suffer from the conventional diseases. You can contribute to the status quo, in which food is fueling torture of animals, destruction of our environment, and cancer for farmworkers as well as for consumers.

Or you can make a change—and set yourself on a new path. You can stand for another possibility and seek greater alignment between what you value for your life and for your world.

The way I see it, with knowledge comes responsibility.

Some things in life are like that. Once you know, you can never go back.

It bears repeating: Cancer doesn't really care what you think, or what you believe. Neither do diabetes, or heart disease, or dementia. But they all do care—a lot—what you eat. They all care how you live.

Eat fewer animal products and processed foods. Eat more whole foods—especially fruits and vegetables. Pay attention to where your food comes from and how it's produced.

And watch your life, and your world, change for the better.

TIME TO SHARE

If you've made any changes or had any success since starting this book, now's a great time to celebrate. You can post your top "win" of the last month on social media, and let your friends and loved ones know that you're making progress on something that matters to you. Did you discover a new way to eat vegetables that you loved? Plant a seed? Give up a junk food you thought you'd be addicted to for life? Did you go organic, give up factory-farmed meat, or swear off sugary sodas?

Use the hashtag #foodrevolution so you can let other food revolutionaries celebrate with you.

You can also share an inspiring book or film, and what it means to you, with people you love. Next time you want to give someone a gift, instead of some trendy new gadget or the iPhone 18 (I've lost track of what number they're on now), what if you gave the gift of learning about health?

Some things are too important, and too beautiful, to keep to ourselves. Personally, I think health is one of those things. So let's learn it. Let's live it. And let's share it.

Imagine with me, for a moment, the implications down the road. Where is your life headed? When you're looking back as you reach the end of your life, who do you want to have been? How do you want to have lived? How do you want to have cared for your body? And how will your food choices have shaped the course of your destiny?

Right now, in this moment, you have a choice. You can continue on the course you've been on, and that will take you where you were headed. And if something more is possible, if some bigger or better or healthier opportunity is open to you, then this is a moment, right now, when you have the opportunity to step forward into the life that can be.

What suffering or disease might you *not* have to experience? What is it worth to you to have your loved ones have the benefit of you, healthy and well, for a long and full life?

And speaking of your loved ones . . . do you know anyone who struggles with excess weight or obesity? Anyone who has high blood pressure or type 2 diabetes, or who is facing cancer? What would it be worth to be able to support them more deeply? What would you give to be able to be a positive influence on the lives of the people you love?

And I'd like to invite you to consider for a moment the fate of our planet. How do you feel, in your heart, about the reality of factory farms? What do you think it does to us, as humans, to be part of a species that forces the animals we raise for food to live in unrelenting misery? And what would it do to your own sense of conscience to help change that? How would it feel to be part of a species mindful of stewardship, that treated animals, and our planet, with respect rather than with cruelty and exploitation?

And do you, like me, fear for the future of our climate, our water supply, and our ability to feed future generations with a constantly expanding population? What would it be worth if you knew that you could contribute to a future in which all people have access to healthy food, in which the climate was stable, and in which there was enough water to go around? How would it feel to live with the deep satisfaction of knowing that your life was making a contribution to the world you want for yourself and for all that you love?

Right here, right now, you and I—and our entire species—face a moment of choice. We know that the path of factory farms, chemicals, antibiotics, added sugars, and processed junk leads not just to suffering, not just to sickness, but also to economic and environmental chaos. It leads to exploitation of animals and farmworkers, to ever more poisons being poured on our land and our food, and to untold suffering for billions.

But we have another option.

When you bring your food choices into alignment with your values, something extraordinary happens. Your health can improve, of course. You can lose weight and have more energy and better sleep and more stable hormones and moods. But you can also start to feel a kind of ebullience. A sense of joy. A feeling, coming from deep inside, that you're on the right path.

Eating becomes an act of love for your body. Food becomes a web of relations, and as you find your place in that web, a kind of congruency takes root. You're more at home in your body, and you're more at home in your world.

When you eat more local food, you deepen your sense of place and of belonging. When you eat more humane food, you expand your heart's capacity for compassion. When you eat more sustainable food, you grow in your connection to the earth's community. And when you eat more healthy food, you're sending your body a signal that you are worth cherishing.

Every bite becomes an opportunity to take a stand for the life, and the world, that you want.

Welcome to the Food Revolution.

ACTION:

Option 1: *Post online about a food or health victory. Have you given up potato chips or fried chicken, or enjoyed a green smoothie seven days in a row? Did you make it through Thanksgiving without falling off the wagon? Did you take a group of friends out to a healthy restaurant or join a CSA program? Share something you've done, large or small. Use the hashtag #foodrevolution.*

Option 2: Go online to all four quizzes in this book to see how your score compares with others, and to connect with a community of kindred spirits, at 31day foodrevolution.com/quizzes. Do you have room for improvement? Decide on a new step to raise your score even higher.

Option 3: Get bulk copies of a book or film you like that you believe could make a positive impact—and share it with friends or loved ones. And here's a trick that should triple the chances that they read or watch what you give them. With a book, insert a Post-it note or two as bookmarks, with comments like "This part made me think of you," or "I'd love to hear your reactions to this chapter!" With a DVD, you can put a Post-it on the front of the case, with a comment like "I loved the part starting at 16:32. It totally made me think of you!"

RECIPES FOR HEALTH

A note about recipe substitutions for our friends on low sugar, oil, and salt (SOS) diets:

Sugar: Most of these recipes are sweetened with fruit only, like dates, but in a few cases, we use a small amount of liquid sweetener such as maple syrup. In general, you can reduce the amount or replace with stevia if desired.

Oil: When a recipe calls for oil, it can often be omitted or replaced with water. When the oil is used in a stir-fry or sauté, you can usually simmer ingredients with a small amount of water or vegetable stock in place of the oil.

Salt: Salt in these recipes is always optional. An acidic ingredient, like lemon juice or vinegar, is a nice way to add flavor without using salt. You'll see tamari/soy sauce and miso in several of the recipes, and these contain sodium. If you're on a low-sodium diet, consider using reduced-sodium soy sauce, adding less, or leaving it out altogether.

A word about GMOs: If you want to avoid GMOs, make sure that all corn, canola, and soy (tamari, edamame, tofu, miso, etc.) products are organic or non-GMO.

About use of animal products: All of the recipes provided here are based on whole foods and are plant-sourced. If you choose to include some consciously sourced animal products in your diet, you can add them in with substitutions or as a garnish.

Breakfasts

My Beloved('s) Smoothie

By Phoenix Robbins

My wife, Phoenix, likes to soak chia seeds in water to create a paste that she stores in the fridge to add to recipes throughout the week. She uses the paste in smoothies, adding more nutrition to an already nutrient-loaded breakfast. Soaking the chia seeds makes them easier to break down in the blender and increases their bioavailability. They provide protein, fiber, and all-important omega-3 fatty acids.

Prep Time: 10 minutes
Serves 2 to 4 (this makes 32 ounces and is great for sharing, or you can store leftovers in the fridge)

Ingredients:

- 2 cups chopped and packed leafy greens, like spinach, kale, Swiss chard, romaine lettuce, bok choy, dandelion greens, or collards
- 2 cups liquid, like water, coconut water, nondairy milk, or sparkling water
- 1–3 cups fresh and/or frozen fruit, like banana, berries, lime, mango, cherries, apple, peach, nectarine, orange, avocado, pear, pineapple, grapes, figs, apricots, or passion fruit
- 2–3 tablespoons chia paste (see note), or 1 tablespoon chia seeds
- Optional flavor and nutrition boosts: hemp seeds, pumpkin seeds, almond butter, cashews, walnuts, nondairy yogurt, protein powder, fresh herbs, ginger root, turmeric root, cacao, cinnamon, vanilla extract

Directions:

Put all ingredients into a high-powered blender and blend for 1 to 2 minutes. Pour into a glass or mason jar or two and enjoy!

(cont.)

Note: To make the chia paste, simply combine 1 part chia seeds and 3 parts water in a sealed container. Soak for at least 2 to 3 hours.

Tip: Many people like to start with a higher volume of fruit and then taper it down to reduce the level of fruit sugar as they become accustomed to the flavors of fresh vegetables.

Blueberry Chia Porridge

By Ocean Robbins

This refreshing porridge is a delightful snack in the afternoon or evening, or it makes a terrific breakfast. It's rich in omega-3 fatty acids, protein, fiber, probiotics, and antioxidants. It's portable. And it's delicious!

Prep Time: 20 minutes, plus 6 hours to set up
Serves 2 to 4

Ingredients:

    6 tablespoons whole chia seeds
    3 cups cold nondairy milk or yogurt
    2 tablespoons maple syrup or other sweetener (optional)
    1 teaspoon vanilla extract
    2–3 cups fresh or frozen blueberries

Directions:

Place chia seeds in a large glass food storage container with a lid (mason jars work great), and pour in milk, syrup, and vanilla. Shake or stir well and let sit for 15 minutes. Add blueberries and stir again.

Put mixture in the refrigerator for at least 6 hours, preferably overnight.

Remove porridge from the refrigerator, stir well, and spoon into serving containers. Remember to chew the chia seeds well so your body absorbs their nutrients.

Sweet Potato Scones

By Dean Ornish, MD, Ornish.com

These scones make a wonderful addition to a brunch spread. Spices, currants, and vitamin-rich orange-fleshed sweet potatoes add delicious flavor, along with plenty of fiber, health-promoting nutrients, and protective antioxidants.

Prep Time: 1 hour and 20 minutes
Cook Time: 20 minutes
Makes 12 scones

Ingredients:

1 pound red-skinned, orange-fleshed sweet potato, washed and pricked with
   a fork
2 cups whole wheat pastry flour or gluten-free flour
2 teaspoons aluminum-free baking powder
½ teaspoon bicarbonate of soda
1½ teaspoons cinnamon
¼ teaspoon freshly ground nutmeg
¾ teaspoon fine sea salt
½ cup plain nondairy yogurt
2 tablespoons liquid sweetener, like maple syrup or honey
1/3 cup dried currants

Directions:

Preheat oven to 400°F.

Wrap sweet potato loosely in aluminum foil. Bake until very soft, about 40 to 50 minutes, depending on size. Remove from oven. Unwrap foil, slice potato open lengthwise, and let cool. (The sweet potato can be baked up to two days ahead of time.)

When sweet potato is cool enough to handle, scoop flesh from skin and, using a fork, mash to a smooth paste. Measure out 1¼ cups mashed sweet potato. (Set aside any remaining sweet potato for other uses.)

Line a roasting tray with parchment paper. In a medium bowl, whisk together flour, baking powder, bicarbonate of soda, cinnamon, nutmeg, and salt. In a small bowl, mix together yogurt and sweetener. Using your fingertips or two forks, cut the sweet potato into the dry ingredients until mixture looks crumbly. Using as few strokes as possible to prevent the scones from being tough, stir in yogurt mixture to make a soft, moist dough. Mix only until there are no more patches of dry flour. Gently fold in currants.

Divide into 12 rounded mounds, about 1/3 cup each, onto prepared roasting tray. Bake for 20 minutes, until puffed and lightly browned. Remove from oven and let cool on a rack.

Since these contain no oil, they're best eaten fresh, within a few hours of being made.

Oyster Mushroom Frittata

By Chef Jason Wyrick, thevegantaste.com, for Neal Barnard, MD,
from Power Foods for the Brain

The frittata, which is an Italian-style omelet, gets a healthy makeover with the use of tofu and the addition of nutrient powerhouses like spinach and oyster mushrooms.

Prep Time: 20 minutes
Cook Time: 25 minutes
Serves 2 to 4

Ingredients:

12 ounces extra-firm tofu
½ teaspoon ground turmeric
½ teaspoon sea salt or black salt, divided
2 small red potatoes, scrubbed and diced
½ teaspoon olive oil
2 cloves garlic, minced
4 cups baby spinach leaves, washed and chopped
6 green onions, sliced
Nonstick cooking spray
1 cup chopped oyster mushrooms
Minced parsley for garnish

Directions:

Preheat oven to 375°F.

Put tofu in a blender and add turmeric and ¼ teaspoon of the salt. Blend until smooth and creamy, stopping to scrape sides as needed. Transfer to a bowl.

Toss potatoes in oil and sprinkle lightly with salt. Roast potatoes for 10 minutes. Remove from oven and set aside.

While potatoes are roasting, spray a frying pan with nonstick cooking spray and cook garlic, spinach, and green onions until the spinach has wilted, about 3 minutes.

In a large bowl, combine tofu, potatoes and spinach mixture. Spray a 6-by-6 baking dish or cast iron frying pan with cooking spray and transfer tofu mixture to dish. Cover with foil and bake for 25 minutes.

When the frittata has just a few more minutes left to cook, toss mushrooms with the remaining ¼ teaspoon salt. Coat a sauté pan with cooking spray and heat over high heat; add mushrooms and sear them until they turn brown and slightly crisp, stirring occasionally, about 5 to 6 minutes.

Remove frittata from oven, top it with the oyster mushrooms and minced parsley, and serve.

Mighty Carrot Raisin Muffins

By Brenda Davis, RD, BrendaDavisRD.com

Commercial muffins are like little cakes with lots of fat, sugar, and white flour, often containing up to 500 calories. Make these whole-food muffins instead, using dried and fresh fruit for sweetness and nut or seed butter instead of oil.

Using a blender makes these fast and easy! They are best right out of the oven, or freeze any you aren't using within two days.

Prep Time: 15 minutes
Cook Time: 25 minutes
Makes 12 muffins

Ingredients:

2 cups rolled oats
¼ cup ground flaxseed
2 teaspoons baking powder
½ teaspoon bicarbonate of soda
½ teaspoon salt (optional)
2 teaspoons cinnamon
½ teaspoon ginger
¼ teaspoon ground clove
¼ teaspoon ground nutmeg
1½ cups nondairy milk
1/3 cup tahini or almond butter
1 large carrot, coarsely chopped (about 1 cup)
½ cup unsweetened applesauce
¾ cup dates (soften with boiling water or steam if very hard)
1 tablespoon lemon juice or apple cider vinegar
1 teaspoon vanilla extract
¾ cup raisins
1 cup coarsely chopped walnuts

(cont.)

Directions:

Preheat oven to 350°F. Spray or line a 12-cup muffin tin and set aside.

In a blender, pulse together oats, flaxseed, baking powder, bicarbonate of soda, salt, cinnamon, ginger, clove, and nutmeg. Remove mixture to a large bowl.

Place milk, tahini, carrot, applesauce, dates, lemon juice, and vanilla in the blender and process on low speed, gradually increasing speed until smooth.

Add wet ingredients into dry ingredients and stir just until mixed. Fold in raisins and walnuts. Divide mixture evenly (about ½ cup) into muffin cups and bake for 25 to 30 minutes, or until an inserted cocktail stick comes out clean. Remove muffins from pan, place on cooling rack, and serve immediately.

Millet Cereal with Apricot-Apple Compote and Warm Coconut Milk

By Caryn Hartglass and Gary De Mattei,
responsibleeatingandliving.com

Millet is a healthy, gluten-free grain that is a good source of important nutrients, like magnesium.

Prep Time: 5 minutes
Cook Time: 40 minutes
Serves 2

Ingredients:

Millet
1 cup millet
2 cups water

Compote
1 apple, diced
8 dried apricots, diced
2 cinnamon sticks
¼ teaspoon freshly grated nutmeg
½ cup boiling water

Garnish
1 cup coconut milk, warmed
1–2 tablespoons ground flaxseed or ground nuts

Directions:

In a medium saucepan, bring the 2 cups water to a boil and stir in the millet. Reduce heat to a simmer and cover, leaving the lid on until all water is absorbed and millet is soft, about 30 minutes. Turn heat off but leave the lid on for at least 5 minutes.

While the millet is cooking, place apple and apricots in a sauté pan and add cinnamon sticks, nutmeg, and ½ cup boiling water. Bring to a boil over medium-high heat. Lower heat and simmer about 8 minutes, or until all water is absorbed and apples and apricots are soft but not mushy. There should be a little syrup in the bottom of the pan.

Spoon millet into bowls and add the compote on top. Drizzle warm coconut milk on top and serve with a touch more grated nutmeg and ground flaxseed.

Ginger Spice Smoothie

By Mark Hyman, MD, from Eat Fat, Get Thin, *DrHyman.com*

This creamy, slightly spicy (in a good way!) drink is great to start your day; ginger is excellent for digestion.

Prep Time: 10 minutes
Serves 2

Ingredients:

1½ cups nondairy milk
2 tablespoons raw almond butter
2 teaspoons grated ginger
¼ teaspoon grated nutmeg
1 handful baby spinach or greens of choice

Directions:

Place all ingredients in a blender and blend until smooth and creamy. Serve immediately.

Snacks and Shares

Deo's Cashew Cream Cheeze

By Deo Robbins

My mom has outdone herself with this one! This versatile dip and spread tastes better than regular cream cheese and has a healthy dose of probiotics in every bite. Use as a dip for veggies, spread on bread, bagels, or crackers, or add to scrambled tofu for extra richness. It also makes a great salad dressing when thinned with a bit of water.

Prep Time: 10 minutes, plus 15 to 18 hours for soaking and fermenting
Makes 1½ cups

Ingredients:

1½ cups raw cashews, soaked overnight
6 capsules good-quality probiotic or acidophilus powder
1–2 tablespoons mild white miso (miso is salty—start with 1 tablespoon and add as needed)
1½ tablespoons nutritional yeast
1 teaspoon onion powder
½ teaspoon salt

Directions:

Rinse and drain soaked cashews. Place in a high-speed blender with enough water to blend until silky. Remove to a bowl with a lid.

Open probiotic capsules and stir in probiotic powder.

Cover bowl with cheesecloth (to breathe but not dry out—you could also use a light tea towel) and keep in a warm place (such as in the oven with just the oven light on or with a jar of hot water) for 7 to 10 hours, until nice and tangy. You'll know the cheeze is ready when it has a rich yogurty flavor.

After it is cultured, put a ½ cup of the cheeze in a bowl and stir in miso, nutritional yeast, onion powder, and salt, mashing to thoroughly combine. Stir the mixture back into the larger batch. Cover with a lid, and let set at room temperature for 3 to 4 hours.

Keeps for about a week in the refrigerator.

Roasted Red Pepper Hummus

By Deo Robbins

Preparing your hummus at home will save you loads of money and give you options for a variety of flavors.

Prep Time: 10 minutes
Makes 2 cups

Ingredients:

One 15-ounce can chickpeas or 1½ cups cooked chickpeas
½ cup roasted red peppers packed in water
1 tablespoon tahini
¼ cup lemon juice
3 tablespoons chopped green onions
1 tablespoon chopped garlic (about 3 cloves—or less to taste)
1 teaspoon ground cumin
½ teaspoon black pepper
Vegetable broth, for thinning (optional)

Directions:

If using canned chickpeas, drain them, reserving liquid, and rinse beans.

Place beans, roasted peppers, tahini, lemon juice, green onions, garlic, cumin, and black pepper in a food processor or blender and process until smooth.

Add reserved bean liquid, or if using cooked beans, water or vegetable broth, as needed for a smoother consistency.

Variations: Add 1 cup loosely packed coriander, basil, or parsley, or leave out the roasted red peppers and add the herb(s). You can also use cannellini beans instead of chickpeas.

Chive Dip and Spread

By Deo Robbins

You can use this delicious spread on bagels or toast or as a dip for crackers or chips. It's also great anywhere you might otherwise use sour cream.

Prep Time: 10 minutes
Makes about 3 cups

Ingredients:

Two 12-ounce packages firm silken tofu
4½ tablespoons rice vinegar
1½ teaspoons onion powder
1½ teaspoons salt
6 tablespoons olive oil (or less to taste)
¾ cup finely chopped chives or green onions

Directions:

In the bowl of a food processor, place tofu, rice vinegar, onion powder, and salt, and process until well mixed, about 30 seconds.

Continue processing while slowly adding olive oil and process until smooth, about 30 seconds.

Place mixture in a bowl and stir in chives. For optimal results, cover and chill before serving.

Baked Chickpea Nuggets

Adapted from a recipe by Holly Yzquierdo

These protein-packed nuggets make a fantastic snack, appetizer (try with BBQ sauce!), or topping for any kind of salad.

Prep Time: 15 minutes
Cook Time: 30 minutes
Serves 4

Ingredients:

One 15-ounce can chickpeas, drained and rinsed

1 tablespoon nutritional yeast

1 teaspoon granulated onion

½ teaspoon garlic powder

½ teaspoon salt

1 tablespoon bread crumbs or panko (can be gluten-free), plus 1/3 cup for coating

Directions:

Preheat oven to 350°F. Line a roasting tray with parchment paper.

Pour chickpeas into a food processor and process for a few seconds.

Add all other ingredients except the last 1/3 cup bread crumbs. Process a few more seconds until everything is well mixed and has a chunky texture.

Place the 1/3 cup bread crumbs in a bowl. Scoop up a teaspoon of chickpea mixture and roll it into a ball, then form into a nugget shape. Roll each nugget in bread crumbs to coat.

Lay nuggets on prepared roasting tray with space between. Bake for 20 minutes, then flip and bake for 10 more. Allow nuggets to cool before eating.

Wild Mushroom Lettuce Wraps

By Chef Jason Wyrick (thevegantaste.com) for Neal Barnard, MD, from Power Foods for the Brain

These wraps are a delicious, elegant way to eat more wild mushrooms. They are extremely versatile—use any type of mushrooms you desire.

Prep Time: 15 minutes

Cook Time: 5 minutes

Serves 2 to 4

(cont.)

Ingredients:

2 heads baby bok choy, thinly sliced

8 to 10 fresh shiitake mushrooms, thickly sliced

½ cup roughly chopped oyster mushrooms

6 to 8 green onions, sliced

2 cloves garlic, minced

1 teaspoon grated fresh ginger

3 tablespoons diced water chestnuts

¼ teaspoon Chinese five-spice powder, or ¼ teaspoon black pepper plus a
   pinch of cloves

2 teaspoons reduced-sodium tamari or soy sauce

3 tablespoons hoisin sauce mixed with 2 tablespoons water

½ teaspoon chili paste

½ cup bean sprouts

¼ cup chopped enoki mushrooms

¼ cup toasted slivered almonds

4 lettuce leaves (preferably butter lettuce)

Directions:

Heat a wok or wide, shallow sauté pan over high heat. Add bok choy and cook until wilting, about 30 seconds. Add shiitake mushrooms and cook another 30 seconds.

Add oyster mushrooms, green onions, garlic, ginger, and water chestnuts and cook another minute.

Add Chinese five-spice and stir. Immediately stir in tamari or soy sauce and hoison mixture if using. Stir in chili paste and cook for another 15 seconds.

Remove from heat and immediately add bean sprouts, enoki mushrooms, and almonds. Serve in lettuce leaves.

Mini Courgette Pizzas

By Ocean Robbins

Let's face it, since the best part of pizza is the toppings, why not use healthy and low-calorie courgette as your crust?

Prep Time: 10 minutes

Cook Time: 12 minutes

Serves 4

Ingredients:

2 medium courgettes, sliced in strips lengthwise, about ¼ inch thick
¼ cup pizza sauce
½ cup shredded vegan "cheeze"
Diced vegetables, like onions, mushrooms, and peppers, or spices for topping
(optional)

Directions:

Preheat the oven to 375°F and lightly spray a roasting tray with olive oil or non-stick cooking spray.

Lay the courgette slices on the roasting tray. Top each slice with sauce, then sprinkle with cheeze and add your desired toppings. Bake for 10 to 12 minutes and serve immediately.

Satisfying Soups and Stews

Mushroom Barley Soup

By Jessica Meyers Altman, gardenfreshfoodie.com

When it's cold outside, cozy up with a bowl of this warm, hearty soup.

Prep Time: 25 minutes
Cook Time: 2 hours
Serves 6 to 8

Ingredients:

1 large yellow onion, chopped
2 carrots, diced
3 stalks celery, diced
12 ounces mushrooms, sliced (about 3½ cups)
2 or 3 cloves garlic, minced (about 1 tablespoon)
1 cup uncooked barley
1½ tablespoons dried dill (or ¼ cup fresh)
1½ teaspoons dried thyme (or 1 tablespoon fresh)
1½–2 teaspoons salt (optional)
½ teaspoon black pepper
2 smaller bay leaves (or 1 large)
7 to 8 cups vegetable stock or water
3 cups sliced napa cabbage
Juice of 1 lemon (about 2 tablespoons; more or less to taste)
¼ cup chopped fresh parsley, plus more for garnish if desired
Several cups additional greens like spinach or kale

Directions:

In a large pot over high heat, sauté onions with a little water to prevent sticking and cook until translucent. Add carrots, celery, and mushrooms, and sauté for about 3 minutes, until slightly softened.

Add in barley, dill, thyme, salt, pepper, bay leaves, and stock or water. Bring to a boil and reduce to simmer. Cook for 30 minutes.

Add in cabbage, and continue to cook until barley is cooked through, about another 30 to 60 minutes.

Stir in lemon juice, parsley, and greens right before serving. Season to taste with additional lemon juice or salt and pepper.

Lovely Lemon Lentil Soup

By Phoenix Robbins

This soup features nutrition heavy-hitters like lentils and sea vegetables (which can be found at natural-foods stores, Asian markets, and many supermarkets), but the lemon keeps it light and refreshing.

Prep Time: 15 minutes
Cook Time: 60 minutes
Serves 6

Ingredients:

3 tablespoons olive oil
2 teaspoons minced garlic
1 large onion, chopped
4 to 6 cups chopped greens (kale, collards, etc.)
7 cups vegetable stock or water with 3 cubes vegetable bouillon
1 cup uncooked red lentils
1 teaspoon sea vegetables (arame, kombu, etc.)
¼ cup tamari or soy sauce
½ cup lemon juice (more or less to taste)
Lemon slices and chives, for garnish

Directions:

Heat oil in a soup pot over medium heat. Add garlic and onion and sauté for a few minutes, until onion is clear.

(cont.)

Add remaining ingredients except for lemon juice and garnishes and bring to a boil.

Reduce heat and simmer 45 minutes to 1 hour, until lentils and vegetables are thoroughly cooked.

Add lemon juice and serve garnished with lemon slices and chives.

Mulligatawny Soup

By Frances Moore Lappé, from Diet for a Small Planet, SmallPlanet.org

The San Francisco Ecology Center is famous for its soups. Ed Lubin of the Center offers this one, which he says is "a favorite of our lunchtime patrons." It is delicious and easy to make.

Prep Time: 30 minutes
Cook Time: 60 minutes
Serves 6 to 8

Ingredients:

3–4 tablespoons olive oil
2 onions, coarsely chopped
2 or 3 cloves garlic, chopped
1 carrot, chopped
2 stalks celery, chopped
1 green pepper, chopped
1 small turnip or parsnip, grated
1 large or 2 small Pippin or other apples, cored and chopped
3/8 cup tomato paste
2 tablespoons chopped parsley
1 teaspoon curry powder
2 cups cooked chickpeas, or one 15-ounce can, undrained
Salt or vegetable seasoning powder

Directions:

Heat oil in a large pot over medium heat and sauté onions and garlic for a few minutes, until onions are translucent. Add carrot, celery, pepper, turnip, apple, tomato paste, parsley, curry powder, and 5 cups water and simmer for 45 minutes to 1 hour. Purée beans in a blender until smooth and add to soup pot, with more water if the soup is too thick.

Taste and adjust seasoning.

Heat through and serve or continue to simmer, the longer the better.

Creamy Carrot Soup

By John Robbins

Everyone loves carrots. Because they are so widely available and inexpensive, we may not appreciate how nutritious they are. As their name suggests, they're one of the food kingdom's richest sources of carotenoids. Regular carotenoid intake has been linked with an up to 50 percent decrease in cancers of the lung, bladder, cervix, prostate, colon, larynx, and esophagus.

Prep Time: 10 minutes

Cook Time: 15 minutes

Serves 4

Ingredients:

3 large carrots, chopped

1 large yellow onion, chopped

½ cup roasted cashews (preferably dry roasted, unsalted, or low salt)

2 tablespoons soy sauce

2 teaspoons curry powder (more if you like it spicy)

¼ cup chopped fresh parsley

Directions:

In a saucepan, combine carrot, onion, and 3 cups of water. Cover and bring to a boil, then turn down heat and simmer 10 minutes.

Place cooked vegetables, cooking liquid, cashews, soy sauce, and curry powder into a blender and blend until creamy, or use an immersion blender.

Serve hot and garnish with parsley to taste.

Corn Chowder

By Caryn Hartglass and Gary De Mattei, responsibleeatingandliving.com

This chowder is tops on the list of hearty comfort foods. Be sure to add the caraway seeds for the best flavor.

(cont.)

Prep Time: 10 minutes
Cook Time: 20 minutes
Serves 4 to 6

Ingredients:

One 16-ounce package frozen corn, or 3 cups fresh corn kernels
2 medium onions, chopped
2 cloves garlic, minced
2 medium potatoes, cut in small cubes (peel if not organic)
1 carrot, cut in small chunks (peel if not organic)
1 tablespoon dried parsley
1 tablespoon dried sage
1 tablespoon caraway seeds
1 cup unsweetened nondairy milk
Salt
Nondairy yogurt, to garnish

Directions:

In a large soup pot over medium heat, sauté the corn, onions, and garlic in about
½ cup water for about 5 minutes, stirring frequently.

Add in potatoes, carrot, parsley, sage, and caraway seeds along with another
5½ cups water. Bring to a boil, then reduce heat, cover, and let cook until potatoes are
soft, about 30 minutes.

With an immersion blender or regular blender, puree about ⅔ of the soup, so that
the soup has a creamy base with some corn, potato, and carrot chunks.

Add in milk and salt to taste. Let soup simmer until ready to serve. Top each bowl
with a dollop of yogurt.

Mexican Lime Soup

By Rip Esselstyn from The Engine 2 Diet

This hearty and playfully seasoned soup is great for guests. Serve in large bowls and
crumble healthy chips on top.

Prep Time: 20 minutes
Cook Time: 25 minutes
Serves 4 to 6

Ingredients:

1 large onion, chopped

8 ounces mushrooms, quartered

2 bay leaves

2 cloves garlic, chopped or pressed

3 poblano peppers, toasted, seeded, and skinned, cut into thin strips

Two 32-ounce cartons vegetable stock

2 ears of corn, cut into 2-inch rounds

4 medium red potatoes, cooked and cut into 1-inch cubes

1 bunch coriander, rinsed and chopped

Zest of 1 lime

Juice of 3 limes

4 tomatoes, chopped

2 avocados, sliced

Corn tortilla strips

Directions:

In a large soup pot over medium heat, sauté onion, mushrooms, and bay leaves with a little water or low-sodium vegetable broth for 5 minutes, until onions brown.

Add garlic, poblanos, and 1 cup of stock. Stir intermittently for 5 minutes, until peppers begin to soften.

Add remaining stock, corn, and potatoes. Cover and cook for 10 minutes, until potatoes are tender. Remove from heat and let sit, covered, for 5 minutes.

Stir coriander, zest, and lime juice into soup immediately before serving.

Serve garnished with tomatoes, avocado, and healthy chips.

Espresso Black Bean Chili

By Mark Bittman, from How to Cook Everything Vegetarian, *markbittman.com*

Vegetarian chili recipes are easy to find online, but this one deserves special attention. It's easy to make and great for a crowd. The espresso/coffee really adds a special flavor, so if you are sensitive to caffeine, try using decaf.

Prep Time: 20 minutes

Cook Time: 1 to 1½ hours, largely unattended

Serves 6 to 8

(cont.)

Ingredients:

3 tablespoons neutral oil, like grapeseed or corn

2 onions, chopped

2 tablespoons minced garlic

3 cups chopped ripe tomato (about 1½ pounds whole; canned is fine; don't bother to drain)

½–1 cup freshly brewed espresso, 1 to 2 cups brewed coffee, or 2 tablespoons espresso powder

2 tablespoons chili powder

¼ cup dark brown sugar or 3 tablespoons molasses

One 3-inch cinnamon stick

1 pound dried black beans, washed, picked over, and soaked if you like

Salt and black pepper

Directions:

Put oil in a large pot with a tight-fitting lid over medium-high heat. When hot, add onions and cook, stirring occasionally, until soft, about 5 minutes. Add garlic and cook for another minute.

Stir in tomato, espresso, chili powder, brown sugar, cinnamon stick, and black beans and add water to cover. Bring to a boil, then lower the heat so the liquid bubbles steadily but not violently. Cover and cook, stirring occasionally, until beans begin to soften, 30 to 40 minutes. Add a good pinch of salt and pepper.

Continue cooking until beans are tender, anywhere from another 45 minutes to 1½ hours. Taste and adjust the seasoning, adding more salt and pepper. Serve or store, covered, in the refrigerator for up to 3 days.

Salads and Dressings

Spicy No-Mayo Coleslaw

By Mark Bittman, from How to Cook Everything (Completely Revised 10th Anniversary Edition), markbittman.com

This version of coleslaw is more flavorful and has far less oil than a restaurant version. It's on the spicy side, with plenty of Dijon along with spring onions and a little garlic and chili.

Prep Time: 30 minutes
Serves 6 to 8

Ingredients:

- 2 tablespoons Dijon mustard, or to taste
- 2 tablespoons sherry vinegar, red wine vinegar, or freshly squeezed lemon juice
- 1 small clove garlic, minced
- 1 tablespoon minced fresh chili, like jalapeño, Thai, serrano, or habanero, or to taste (optional)
- ¼ cup groundnut oil or extra virgin olive oil
- 6 cups cored and shredded napa, savoy, green, and/or red cabbage
- 1 large red or yellow pepper, cored, seeded, and diced or shredded
- 1/3 cup chopped spring onion, more or less
- Salt and black pepper
- ¼ cup chopped fresh parsley

Directions:

To make the dressing, whisk together the mustard and vinegar in a small bowl along with the garlic and chili. Add the oil a little at a time, whisking all the while.

Combine the cabbage, pepper, and spring onion in a large bowl and toss with the dressing.

Sprinkle with salt and pepper and refrigerate until ready to serve. (It's best to let the slaw rest for an hour or so to allow the flavors to mellow; the cabbage will also

(cont.)

soften a bit and exude some juice. You can let it sit longer, up to 24 hours, if you like. Drain the slaw before continuing.)

Just before serving, toss with parsley.

Cabbage and Carrot Slaw, Mexican Style. Grate 2 medium carrots and use them instead of pepper. Use freshly squeezed lime juice in place of vinegar. Finish with coriander if you like instead of parsley.

Apple Slaw. Use carrots instead of pepper, as in the preceding variation. Use 1 medium onion, grated, in place of the spring onion. Shred or grate 2 medium or 1 large Granny Smith apples (or use any tart, crisp apple) and include them in the mix. Lemon juice or cider vinegar is the best choice of acid here.

Hemp Seed Caesar Salad

By Jenny Brewer, nourishingnutrition.com

Hemp seeds (typically available from natural-foods stores and online grocers) are rich in healthy fats, protein, and nutrients like magnesium. They are wonderful sprinkled on salads, and when you blend them with a liquid, they turn into a creamy base for dressings and dips. Toasted nori crumbled on top adds a light "fishy" flavor, making this recipe reminiscent of a traditional Caesar salad.

Prep Time: 20 minutes
Serves 4 to 6

Ingredients:

¾ cup hemp seeds
2 or 3 cloves garlic, chopped
1 tablespoon nutritional yeast
1 tablespoon Dijon mustard
½ tablespoon tamari
Juice of 1 large lemon
¼ cup fresh parsley
Salt and black pepper

1 head Romaine lettuce, washed and torn into bite-size pieces
4 cups baby spinach, chopped
1 avocado, cut into chunks (optional—but delicious!)
1 .18-ounce package nori snacks (the small package of toasted sheets; optional)

Directions:

Place hemp seeds, garlic, and ¾ cup water into a high-powered blender and blend until mixture is smooth and creamy. Add nutritional yeast, mustard, tamari, lemon juice, and parsley and blend the mixture well. Add salt and pepper to taste.

Place lettuce and spinach in a large bowl and pour dressing overtop. (You will likely have leftover dressing, which is a good thing!) Toss to mix. Place salads on serving plates, and top with avocado chunks. Crumble toasted nori sheets overtop and serve.

Quickest Black Bean Salad

By Ann Crile Esselstyn in Prevent and Reverse Heart Disease,
by Caldwell B. Esselstyn Jr., MD

Dr. Esselstyn has helped tens of thousands of people prevent and reverse heart disease. His wife, Ann, creates many of their recipes and says about this one: "We could eat this for every meal in summer. It is the salad I make when I have to take a dish to an event, because it is so quick to assemble and everyone comes back for more. It is easy to expand by adding more tomatoes or frozen corn. As always, use LOTS of coriander."

Prep Time: 10 minutes
Serves 4 to 6

Ingredients:

Two 15-ounce cans or 3 cups black beans, drained and rinsed well
1 very large tomato, chopped
One 16-ounce package frozen corn
½ Vidalia or red onion, chopped
One 6-ounce can sliced or diced water chestnuts, drained and rinsed
1 bunch coriander or parsley, chopped
Juice and zest from ½ lime
3 tablespoons balsamic vinegar, or more to taste

Directions:

Put beans, tomato, corn, onion, and water chestnuts in a large bowl (glass looks pretty) and mix. Rinsing the beans will keep the salad from looking gray.

Add coriander, lime juice and zest, and vinegar and mix again.

Serve alone or with baked corn tortilla chips.

Kale Salad with Apples and Dried Cherries

By Joel Fuhrman, MD, from drfuhrman.com

Dr. Joel Fuhrman's website features many healthy and tasty recipes, like this one for antioxidant-rich kale combined with apples and dried fruit for a touch of sweetness. This recipe also demonstrates how to massage kale to make it tender—a technique you will want to use over and over.

Prep Time: 15 minutes
Serves 2 to 4

Ingredients:

- 1 bunch kale, tough stalks and center ribs removed
- 1 avocado, chopped
- 2 tablespoons lemon juice
- 1 tablespoon white balsamic vinegar
- 1 cup thinly sliced red cabbage
- 1 large apple, cored and chopped
- 2 tablespoons chopped unsweetened, unsulfured dried cherries, blueberries,
    or currants (see note)
- ½ medium red onion, minced
- 2 tablespoons chopped chives

Directions:

Roll up each kale leaf and slice thinly. Add to a large mixing bowl along with avocado, lemon juice, and vinegar. Using your hands, massage the avocado, lemon juice, and vinegar into the kale leaves until the kale starts to soften and wilt and each leaf is coated, about 2 to 3 minutes.

Mix in cabbage, apple, dried cherries, onion, and chives. Serve immediately.

Note: If you have problems finding unsweetened, unsulfured cherries or blueberries, they can be ordered online from a number of sources.

Terrific Tahini Dressing

By Ocean Robbins

Tahini, or sesame seed paste, makes this dressing rich and creamy. It can be used on just about any kind of salad, as a sauce over quinoa or rice and beans, or in a veggie wrap.

Prep Time: 10 minutes
Makes 3¾ cups

Ingredients:

1 ¼ cup neutral oil, such as canola, sunflower, grape seed, or almond—or if
   you like the flavor, you can use avocado or olive oil

½ cup flax oil, as fresh as possible (if that isn't available, you may use one of
   the oils listed above, or try MCT oil)

1 cup lemon juice

½ cup shoyu or tamari soy sauce or soy-free coconut aminos (depending on
   how salty you want your dressing)

½ medium onion, chopped

1 or 2 cloves garlic

¼ cup tahini

1 tablespoon maple syrup

¼ cup nutritional yeast flakes (optional, but recommended)

Directions:

Place all ingredients in a blender and blend well. Keeps well in the refrigerator for up
to a week.

Entrées and Greens

Steamed Greens with Walnut Parmesan

By Caryn Hartglass and Gary De Mattei,
responsibleeatingandliving.com

Leafy greens are especially delicious topped with this easy-to-make cheesy "parmesan" made with only walnuts, nutritional yeast, and a pinch of salt.

Prep Time: 15 minutes
Cook Time: 30 minutes
Serves 4

Ingredients:

½ pound kale (about 8 to 10 large leaves) or other leafy green like collards,
    spinach, or chard
¼ cup walnuts
2 tablespoons nutritional yeast
Pinch of salt

Directions:

Prepare a pot of water with steamer basket. Place over high heat.
    Wash the greens. Tear the leaves from the stalks. Save stalks for juicing or soup.
    Coarsely chop leaves into 2- to 3-inch-wide pieces.
    When water comes to a boil, add greens and cook for 5 to 10 minutes.
    Chop walnuts fine on a cutting board or in a food processor. Toss with nutritional yeast. Salt to taste.
    Remove greens from steamer when leaves are tender. Place in a bowl. Top with walnut/yeast mixture and mix well. Serve immediately.

Kale with Onions and Pine Nuts

By Michael Pollan, from MichaelPollan.com

The fabulous writer Michael Pollan penned a great phrase about eating when he said: "Eat food. Not too much. Mostly plants." How wonderful that we can follow his advice and eat this delicious plant-based recipe to our heart's (and tummy's) content!

Prep Time: 10 minutes
Cook Time: 20 minutes
Serves 4 to 6

Ingredients:

1/3 cup pine nuts
1½ tablespoons extra virgin olive oil
2 yellow onions (about ¾ pound total), cut into thin wedges
2 bunches Tuscan or lacinato kale (about 1½ pounds total), stalks removed, leaves chopped
1 tablespoon fresh lemon juice
½ teaspoon crushed red pepper flakes
¾ teaspoon kosher salt

Directions:

Heat a large, deep frying pan over medium heat. Add pine nuts and cook, stirring often, until golden brown, 3 to 4 minutes; set aside.

In same frying pan, heat oil over medium heat. Add onions and cook, stirring occasionally, until deep golden brown and tender, 12 to 14 minutes. Add kale, lemon juice, and ¼ cup water and toss gently. Cover and cook until just wilted, 3 to 4 minutes.

Remove from heat and add reserved pine nuts, red pepper flakes, and salt. Toss well and serve.

Quinoa with Walnuts

By Deo Robbins

Mushrooms, walnuts, and high-protein quinoa are combined to make a filling, pilaf-type dish that can be enjoyed as is or stuffed inside a courgette or aubergine.

Prep Time: 10 minutes
Cook Time: 30 minutes
Serves 4

(cont.)

Ingredients:

1–2 tablespoons olive oil

1 medium onion, chopped small

1 celery stalk, chopped small

1 medium carrot, chopped small

6 button mushrooms, sliced thin

1 cup uncooked quinoa, soaked 5 minutes, rinsed, and drained

½ teaspoon black pepper

½ teaspoon dried rosemary

1–2 tablespoons soy sauce or coconut aminos

½ cup chopped walnuts

¼ cup chopped fresh parsley

Directions:

Heat oil in a saucepan over medium-high heat. Add onion, celery, and carrot and cook about 5 minutes, stirring occasionally. Add mushrooms and continue stirring 1 more minute.

Stir in quinoa, 2 cups water, pepper, rosemary, and soy sauce. Cover and bring to boil. Then turn down heat and simmer 25 minutes.

Toss cooked quinoa in a bowl with walnuts and parsley. Serve hot or cold.

Spicy Sweet Potato Bakes

By Deo Robbins

Sweet potatoes are traditional holiday fare, but these naturally tasty tubers can easily go on menus throughout the year. Their nutritive profile, including manganese, potassium, dietary fiber, and vitamins C, B_1, B_2, and B_6, makes them part of any nutritional all-star team.

Prep Time: 10 minutes

Cook Time: 40 minutes

Serves 4

Ingredients:

4 long, thin sweet potatoes, washed well

2 tablespoons olive oil

2 tablespoons paprika

½ teaspoon black pepper

½ teaspoon onion powder

½ teaspoon garlic powder

½ teaspoon dried thyme

½ teaspoon dried rosemary

¼ teaspoon cayenne pepper

½ teaspoon salt (optional)

Directions:

Preheat oven to 375°F. Lightly oil a roasting tray or shallow pan.

Cut sweet potatoes in quarters lengthwise, then in half across the middle. Place in a large bowl. Add olive oil and toss with your hands, coating the potatoes.

Sprinkle in spices and salt and mix in so that potatoes are coated with spice mix.

Lay pieces on the prepared roasting tray. Bake for 20 minutes on one side. Flip pieces over and bake for about 15 minutes more, or until lightly browned.

Stir-Fried Cauliflower Couscous

From Grain Brain: The Surprising Truth about Wheat, Carbs, and Sugar: Your Brain's Silent Killers, by David Perlmutter, MD, with Kristin Loberg, copyright © 2013. Reprinted by permission of Little, Brown and Company, an imprint of Hachette Book Group, Inc.

Move over, kale—cauliflower is enjoying its time in the spotlight as a #1 celebrity vegetable! It's a cruciferous vegetable with a multitude of health benefits. Plus, when processed, it has a texture that's similar to rice, so it can be a great substitute in stir-fry dishes. Use this as a side dish, or for a heartier meal, add beans, nuts, and greens.

Prep Time: 10 minutes

Cook Time: 10 minutes

Serves 4

(cont.)

Ingredients:

1 head cauliflower

2 tablespoons olive oil

1 onion, finely diced

1 clove garlic, minced

Salt and black pepper

1 tablespoon fresh herbs of choice, minced

1 tablespoon lemon juice

Directions:

Cut the cauliflower into 2- to 3-inch pieces and place them in the bowl of a food pro-cessor. Pulse until cauliflower looks like tiny nuggets. Watch carefully, as it doesn't take long to turn nuggets into purée.

If you don't have a food processor, grate the cauliflower on the large holes of a box grater or chop it using a very sharp chef's knife.

(Optional: Place cauliflower nuggets in clean tea towels or kitchen paper and wring out moisture. This will result in a less mushy stir-fry.)

Heat olive oil in a large sauté pan. Add onion and garlic and cook, stirring, just until soft, about 3 minutes. Add the raw cauliflower nuggets, season with salt and pepper to taste, and cook, stirring, until the cauliflower begins to color, about 5 minutes.

Remove from the heat and stir in fresh herbs and lemon juice. Taste to adjust seasoning.

Note: Many people discard the core of the cauliflower and use only the florets to make couscous, yet there is absolutely no sound reason for doing this. The core tastes only a bit stronger than the florets, and adds at least one serving to the mix.

Marinated Tempeh

By Caryn Hartglass and Gary De Mattei,
responsibleeatingandliving.com

Tempeh is a fermented, whole-food source of soy that is rich in nutrients. Once cooked, this tempeh can be used in a variety of dishes, like stir-fries or even sliced for a sand-wich. Tempeh Reubens, anyone?

Prep Time: 10 minutes

Cook Time: 45 minutes

Serves 4

Ingredients:

Marinade

2 cups vegetable stock or water

1 cup dry white wine or vermouth (you may use nonalcoholic wine, or additional vegetable stock or water if you prefer)

½ cup fresh-squeezed lemon juice

1 teaspoon onion powder

1 teaspoon dried parsley

1 teaspoon dried sage

1 teaspoon dried rosemary

1 teaspoon dried thyme

1 teaspoon paprika

1 bay leaf

1 teaspoon black pepper

4 cloves garlic, smashed

Salt

Two 8-ounce packages tempeh

Directions:

Preheat oven to 375°F.

In a large bowl, thoroughly mix the marinade ingredients.

Place the tempeh on a large roasting tray with high sides. Pour the marinade over the tempeh. Cover with a sheet of parchment paper and then cover that with a sheet of aluminum foil.

Bake for 45 minutes. Remove from oven and let cool before serving.

Deo's Delicious Greens

By Deo Robbins

In addition to all the things I love about my mom, she also makes a seriously mean pot of greens!

Prep Time: 10 minutes
Cook Time: 15 minutes
Serves 4

(cont.)

Ingredients:

1 tablespoon coconut or olive oil

2 yellow onions, sliced

2 cloves garlic, minced

2 bunches kale, washed, stalks removed, leaves thinly sliced

1 teaspoon soy sauce

Salt and black pepper

Directions:

Heat coconut oil in a frying pan over medium heat. Add onions and stir frequently until they begin to soften, about 5 minutes. Stir in garlic and kale. Add soy sauce and cover the frying pan. The salt in the soy sauce will draw out some juices, and the cover will hold in the steam to tenderize the veggies. After 3 minutes or so, remove the lid to stir, then replace it so the veggies can steam in their own juices.

Continue stirring and re-covering a few times, until the kale reaches the desired tenderness, approximately 10 minutes. If it begins to stick, you can add more soy sauce or a small amount of water. Season to taste with salt and pepper and serve.

Black Thai Peas

By Caryn Hartglass and Gary De Mattei,
responsibleeatingandliving.com

Some believe that eating black-eyed peas on New Year's Day will bring good luck. Black-eyed peas in a rich and spicy coconut curry sauce? Who needs good luck when there's good eating?

Prep Time: 10 minutes
Cook Time: 30 minutes
Serves 8 to 10

Ingredients:

5 cups cooked black-eyed peas, or three 15-ounce cans
1 red onion, chopped
1 cinnamon stick
1 teaspoon mustard powder
1 teaspoon cumin
1 teaspoon turmeric
1 teaspoon red pepper flakes
½ teaspoon chili powder
½ teaspoon ground coriander
¼ teaspoon cayenne pepper
1 cup strained tomatoes
1 cup coconut milk
Salt and pepper

Directions:

Place all ingredients in a large saucepan over medium heat with 1 cup water.

Cook, stirring occasionally, until the liquid reduces down to make a thick stew, about 30 minutes. Remove the cinnamon stick.

Delicious as is or served with greens over quinoa.

Pasta and Yeast "Cheeze" Casserole

By Deo Robbins

Nutritional yeast is a terrific addition to almost anyone's diet. It's an excellent source of protein and contains all the essential amino acids. Particularly rich in lysine and tryptophan, it's a welcome complement to most grains.

Prep Time: 15 minutes
Cook Time: 30 minutes
Serves 6

(cont.)

Ingredients:

12–14 ounces brown (or other) rice, or penne pasta
¾ cup canola/coconut/other vegetable oil
½ cup whole wheat pastry flour or all-purpose gluten-free flour
1 onion, chopped
2 cloves garlic, crushed
2 tablespoons soy sauce or tamari
1½ teaspoons salt
Pinch of turmeric
Black pepper
1 cup nutritional yeast flakes

Directions:

Preheat oven to 350°F. Oil a 9-by-13-inch baking dish.

Cook pasta to al dente according to package directions; rinse, drain, and set aside in a mixing bowl.

Bring 3½ cups water to a boil in a covered pot, reduce heat, and keep simmering.

Heat ½ cup of the oil in a large saucepan over medium heat. Gradually stir flour into the heated oil and whisk over medium heat until the mixture is smooth and bubbling. Whisk in heated water, then stir in onion, garlic, soy sauce, salt, turmeric, and black pepper to taste. Continue stirring for 5 minutes as mixture thickens and boils. Whisk in nutritional yeast and remaining ¼ cup oil.

Mix ¾ of the sauce into the cooked pasta, then spread the pasta into the prepared baking dish. Pour the remainder of the sauce on top. Bake for 15 minutes. Broil the top until light brown, 1 to 3 minutes.

Treats and Desserts

Peachy Keen "Ice Cream"

By Ocean Robbins

This is our go-to dessert when we want something fast, tasty, and nutritious. There are infinite variations and they're all delicious! Most people enjoy it "soft serve" style, in a dish, while others eat it in a cone. You'll want to start freezing bananas today so you always have them on hand to make this delicious treat.

Prep Time: 10 minutes
Serves 4

Ingredients:

2 large ripe bananas, peeled, sliced, and frozen (about ¾ cup sliced bananas)
½ to ¾ cup nondairy milk
1 seedless navel orange, peeled and chopped
½ cup frozen peach slices
¼ cup frozen mango slices
1 teaspoon vanilla extract
¼ cup raw walnuts or cashews (optional if you want a creamier texture)

Directions:

Put all ingredients in blender, and blend until everything has been pulverized. (If you have a Vitamix, use the plunger to help mix all the ingredients while maintaining a thick consistency).

This is best eaten immediately, as refreezing will leave you with a solid icy block.

Variations: You may add other frozen fruit such as blueberries, or a teaspoon of raw cacao powder, or a tablespoon of peanut butter. Or cut out the frozen peach and mango, and instead sprinkle each serving with a dash of cinnamon, nutmeg, and/or pumpkin pie spice.

Peanut Butter Fudge Balls

By Ocean Robbins

These aren't the healthiest recipe you'll find in this book—but they sure are delicious!

Prep Time: 35 minutes
Makes about 20 balls

Ingredients:

Peanut Butter Balls
¾ cup unsalted peanut butter
6 large ripe Medjool dates, pitted
2 teaspoons vanilla extract
¼ teaspoon salt
2 tablespoons oat flour

Fudge Coating
1/3 cup coconut butter (not the same thing as coconut oil)
¼ cup unsweetened cocoa powder
1 teaspoon vanilla extract
¼–½ cup maple syrup (depending on desired sweetness)

Directions:

Line a small roasting tray with parchment paper.

Place peanut butter, dates, vanilla, and salt in a food processor and blend well. Remove mixture to a bowl, add flour, and mix with your hands until flour is absorbed into mixture.

Roll mixture into 1-inch balls and place on prepared roasting tray, and put in the freezer while making the fudge coating.

Melt the coconut butter in a medium glass bowl in the microwave (about 1 minute) or in a saucepan over the hob. Whisk cocoa powder, vanilla, and maple syrup into melted coconut butter until smooth.

Remove peanut butter balls from freezer. Drop them, one at a time, into fudge and use a spoon to coat. Place back onto roasting tray and put into freezer for at least 15 minutes for the fudge to set. These are best kept refrigerated or frozen.

Walnut Cookies

By Brenda Davis, RD, BrendaDavisRD.com

These cookies are wondrous! They contain no oil or added sugar and are gluten-free. Plus they're an amazing source of omega-3 fatty acids!

Prep Time: 45 minutes
Cook Time: 20 minutes
Makes: 3 dozen small cookies

Ingredients:

2 cups pitted dates, loosely packed
¼ cup tahini or almond butter
¼ cup ground flaxseed
1 teaspoon vanilla extract
¼ teaspoon salt (optional)
2 cups walnuts, finely chopped (or coarsely ground in blender)
1 cup rolled oats, ground into flour
Walnut or pecan halves (optional)

Directions:

Preheat oven to 300°F. Lightly oil two roasting trays, or line with silicone baking mats.

Place dates in a small saucepan with ¾ cup water and simmer until dates are tender, about 5 minutes. When dates are tender, mash them with a fork.

Put dates in a large bowl and stir in tahini, flaxseed, vanilla, and salt. Add nuts and ground oats. Stir until mixed.

Drop by teaspoon onto prepared roasting trays and press down with a fork. (Dip fork in water after each cookie to prevent sticking.) Top with a walnut or pecan half.

Bake for about 20 minutes, until browned.

Food Babe's Coconut Creamsicle Berry Pops

By Vani Hari, FoodBabe.com

Be sure to use pure coconut milk—canned or fresh—to make these luscious popsicles.

Prep Time: 5 minutes, plus 2 hours for freezing
Makes 4 pops

(cont.)

Ingredients:

1¼ cups coconut milk

½ cup mixed berries (you might want to dice the strawberries if they're big)

1 teaspoon orange zest

¼ cup freshly squeezed orange juice

2 tablespoons maple syrup, coconut nectar, or honey

Pinch of sea salt

Directions:

Place all ingredients into a large pitcher or bowl and mix well to combine.

Fill popsicle molds to the top and place popsicle sticks in the molds. Freeze for at least 2 hours, or overnight. Enjoy!

Baked Apples and Cashew Cream

By Jenny Brewer, nourishingnutrition.com

This creamy, sweet apple dessert is so fabulous you'll want to make enough for leftovers! Apples are a good source of vitamin C and healthy fibers, like pectin.

Prep Time: 15 minutes

Cook Time: 30 minutes

Serves 4

Ingredients:

6 dates, pitted and soaked in hot water for at least 10 minutes

1½ tablespoons coconut oil

1½ teaspoons cinnamon

Pinch of salt (optional)

4 baking apples, like Honeycrisp or Fuji, washed and cored, leaving bottoms intact to hold in date mixture

Directions:

Preheat oven to 375°F.

Place dates, coconut oil, cinnamon, and salt into a food processor and puree until dates are completely broken down and mixture is combined.

Fill the cavity of each apple with the date mixture. Stand the apples in a shallow baking dish. Add enough water to measure about ½ inch from the bottom of the pan. Bake for about 30 minutes, until apples are tender but still hold their shape.

Serve with a large dollop of cashew cream (recipe follows).

Cashew Cream

Prep Time: 35 minutes
Makes about 1 cup

Ingredients:

1 cup raw unsalted cashews, soaked at least 30 minutes (the longer the better—ideally overnight)
¼ cup water or unsweetened nondairy milk (milk makes it creamier)
1 tablespoon maple syrup
1 teaspoon vanilla extract

Directions:

Drain and rinse cashews. Place in a food processor and pulse until cashews are a fine consistency. With motor running, add remaining ingredients and continue processing until mixture is creamy, stopping to scrape sides as needed. Add more liquid if needed to achieve desired consistency. Taste and add additional maple syrup if desired. Serve spooned atop baked apples.

Store any leftover cream in the refrigerator and eat within 5 days. It is wonderful on a variety of fruits and stirred into porridge.

Turmeric Milk

By Kris Carr, Crazy Sexy Juice: 100 Simple Juice, Smoothie & Nut Milk Recipes to Supercharge Your Health, KrisCarr.com

Turmeric has incredible anti-inflammatory properties. This golden turmeric milk can be served cold, or warmed for a bedtime treat.

Prep Time: 10 minutes
Serves 3 to 4

(cont.)

Ingredients:

3 cups almond milk

½ cup canned coconut milk (full or reduced fat)

1½ teaspoons turmeric powder or 1-inch piece fresh turmeric root, peeled

½-inch piece ginger, peeled

½ teaspoon ground cinnamon

¼ teaspoon ground cardamom

2 tablespoons maple syrup

Directions:

Place all ingredients in a blender and blend until smooth. Serve immediately or store in an airtight container in the fridge for up to 4 days.

FOOD REVOLUTION
MEAL PLAN

Following this five-day meal plan will help you start your Food Revolution strong! You'll find expanded meal plans online, complete with shopping lists and chef tips for making your time in the kitchen more efficient and enjoyable, at 31dayfoodrevolution.com/mealpan.

Food Revolution Meal Plan

	Day 1	Day 2	Day 3	Day 4	Day 5
Breakfast	My Beloved(s) Smoothie*	Blueberry Chia Porridge*	Porridge with cinnamon, raisins, walnuts, and banana	Millet Cereal with Apple-Apricot Compote and Warm Coconut Milk*	Oyster Mushroom Frittata*
Lunch	Green salad with dressing of choice, an avocado, and your favorite crackers	Kale Salad with Apples and Dried Cherries* and leftover Corn Chowder*	Leftover Kale Salad* with your favorite cracker, topped with Deo's Cashew Cream Cheeze*, sliced tomato, and spices	Green salad topped with leftover Quinoa and Walnuts* and dressing of choice	Leftover Black Thai Peas*
Dinner	Corn Chowder*	Quinoa with Walnuts* and Deo's Delicious Greens*	Creamy Carrot Soup* (sprinkle with toasted pumpkin seeds)	Black Thai Peas* with a baked sweet potato	Hemp Seed Caesar Salad* topped with Marinated Tempeh*
Snack Ideas	Apple slices with almond or peanut butter	Celery with Deo's Cashew Cream Cheeze*	Leftover Blueberry Chia Porridge*	Carrots with Deo's Cashew Cream Cheeze* or nut butter	Mighty Carrot Raisin Muffins*

* Recipe found in this book

Acknowledgments

My gratitude goes to my beloved life partner, Phoenix, who has nurtured, challenged, loved, and inspired me for 24 years (and we're just getting started!). You are the greatest miracle in my life. To my twin sons, River and Bodhi, who humble and amaze me, and who have taught me so much about who I am, what I value, and what truly matters.

I am so infinitely grateful to my dad, John—my colleague and one of my dearest friends, who has blazed a trail that's inspired millions (including me!), and my mom, Deo, whom I consider to be the most loving human I've ever known.

Gratitude to my agent, Doug Abrams, and to Lara Love Hardin and the whole team at Idea Architects for your brilliant partnership in bringing this book to manifestation. Huge thanks to my extraordinary Idea Architects developmental editor, Katherine Vaz. Your keen insights and steady support were exquisite and fundamental. Readers have you to thank for helping to shape, clarify, and polish every page.

And deep appreciation to Karen Murgolo and everyone at Grand Central for believing in me, and in this book, and for your support and commitment to our shared mission.

I'm thankful to Dr. Joel Fuhrman, Jennifer Brewer, Lauren Kretzer, AnnMarie Roth, Emily Honeycutt, Stacey Murphy, Kris Carr, Sage Lavine, Dr. Susan Peirce Thompson, and Ryan Eliason for your potent insights, your steady guidance, and your editorial support.

Thank you to Michael Carwile, Sierra Kohlruss, and the whole team at Food Revolution Network for your partnership in changing this world. I particularly want to thank Alysha Vandergriff, Amy Smith, Carly Verble, Carrie Weaver, Chelsea Chapman, Emily Cohn, Gregg Boggs, Janna Fackrell, Jon More, Kaia Alexander, Liana Minassian, Lindsay Oberst, Lionel Church, Mark Romero, Rachel Chernick, Sarah Warbuck, Stefan Vintila, Veronica Monet, Victoria Carwile, and Zach

Edwards. You've all brought immense talent, passion, and dedication to our shared endeavors, and I am forever grateful.

Thanks to Amie Hamlin, Angela D'Amico, Anne Swan, Aryana and Aaran Solh, Carol Brinkman, Craig Watts, Dorothy Prabhu, Emily Iaconelli, Francine Regan-Pollock, Gina Lemos, Ginny Trierweiler, Heather Fleming, Kate McGoey-Smith, Mabel Pais, Marianne Bradley-Kopec, Dr. Pat Spensley, Paul Figueroa, Rhonda Hogan, Ron Finley, Sarah Medlicott, Shannon Briggs, and Stephanie Prima for sharing so generously of your stories and your wisdom.

Thank you to all the generous recipe contributors, including Ann and Dr. Caldwell Esselstyn, Brenda Davis, Caryn Hartglass, Dr. David Perlmutter, Dr. Dean Ornish, Deo Robbins, Francis Moore Lappé, Gary De Mattei, Holly Yzquierdo, Jason Wyrick, Jenny Brewer, Jessica Meyers Altman, Dr. Joel Fuhrman, John Robbins, Kris Carr, Mark Bittman, Dr. Mark Hyman, Michael Pollan, Dr. Neal Barnard, Phoenix Robbins, Rip Esselstyn, and Vani Hari.

Thanks to my generous book support team for your honest feedback and caring attention, helping to advise and advance the shaping of this book. I'm especially grateful to Alice Helscher, Anne Becker, Anne Meng, Barb Dennis, Bettie Banks, Cecilia Jones, Claire Zammit, Delisa Renideo, Francine Regan-Pollock, Gail Cooper, Kari Hamerschlag, Kathleen Elliot, Kathy Bottroff, Leonny Priest, Lily Clair, Sarah Higdon, Sheila Clark-Edmands, Stella Montane, Stephanie Prima, Veronica Monet, Yvonne Williams-McMillan, Zoe Putnam, and everyone else who has given so abundantly of your time and your attention.

And thank you to you, dear reader, for caring about what you eat, and about how it impacts your health and your planet. Together, one bite at a time, we are shifting the course of food history and taking a stand for the health that we and our world deserve.

Converting to Metrics

Volume Measurement Conversions

Cups	Tablespoons	Teaspoons	Milliliters
		1 tsp	5 ml
1/16 cup	1 tbsp	3 tsp	15 ml
1/8 cup	2 tbsp	6 tsp	30 ml
¼ cup	4 tbsp	12 tsp	50 ml
1/3 cup	5 1/3 tbsp	16 tsp	75 ml
½ cup	8 tbsp	24 tsp	125 ml
2/3 cup	10 2/3 tbsp	32 tsp	150 ml
¾ cup	12 tbsp	36 tsp	150 ml
1 cup	16 tbsp	48 tsp	250 ml

Weight Conversion Measurements

US	Metric
1 ounce	28.4 grams (g)
8 ounces	227.5 g
16 ounces (1 pound)	455 g

Cooking Temperature Conversions

Celsius/Centigrade	$F = (C \times 1.8) + 32$
Fahrenheit	$C = (F-32) \times 0.5555$

Zero degrees Celsius and 100°C are arbitrarily placed at the melting and boiling points of water, while Fahrenheit establishes 0°F as the stabilized temperature when equal amounts of ice, water, and salt are mixed. So, for example, if you are baking at 350°F and want to know that temperature in Celsius, the following calculation will provide it: $C = (350-32) \times 0.5555 = 176.66°C$.

Organizations Doing Good

BUY HEALTHY FOOD

- **Thrive Market** (31dayfoodrevolution.com/thrive) is an American membership-based e-commerce retailer offering nonperishable natural and organic food products at reduced costs.
- **Local Harvest** (localharvest.org/csa/) provides a directory of community-supported agriculture (CSA) programs in the United States.
- **Eat Well Guide** (eatwellguide.org) offers a searchable (and growing) database of more than 25,000 hand-picked restaurants, farms, markets and other sources of local, sustainable food.
- **International Community Supported Agriculture Network** (urgenci.net) brings together citizens, small farmers, consumers, and activists to spread sustainable agriculture programs worldwide.

GROW HEALTHY FOOD

- **Food Not Lawns** (foodnotlawns.com) is a network of gardeners and activists sharing food, seeds, tools, land, skills, and other resources in neighborhood-based, friendship-driven communities.
- **Socially Responsible Agriculture Project** (sraproject.org) helps communities stand up to factory farms, and helps farmers transition to more sustainable and humane farming systems.
- **Tower Garden** (towergarden.com) is a vertical growing system that can incorporate containers filled with potting mix or can function as a hydroponic or aeroponic system.

- **Food Is Free Project** (foodisfreeproject.org) teaches people how to connect with their neighbors and line their street with front-yard community gardens, providing free harvests to anyone. More than 300 cities around the world have started Food Is Free Projects in elementary schools, community arts spaces, churches, and small businesses.
- **Grow Your Own Vegetables** (31dayfoodrevolution.com /garden) provides online courses and trainings to help backyard gardeners succeed.

SPREAD HEALTHY FOOD

- **Wholesome Wave** (wholesomewave.org) is a nonprofit that secures funding to double the value of food stamps when used to purchase fruits and vegetables. They're serving more than 500,000 people and 1,400 farmer's markets in 49 U.S. states (and counting!). Find out if they're in your community, or make a donation, at the website above.
- **Opportunity International** (opportunity.org) provides micro-credit loans to help millions of people worldwide start businesses and climb out of poverty. Ninety-five percent of their loans go to women, and they boast a 99 percent loan repayment rate. They have a vibrant agricultural loan portfolio that helps build food security and sustainability.
- **Planting Justice** (plantingjustice.org) empowers people impacted by mass social inequality with the skills and resources to cultivate food sovereignty, economic justice, and community healing. With a focus on jobs and healthy food, they operate an organic nursery that ships more than 1,100 plants across the U.S., and train budding community leaders to grow, harvest, and prepare healthy food.
- **Food Empowerment Project** (foodispower.org) seeks to create a more just and sustainable world by providing education and advocacy for healthy food in the communities that need it most.
- **Trees for the Future** (31dayfoodrevolution.com/trees) has planted more than 145 million trees in dozens of countries and revitalized hundreds of thousands of acres of soil while improving the lives of

people in thousands of communities. They focus on organic fruit and nut trees, providing a healthy source of nourishment for generations to come. Food Revolution Network works with them to fund the planting of a fruit or nut tree for every product sold (including every copy of this book!).

KEEP ON LEARNING

- **NutritionFacts.org**, founded by Michael Greger, MD, provides thousands of educational videos and articles offering seasoned advice on the major food issues of our times.
- **Physician's Committee for Responsible Medicine** (pcrm .org), founded by Neal Barnard, MD, provides research-backed education and potent advocacy for nutrition and research.
- **ChrisBeatCancer.com** is the online portal set up by cancer survivor turned natural health educator Chris Wark. When someone I love is facing cancer and asking for guidance, this is usually the first place I send them.
- **Ornish.com** offers a treasure trove of free guidance and information from one of the world's leading lifestyle medicine experts.
- **DrFuhrman.com**, founded by bestselling *Eat to Live* author Joel Fuhrman, MD, offers personalized guidance for vitamins and supplements, recipes, and a vast library of knowledge on how you can leverage excellent nutrition for lasting wellness.
- **The Truth About Cancer** (thetruthaboutcancer.com) provides outside-the-box resources for natural and alternative approaches to cancer treatment, prevention, causes, and solutions.

LIFESTYLE APPLICATION

- **Forks Over Knives** (forksoverknives.com) provides a whole-foods, plant-based online cooking school and meal planner to help you put the lessons from the wildly popular film series into action.
- **Green Smoothie Girl** (greensmoothiegirl.com) provides courses, trainings, and seminars to support detoxification, micronutrient saturation, and overall health.

- **Crazy Sexy Wellness** (kriscarr.com) was founded by bestselling author and "cancer thriver" Kris Carr. Kris provides wellness tips, nutritional guidance, and inspirational wisdom to help you live with passion, purpose, and vitality.
- **Well.org**, founded by Dr. Pedram Shojai, provides a suite of programs, trainings, films, and other resources to support a healthy body, inner peace, global sustainability, and a conscious and healthy economy.
- **Bright Line Eating** (brightlineeating.com) was founded by Susan Peirce Thompson, PhD, with the simple goal of ending the obesity epidemic forever. Take her quiz at 31dayfoodrevolution .com/foodquiz to find out if you're addicted to food and how you can apply her breakthrough insights.

EDUCATION AND ADVOCACY

- **American College of Lifestyle Medicine** (lifestylemedicine .org) offers training, certifications, and support to help health care professionals leverage food and lifestyle on behalf of their patients' health.
- **Foodbabe.com**, founded by bestselling author Vani Hari, investigates food industry shenanigans and offers articles and guides for healthy dining, healthy shopping, and menu planning to keep your family safe and well.
- **Center for Food Safety** (centerforfoodsafety.org) is at the forefront of organizing a powerful food movement that's fighting the industrial model and promoting organic, ecological, and sustainable alternatives. They offer education for the public, and have a staff of two dozen attorneys standing up for safe food for all.
- **Environmental Working Group** (ewg.org) provides breakthrough research and education to drive informed consumer choice and civic action.
- **Organic Consumers Association** (organicconsumers.org) mobilizes consumers for the integrity and growth of organic agriculture, and for children's health, corporate accountability, fair trade, and environmental sustainability.

- **Green America** (greenamerica.org) seeks to harness the strength of consumers, investors, businesses, and the marketplace to create a socially just and environmentally sustainable society. They bridge conscious consumers with ethical businesses to support a clean, green, vibrant economy.
- **Roots & Shoots** (rootsandshoots.org), founded by Jane Goodall, PhD, offers tools, community, and support to help young people of all ages launch initiatives that change the world for the better.
- **Mercy For Animals** (mercyforanimals.org) is on the front lines of the movement to expose animal cruelty and to protect farmed animals. From factory farms to corporate boardrooms, courts of justice to courts of public opinion, Mercy For Animals speaks up against cruelty and stands for compassion.

Endnotes

FOREWORD

1. See K. Northstone, C. Joinson, P. Emmett, et al., "Are Dietary Patterns in Childhood Associated with IQ at 8 Years of Age? A Population-Based Cohort Study," *Journal of Epidemiology and Community Health* 66, no. 7 (2012): 624–28; D. B. Jackson and K. M. Beaver, "The Role of Adolescent Nutrition and Physical Activity in the Prediction of Verbal Intelligence During Early Adulthood: A Genetically Informed Analysis of Twin Pairs," *International Journal of Environmental Research and Public Health* 12, no. 1 (2015): 385–401; and K. M. Purtell and E. T. Gershoff, "Fast Food Consumption and Academic Growth in Late Childhood," *Clinical Pediatrics* 54, no. 9 (2015): 871–77.
2. T. N. Akbaraly, E. J. Brunner, J. E. Ferrie, et al., "Dietary Pattern and Depressive Symptoms in Middle Age," *British Journal of Psychiatry* 195, no. 5 (2009): 408–13.
3. S. C. Moore, L. M. Carter, and S. van Goozen, "Confectionery Consumption in Childhood and Adult Violence," *British Journal of Psychiatry* 195 (2009): 366–67; M. B. Liester and J. D. Moore-Liester, "Is Sugar a Gateway Drug?," *Journal of Drug Abuse* 1, no. 1 (2015): 8.
4. See, respectively, S. M. Booker, "Headliners: Maternal Nutrition and Child Cancer: Mother's Pre-pregnancy Diet May Influence Child Cancer Risk," *Environmental Health Perspectives* 112, no. 15 (2004): A877; M. R. Keleher, R. Zaidi, S. Shah, et al., "Maternal High-Fat Diet Associated with Altered Gene Expression, DNA Methylation, and Obesity Risk in Mouse Offspring," *PLoS ONE* 13, no. 2 (2018): e0192606; University of Granada, "Diet During Pregnancy and Early Life May Affect Children's Behavior and Intelligence," *ScienceDaily*, September 13, 2013.
5. "Obesity and Cancer," National Cancer Institute, 2017.
6. C. A. Thomson, T. E. Crane, D. O. Garcia, et al., "Association Between Dietary Energy Density and Obesity-Associated Cancer: Results from the Women's Health Initiative," *Journal of the Academy of Nutrition and Dietetics* 118, no. 4 (2018): 617–26.
7. A. Sánchez-Villegas, E. Toledo, J. de Irala, et al., "Fast-Food and Commercial Baked Goods Consumption and the Risk of Depression," *Public Health Nutrition* 15, no. 3 (2011): 424.
8. S. Mahabir, "Association Between Diet During Preadolescence and Adolescence and Risk for Breast Cancer During Adulthood," *Journal of Adolescent Health* 52, no. 5 (2013): S30–S35.
9. M. A. Makary and M. Daniel, "Medical Error—The Third Leading Cause of Death in the US," *BMJ* 353 (2016): i2139.

INTRODUCTION

1. Aaron Foley, "City of Detroit Hits Record Unemployment Rate: Almost 30 Percent," *MLive*, August 28, 2009.

2. Tom Philpott, "From Motown to Growtown: The Greening of Detroit," *Grist*, August 25, 2010.

3. Stephanie Held, "10 Detroit Urban Farms Rooting Goodness into the City," *Daily Detroit*, July 6, 2015.

CHAPTER 1

1. "Food Availability (Per Capita) Data System," U.S. Department of Agriculture, last updated 2017.

2. Sharon Basaraba, "Protein Needs for People over 70," VeryWell Fit, April 17, 2018.

3. Sophie Egan, "How Much Protein Do We Need," *New York Times*, July 28, 2017.

4. "EFSA Sets Population Reference Intakes for Protein," European Food Safety Authority, February 9, 2012.

5. "2018 Protein Powder Study," Clean Label Project.

6. I. Delimaris, "Adverse Effects Associated with Protein Intake Above the Recommended Dietary Allowance for Adults," *ISRN Nutrition* 13 (July 2013): http://dx.doi .org/10.5402/2013/126929.

7. M. E. Levine et al., "Low Protein Intake Is Associated with a Major Reduction in IGF-1, Cancer, and Overall Mortality in the 65 and Younger But Not Older Population," *Cell Metabolism* 19, no. 3 (2014): 407–17.

CHAPTER 2

1. J. Hallmayer et al., "Genetic Heritability and Shared Environmental Factors Among Twin Pairs with Autism," *Archives of General Psychiatry* 68, no. 11 (2011): 1095–1102.

2. Hannah Furfaro, "Children of Smart Fathers Have Higher Risk of Autism," *Scientific American*, May 14, 2017.

3. Carey Reed, "Genius and Autism May Share Genetic Link, Study Finds," *PBS*, May 2, 2015.

4. Keith Matheny, "Can Men Pass Exposure to PBBs to Kids? Emory U. Study Seeks Volunteers," *Detroit Free Press*, March 12, 2018.

5. "Birth Defects and Environmental Causes," Oshman & Mirisola, LLP, 2018.

6. M. J. Carvan III et al., "Mercury-Induced Epigenetic Transgenerational Inheritance of Abnormal Neurobehavior Is Correlated with Sperm Epimutations in Zebrafish," *PLoS ONE* 12, no. 5 (2017): e0176155.

7. D. Zeevi et al., "Personalized Nutrition by Prediction of Glycemic Responses," *Cell* 163, no. 5 (2015): 1079–94.

CHAPTER 3

1. "Dietary Risks Are Leading Cause of Disease Burden in the US and Contributed to More Health Loss in 2010 than Smoking, High Blood Pressure, and High Blood Sugar," Institute for Health Metrics and Evaluation, July 10, 2013.

2. Ibid.

3. See M. Mekonnen and A. Hoekstra, "A Global Assessment of the Water Footprint of Farm Animal Products," *Ecosystems* 15 (2012): 401–15; "How Does Meat in the Diet Take an Environmental Toll?," *Scientific American*; and Food and Agriculture Organization of the United Nations, *Livestock's Long Shadow—Environmental Issues and Options* (Rome: 2006).

4. For diabetes, see Jonathan Shaw, "A Diabetes Link to Meat," *Harvard Magazine*, January–February 2012. For Alzheimer's, see W. B. Grant, "Using Multicountry Ecological and Observational Studies to Determine Dietary Risk Factors for Alzheimer's Disease," *Journal of the American College of Nutrition* 35, no 5 (2016): 476–89. For cancer, see V. Bouvard et al., "Carcinogenicity of Consumption of Red and Processed Meat," International Agency for Research on Cancer Monograph Working Group, *Lancet Oncology*, October 2015.

CHAPTER 4

1. See "The Industry," Natural Foods Investor; *Natural and Organic Foods in the U.S., 5th Edition.*
2. "European Organic Market Growth in Double Digits," Fresh Plaza, February 16, 2017.
3. Nicole Pierce, "Organic Food Companies Who Sold Out to Mega Food Corporations," Trace Botanicals, January 19, 2016.
4. "Amazon Plans to Buy Whole Foods: What Does This Mean for the Future of Food?," Food Revolution Network, June 21, 2017.
5. Katherine Paul and Ronnie Cummins, "Here's How to Boycott Organic Imposters," Organic Consumers Association, July 21, 2017.
6. Ben Blatt, "Unacceptable Ingredients," Slate.com, February 18, 2014.
7. "Unacceptable Ingredients for Food," Whole Foods Market.
8. Amy Lebrock, "Good Growth: Farmers Markets Still On the Rise," *Sustainable America Blog*, August 6, 2014.
9. Diane Quagliani, "Survey Reveals Farmers Market Growth Trends," Progressive Grocer, August 24, 2015.
10. European CSA Research Group, *Overview of Community Supported Agriculture in Europe*, May 2016.
11. "Celeriac: This Ugly Root Is a Superfood for Cleansing Your Kidneys," Juicing for Health, November 22, 2017.
12. Jason Mathers, "Is Online Shopping Better for the Environment?," Environmental Defense Fund, December 21, 2013.

CHAPTER 5

1. For European data, see "The Challenge of Obesity in the WHO European Region and the Strategies for Response," World Health Organization, 2007. For American data, see Christopher J. L. Murray, "The Vast Majority of Americans Are Overweight or Obese, and Weight Is a Growing Problem Among US Children," Institute for Health Metrics and Evaluation.
2. Sarah Schmidt, "U.S. Weight Loss & Diet Industry: Stuck in Survival Mode?," Market Research Blog, January 23, 2017.
3. "Obesity: 'Slim Chance' of Return to Normal Weight," *BBC News*, July 17, 2015.
4. L. Yazdanpanah et al., "Literature Review on the Management of Diabetic Foot Ulcer," *World Journal of Diabetes* 6, no. 1 (2015): 37–53.
5. Jordan Gaines Lewis, "What Happens to Your Brain When You Give Up Sugar," *Chicago Tribune*, March 1, 2015.
6. Alyssa Raiola, "Here's Exactly How Many Pounds (!) of Sugar Americans Eat in a Year," *Greatist*, December 19, 2016.
7. "What Is Food Addiction?" Food Addiction Institute.

CHAPTER 6

1. "Key Safety Questions About Teflon Nonstick Coatings," Chemours.
2. "Healthy Home Tip 6: (Still) Skipping the Nonstick," Environmental Working Group, November 12, 2009.
3. Susan Chamberlain, "Bird-Safe Cookware: Is There a Killer in Your Kitchen?," Petcha.
4. Steve Dale, "Fatal Fumes," *Chicago Tribune*, March 26, 1995.
5. Kamal Patel, "Are Cast Iron Pans Unsafe?," Examine.com, December 12, 2017.
6. Matthew Hoffman, "Pots, Pans, and Plastics: A Shopper's Guide to Food Safety," WebMD, December 19, 2008.
7. For diabetes and obesity, see Fiona Macdonald, "BPA Exposure Has Been Linked to an Increase in Diabetes and Obesity," Science Alert, September 29, 2015. For heart disease, see Daniel J. DeNoon, "BPA May Be Linked to Heart Disease Risk," WebMD, January 12, 2010. For asthma, see Mandy Oaklander, "The Link Between Asthma and This Chemical," Time Health, October 7, 2014. For cancer and reproductive problems, see A. Konieczna et al., "Health Risk of Exposure to Bisphenol A (BPA)," *Roczniki Panstwowego Zakladu Higieny* 66, no. 1 (2015): 5–11. For liver problems, see K. M. Min et al., "Bisphenol A Impairs Mitochondrial Function in the Liver at Doses Below the No Observed Adverse Effect Level," *Journal of Korean Medical Science* 27, no. 6 (2012): 644–52. For ADHD, see S. Tewar et al., "Association of Bisphenol A Exposure and Attention-Deficit/ Hyperactivity Disorder in a National Sample of U.S. Children," *Environmental Research* 150 (2016): 112–18.
8. C. Z. Yang et al., "Most Plastic Products Release Estrogenic Chemicals: A Potential Health Problem That Can Be Solved," *Environmental Health Perspectives* 119 (2011): 989–96.
9. "Global WASH Fast Facts," Centers for Disease Control and Prevention, April 11, 2016.
10. M. T. Do et al., "Chlorination Disinfection By-Products and Pancreatic Cancer," *Environmental Health Perspectives* 113, no. 4 (2005): 418–24.
11. R. D. Morris et al., "Drinking Water and Cancer," *Environmental Health Perspectives* 103, no. 8S (1995): 225–31.
12. BioMed Central/Environmental Health, "Drinking Tap Water Disinfected with Chlorine May Harm Fetus, Study Suggests," *ScienceDaily*, June 5, 2008.
13. Joseph Hattersley, "Chlorine on Tap: Don't Drink It," What Doctors Don't Tell You, February 2004.
14. "Flint Water Crisis Fast Facts," CNN Library, April 8, 2018.
15. Darryl Fears, "It's Not Just Flint. Lead Taints Water Across the U.S., EPA Records Show," *Washington Post*, March 17, 2016.
16. Olivia Kelly, "The 20 Dublin Homes with the Highest Levels of Lead in Water," *Irish Times*, May 5, 2015.
17. Esa Nummi, "An Update on the 'Lead-Free by 2014' Mandate—Europe," ThermoFisher Scientific, September 29, 2015.
18. David Andrews and Bill Walker, "Erin Brockovich Carcinogen in Tap Water of More Than 200 Million Americans," EWG.org, September 20, 2016.
19. "Drugs in the Drinking Water? Don't Ask and Officials Won't Tell," Food Revolution Network, March 25, 2016.
20. Sandra Laville and Matthew Taylor, "A Million Bottles a Minute: World's Plastic Binge 'As Dangerous as Climate Change'," *Guardian*, June 28, 2017; "Global Bottled Water Market to Reach $280 Billion by 2020," Water Quality Products, September 21, 2016.

21. H. H. Le et al., "Bisphenol A Is Released from Polycarbonate Drinking Bottles and Mimics the Neurotoxic Actions of Estrogen in Developing Cerebellar Neurons," *Toxicology Letters* 176, no. 2 (2008): 149–56.

22. Laville and Taylor, "A Million Bottles a Minute."

CHAPTER 7

1. "America's $165 Billion Food-Waste Problem," *CNBC*, April 22, 2015.

2. "Food Waste: Britons Are Worst Offenders in Europe," *Week UK* August 12, 2015.

3. "12 Ways to Save Big on Groceries and Shop on a Budget," My Money Coach.

PART 2: Nourish

1. K. Adams, W. S. Butsch, and M. Kohlmeier, "The State of Nutrition Education at US Medical Schools," *Journal of Biomedical Education* 2015: http://dx.doi.org/10.1155/2015/357627.

CHAPTER 8

1. P. Anand et al., "Cancer Is a Preventable Disease That Requires Major Lifestyle Changes," *Pharmaceutical Research* 25, no. 9 (2008): 2097–2116.

2. David Chan, "Where Do the Millions of Cancer Research Dollars Go Every Year?," *Slate*, February 7, 2013.

3. Kimberly Leonard, "Global Cancer Spending Reaches $100 Billion," *US News and World Report*, May 5, 2015.

4. American Institute for Cancer Research, *The AICR 2015 Cancer Awareness Survey Report*, 2015.

5. Rick Mullin, "Cost to Develop New Pharmaceutical Drug Now Exceeds $2.5 Billion," *Scientific American*, November 24, 2014.

6. "Food Fight! The Association vs. the Institute," Block Center, April 28, 2014.

7. Kat Kinsman, "Activists Call Foul on KFC Bucket Campaign," *CNN*, April 28, 2010.

8. John Robbins, "Greed, Cancer and Pink KFC Buckets," *Huffington Post*, May 17, 2010.

9. "Chemicals in Meat Cooked at High Temperatures and Cancer Risk," National Cancer Institute, July 11, 2017.

10. Anand et al., "Cancer Is a Preventable Disease."

11. "Eating Mushrooms Daily 'May Cut Breast Cancer Risk by Two Thirds,'" *Telegraph*, March 16, 2009.

12. M. Zhang et al., "Dietary Intake of Mushrooms and Green Tea Combine to Reduce the Risk of Breast Cancer in Chinese Women," *International Journal of Cancer* 124, no. 6 (2009): 1404–8.

13. Joel Fuhrman, "Mighty Mushrooms: Boost Immune Function and Guard Against Cancer," Dr. Fuhrman, May 31, 2017.

14. S. Patel and A. Goyal, "Recent Developments in Mushrooms as Anti-Cancer Therapeutics: A Review," *3 Biotech* 2, no. 1 (2012): 1–15.

15. Fuhrman, "Mighty Mushrooms."

16. Eric Metcalf, "The Anti-Cancer Diet: Foods That Prevent Cancer," Everyday Health.

17. Linus Pauling Institute, "Cruciferous Vegetables," April 2017, Oregon State University.

18. J. V. Higdon et al., "Cruciferous Vegetables and Human Cancer Risk: Epidemiologic Evidence and Mechanism Basis," *Pharmacological Research* 55, no. 3 (2007): 224–36.

19. "Celery First Used as a Medicine," Texas AgriLife Extension Service.

20. S. Madhusudhan, "7 Incredible Benefits of Celery in Fighting the Risk of Cancer," NDTV Food, January 23, 2017.

21. Christina Sarich, "Compound in Celery Found to Destroy 86% of Lung Cancer Cells," Natural Society, September 28, 2014.

22. E. J. Choi and G. H. Kim, "Apigenin Induces Apoptosis Through a Mitochondria/Caspase-Pathway in Human Breast Cancer MDA-MB-453 Cells," *Journal of Clinical Biochemistry and Nutrition* 44, no. 3 (2009): 260–65.

23. X. Pan et al., "Effect of Apigenin on Proliferation and Apoptosis of Human Lung Cancer NCI-H460 Cells," *Nan Fang Yi Ke Da Xue Xue Bao (Journal of Southern Medical University)* 33, no. 8 (2013): 1137–40.

24. J. H. Lee et al., "Anti-inflammatory Mechanisms of Apigenin: Inhibition of Cyclooxygenase-2 Expression, Adhesion of Monocytes to Human Umbilical Vein Endothelial Cells, and Expression of Cellular Adhesion Molecules," *Archives of Pharmacal Research* 30, no. 10 (2007): 1318–27.

25. D. Y. Lim et al., "Luteolin Decreases IGF-II Production and Downregulates Insulin-Like Growth Factor-I Receptor Signaling in HT-29 Human Colon Cancer Cells," *BMC Gastroenterology* 12 (2012): 9.

26. V. Elangovan et al., "Chemopreventive Potential of Dietary Bioflavonoids Against 20-Methylcholanthrene-Induced Tumorgenesis," *Cancer Letters* 87, no. 1 (1994): 107–13.

27. Shubra Krishan, "11 Super Health Benefits in Just One Celery Stalk," Care 2; "Celery and Celery Seed Are Powerful, Proven Healers," DoctorMurray.com.

CHAPTER 9

1. Michael Greshko, "How Many Cells Are in the Human Body—and How Many Are Microbes?," *National Geographic*, January 13, 2016.

2. M. Lyte, "Microbial Endocrinology in the Microbiome-Gut-Brain Axis: How Bacterial Production and Utilization of Neurochemicals Influence Behavior," *PLoS Pathogens* 9, no. 11 (2013): e1003726.

3. Jane Brody, "Unlocking the Secrets of the Microbiome," *New York Times*, November 6, 2017.

4. Rachel O'Regan, "What's the Link Between Sugar and Gut Health?," I Quit Sugar, April 10, 2017.

5. A. Moshfegh, J. Goldman, and L. Cleveland, "What We Eat in America, NHANES 2001–2002: Usual Nutrient Intakes from Food Compared to Dietary Reference Intakes," U.S. Department of Agriculture, Agricultural Research Service, 2005.

6. S. B. Eaton, "The Ancestral Human Diet: What Was It and Should It Be a Paradigm for Contemporary Nutrition?," *Proceedings of the Nutrition Society* 65, no. 1 (2006): 1–6.

7. For British data, see "Dietary Fibre," British Nutrition Foundation, January 2017. For U.S. data, see Kathleen Zelman, "Fiber: How Much Do You Need?," WebMD, April 7, 2016.

8. Martha Stewart, "4 Habits for a Healthy Gut," CNN Health, June 18, 2014.

9. For WHO, see International Agency for Research on Cancer, "IARC Monographs Volume 112: Evaluation of Five Organophosphate Insecticides and Herbicides," World Health Organization, March 20, 2015. For California, see Cheryl Hogue, "California to List Glyphosate as a Carcinogen," *Chemical and Engineering News*, July 3, 2017.

10. "Glyphosate Formulations and Their Use for the Inhibition of 5-Enolpyruvylshiki-mate-3-phosphate Synthase," Google Patents, August 30, 2002.

11. C. Benbrook, "Trends in Glyphosate Herbicide Use in the United States and Globally," *Environmental Sciences Europe* 28 (2016): 3.

12. "Monsanto Caught Ghostwriting Stanford University Hoover Institution Fellow's Published Work," *CBS SFBay Area,* August 4, 2017.

13. M. A. Faria, "Glyphosate, Neurological Diseases—and the Scientific Method," *Surgical Neurology International* 6 (2015): 132.

14. V. Tzin and G. Galili, "New Insights into the Shikimate and Aromatic Amino Acids Biosynthesis Pathways in Plants," *Molecular Plant* 3, no. 6 (2010): 956–72.

15. "IARC's Report on Glyphosate," Monsanto, April 21, 2017.

16. B. Cohn et al., "DDT Exposure in Utero and Breast Cancer," *Journal of Clinical Endocrinology & Metabolism* 100, no. 8 (2015): 2865–72.

17. "CDC: 4 out of 5 Americans Prescribed Antibiotics Each Year," *CBS News,* April 11, 2013.

18. Maryn McKenna, "The Coming Cost of Superbugs: 10 Million Deaths per Year," *Wired,* December 15, 2014.

19. Review on Antimicrobial Resistance, *Antimicrobial Resistance: Tackling a Crisis for the Health and Wealth of Nations,* 2014.

20. "Fact Sheet: Antibiotic Resistance," World Health Organization, February 5, 2018.

21. T. Van Boeckel et al., "Global Trends in Antimicrobial Use in Food Animals," *Proceedings of the National Academy of Sciences* 112, no. 18 (2015): 5649–54.

22. "CDC: 1 in 3 Antibiotic Prescriptions Unnecessary," Centers for Disease Control and Prevention, May 3, 2016.

23. Jane Brody, "Unlocking the Secrets of the Microbiome," *New York Times,* November 6, 2017.

24. "Probiotics," WebMD, July 18, 2017.

25. T. A. Tompkins, I. Mainville, and Y. Arcand, "The Impact of Meals on Probiotic Transit Through a Model of the Human Upper Gastrointestinal Tract," *Beneficial Microbes* 2, no. 4 (2011): 295–303.

26. K. Y. Park, J. K. Jeong, Y. E. Lee, and J. W. Daily III, "Health Benefits of Kimchi (Korean Fermented Vegetables) as a Probiotic Food," *Journal of Medicinal Food* 17, no. 1 (2014): 6–20.

27. "In 2018, Kombucha Is Getting Big—and Craftier," Well and Good, December 7, 2017.

28. D. Banerjee et al., "Comparative Healing Property of Kombucha Tea and Black Tea Against Indomethacin-Induced Gastric Ulceration in Mice: Possible Mechanism of Action," *Food & Function* 1, no. 3 (2010): 284–93.

29. P. Dipti et al., "Lead Induced Oxidative Stress: Beneficial Effects of Kombucha Tea," *Biomedical Environment Sciences* 16, no. 3 (2003): 276–82.

CHAPTER 11

1. "6 Scientifically Proven Fruits That Can Reverse Hair Loss," Natural Living Ideas, November 6, 2016.

2. Jessica Maki, "Berries Keep Your Brain Sharp," *Harvard Gazette,* April 26, 2012.

3. Catherine Pearson, "Cognitive Impairment Study Shows Berries Significantly Slow Degeneration," *Huffington Post,* April 26, 2012.

4. "World Alzheimer Report 2015 Reveals Global Cost of Dementia Set to Reach US $1 Trillion by 2018," Alzheimer's Disease International, August 25, 2015.

5. A. Cassidy et al., "High Anthocyanin Intake Is Associated with a Reduced Risk of Myocardial Infarction in Young and Middle-Aged Women," *Circulation* 127 (2013): 188–96.

6. Ruth Schuster, "Archaeologists Find 780,000-Year-Old Remains of Prehistoric Man's Meal," *Haaretz*, December 6, 2016.

7. Emilio Ros, "Health Benefits of Nut Consumption," *Nutrients* 2, no. 7 (2010): 652–82.

8. D. Jenkins et al., "Possible Benefit of Nuts in Type 2 Diabetes," *Journal of Nutrition* 138, no. 9 (2008): 1752S–56S.

9. Emily Esfahani Smith, "The Lovely Hill: Where People Live Longer and Happier," *Atlantic*, February 4, 2013.

10. M. Aldemir et al., "Pistachio Diet Improves Erectile Function Parameters and Serum Lipid Profiles in Patients with Erectile Dysfunction," *International Journal of Impotence Research* 23 (2011): 32–38.

11. "Worldwide Revenue of Pfizer's Viagra from 2003 to 2017 (in Million U.S. Dollars)," Statistica, February 2018.

12. "Food Allergy Facts and Statistics for the U.S.," Food Allergy Research and Education.

CHAPTER 12

1. Federation of American Societies for Experimental Biology, "Eating Green Leafy Vegetables Keeps Mental Abilities Sharp," *Science Daily*, March 30, 2015.

2. Richard Alleyne, "Spinach Boosts Muscle Strength, Just as Popeye Always Said," *Telegraph*, June 26, 2012.

3. A. Olsen, C. Ritz, L. Kramer, and P. Møller, "Serving Styles of Raw Snack Vegetables. What Do Children Want?," *Appetite* 59, no. 2 (2012): 556–62.

4. Emily Honeycutt, "How to Teach Your Kids to Love Healthy, Plant-Powered Foods (from a Mother Who Knows)," Food Revolution Network, July 7, 2017.

CHAPTER 13

1. "Cause of Death: Alzheimers-Dementia by Country," World Life Expectancy.

2. For dementia, see Y. Pu et al., "Dietary Curcumin Ameliorates Aging-Related Cerebrovascular Dysfunction Through the AMPK/Uncoupling Protein 2 Pathway," *Cellular Physiology and Biochemistry* 32, no. 5 (2013): 1167–77; and S. Mishra and K. Palanivelu, "The Effect of Curcumin (Turmeric) on Alzheimer's Disease: An Overview," *Annals of Indian Academy of Neurology* 11, no. 1 (2008): 13–19. For heavy metals, see W. Garcia-Nino and J. Pedraza-Chaverri, "Protective Effect of Curcumin Against Heavy Metals-Induced Liver Damage," *Food Chemisty Toxicology* no. 69 (2014): 182–201. For heart disease, see W. Wongcharoen and A. Phrommintikul, "The Protective Role of Curcumin in Cardiovascular Diseases," *International Journal of Cardiology* 133, no. 2 (2009): 145–51.

3. "Curcumin," UCLA Alzheimer Translation Center.

4. "Turmeric," Cancer Research UK, August 6, 2015.

5. K. A. Steinmetz et al., "Vegetables, Fruit, and Colon Cancer in the Iowa Women's Health Study," *American Journal of Epidemiology* 139, no. 1 (1994): 1–15.

6. H. Li et al., "An Intervention Study to Prevent Gastric Cancer by Micro-Selenium and Large Dose of Allitridum," *Chinese Medical Journal (English)* 117, no. 8 (2004): 1155–60.

7. E.A. Lissiman et al., "Garlic for the Common Cold," *Cochrane Database of Systematic Reviews* 11 (2014).

8. M. Maghbooli et al., "Comparison Between the Efficacy of Ginger and Sumatriptan in the Ablative Treatment of the Common Migraine," *Phytotherapy Research* 28, no. 3 (2014): 412–15.

9. Pasupuleti Visweswara Rao and Siew Hua Gan, "Cinnamon: A Multifaceted Medicinal Plant," *Evidence-Based Complementary and Alternative Medicine* 2014.

10. A. K. Maji and P. Banerji, "Phytochemistry and Gastrointestinal Benefits of the Medicinal Spice, Capsicum Annuum L. (Chilli): A Review," *Journal of Complementary and Integrative Medicine* 13, no. 2 (2016): 97–122.

11. C. Kang, "Gut Microbiota Mediates the Protective Effects of Dietary Capsaicin Against Chronic Low-Grade Inflammation and Associated Obesity Induced by High-Fat Diet," *mBio* 8, no. 3 (2017): e00470-17.

12. M. Chopan and B. Littenberg, "The Association of Hot Red Chili Pepper Consumption and Mortality: A Large Population-Based Cohort Study," *PloS ONE* 12, no. 1 (2017): e0169876.

CHAPTER 14

1. "Calories in Beverages: Salted Caramel Mocha with Nonfat Milk Without Whipped Cream," Calorie King.

2. Kris Gunnars, "Why Is Coffee Good for You? Here Are 7 Reasons," Authority Nutrition, April 30, 2018.

3. M. H. Eskelinen and M. Kivipelto, "Caffeine as a Protective Factor in Dementia and Alzheimer's Disease," *Journal of Alzheimer's Disease* 20, no. S1 (2010): S167–74.

4. M. H. Eskelinen et al., "Midlife Coffee and Tea Drinking and the Risk of Late-Life Dementia: A Population-Based CAIDE Study," *Journal of Alzheimer's Disease* 16, no. 1 (2009): 85–91.

5. "Starbucks, Others Must Carry Cancer Warning in California, Judge Rules," *CBS News*, March 30, 2018.

6. David Katz, "What You Need to Know About the Coffee Cancer Warning in California," *Vice News*, April 2, 2018.

7. Catherine Paddock, "Coffee Drinking May Halve Risk of Mouth and Throat Cancer," *Medical News Today*, December 12, 2012.

8. See, respectively, "Study: Coffee Reduces Uterine Cancer Risk," video, *CBS News*, May 3, 2010; American Association for Cancer Research, "Coffee Consumption Associated with Reduced Risk of Advanced Prostate Cancer," *ScienceDaily*, December 8, 2009; C. Holick et al., "Coffee, Tea, Caffeine Intake, and Risk of Adult Glioma in Three Prospective Cohort Studies," *Cancer Epidemiology, Biomarkers & Prevention* 19, no. 1 (2010): 39–47; Lund University, "Coffee May Protect Against Breast Cancer, Study Shows," *ScienceDaily*, April 25, 2008; Hannah Osborne, "Coffee Reduces Liver Cancer Risk," *Newsweek*, May 25, 2017; Gan Weng et al., "The Effect of Caffeine on Cisplatin-Induced Apoptosis of Lung Cancer Cells," *Experimental Hematology & Oncology* 4 (2015): 5; and Erikka Loftfield et al., "Coffee Drinking and Cutaneous Melanoma Risk in the NIH-AARP Diet and Health Study," *Journal of the National Cancer Institute* 107, no. 2 (2015).

9. Harvard T.H. Chan School of Public Health, "Increasing Daily Coffee Consumption May Reduce Type 2 Diabetes Risk," Harvard University.

10. S. Bidel et al., "Coffee Consumption and Risk of Total and Cardiovascular Mortality Among Patients with Type 2 Diabetes," *Diabetologia* 49, no. 11 (2006): 2618–26.

11. "Coffee Is Number One Source of Antioxidants," Phys.org, August 29, 2005.

12. "Does Caffeinated Coffee Have More Antioxidants than Decaffeinated Coffee?," Dr. Gourmet.

13. Lorenzo Emden, "Decaffeination 101: Four Ways to Decaffeinate Coffee," Coffee Confidential.

14. "The Economics of Coffee," PBS Independent Lens.

15. Garrett Oden, "Cold Brew Coffee—Everything You Need to Know," Coffee Brew Guides, September 28, 2015.

16. "Tea—A Brief History of the Nation's Favourite Beverage," UK Tea & Infusions Association.

17. "Green Tea Cancer Treatment," Cancer Tutor, February 26, 2017.

18. Chris Irvine, "Three Cups of Tea Can Cut Breast Cancer Risk by a Third," *Telegraph*, January 22, 2009; Laura Newcomer, "13 Reasons Tea Is Good for You," *Time*, September 4, 2012.

19. T. Murase et al., "Green Tea Extract Improves Endurance Capacity and Increases Muscle Lipid Oxidation in Mice," *American Journal of Physiology: Regulatory, Integrative, and Comparative Physiology* 288, no. 3 (2005): R708–15.

20. C. L. Shen et al., "Green Tea Polyphenols Benefits Body Composition and Improves Bone Quality in Long-Term High-Fat Diet-Induced Obese Rats," *Nutrition Research* 32, no. 6 (2012): 448–57.

21. D. Grassi et al., "Black Tea Consumption Dose-Dependently Improves Flow-Mediated Dilation in Healthy Males," *Journal of Hypertension* 27, no. 4 (2009): 774–81.

22. M. W. Ho, "Green Tea, the Elixir of Life?," Science in Society, January 7, 2018.

23. "Black Iced Tea with Lemon," Lipton.com.

24. World Health Organization, *Global Status Report on Alcohol and Health 2014*, May 12, 2014.

25. W. Y. Chen et al., "Moderate Alcohol Consumption During Adult Life, Drinking Patterns, and Breast Cancer Risk," *JAMA* 306, no. 17 (2011): 1884–90.

26. "17 Surprising Benefits of Grapes," Organic Facts, January 18, 2018.

27. See, respectively, "Not Just for the Heart, Red Wine Shows Promise as a Cavity Fighter," American Chemical Society, May 21, 2014; W. Dunn et al., "Modest Wine Drinking and Decreased Prevalence of Suspected Nonalcoholic Fatty Liver Disease," *Hepatology* 47, no. 6 (2008): 1947–54; A. Gea et al., "Alcohol Intake, Wine Consumption and the Development of Depression: The PREDIMED Study," *BMC Medicine* 11 (2013): 192; and E. J. Neafsey and M. A. Collins, "Moderate Alcohol Consumption and Cognitive Risk," *Neuropsychiatric Disease and Treatment* 7 (2011): 465–84.

28. "Foods That Fight Cancer: Grapes and Grape Juice," American Institute for Cancer Research.

29. "Resveratrol—Many Actions Against Cancer," CANCERactive.

30. C. Gupta et al., "Chemosensitization of Tumors by Resveratrol," *Annals of the New York Academy of Sciences* 1215, no. 1 (2011): 150–60.

31. "Moderate Red Wine Consumption May Reduce Prostate Cancer Risk," CABI, September 24, 2004.

32. "Resveratrol—Many Actions Against Cancer."

33. Katherine Zeratsky, "Does Grape Juice Offer the Same Heart Benefits as Red Wine?," Mayo Clinic, July 18, 2017.

34. Amanda Fiegl, "A Brief History of Chocolate," *Smithsonian*, March 1, 2008.

35. William J. Cromie, "Cocoa Shows Promise as Next Wonder Drug," *Harvard Gazette*, February 22, 2007.

36. Brierley Right, "11 Anti-Aging Drinks," Eating Well.

37. N. Hollenberg et al., "Flavanols, the Kuna, Cocoa Consumption, and Nitric Oxide," *Journal of the American Society of Hypertension* 3, no. 2 (2009): 105–12.

38. Linda Rao, "Dark Chocolate Can Pack a Big Antioxidant Wallop," *Prevention*, November 3, 2011.

39. I. Janszky et al., "Chocolate Consumption and Mortality Following a First Acute Myocardial Infarction: The Stockholm Heart Epidemiology Program," *Journal of Internal Medicine* 266, no. 3 (2009): 248–57.

40. "Cocoa, the Health Miracle," Medicine Hunter.

41. Michael Joseph, "Dark Chocolate vs. Milk Chocolate: Which Is Better?," Nutrition Advance, October 28, 2016.

42. "Cocoa Production in a Nutshell," Make Chocolate Fair.

43. Brian O'Keefe, "Inside Big Chocolate's Labor Problem," *Fortune*, March 1, 2016.

CHAPTER 15

1. "Staple Foods: What Do People Eat," FOA.org.

2. "Whole Grains," American Heart Association, May 1, 2017; "Nutrition and Healthy Eating," Mayo Clinic, July 18, 2017; "Whole Grains," European Food Information Council, July 9, 2015.

3. "What's Wrong with Grains," Paleo Hacks.

4. Jane Brody, "The Fats You Do Not Need to Fear, and the Carbs That You Do," *New York Times*, October 19, 2015.

5. For heart disease, see "Whole Grains and Fiber," American Heart Association. For gum disease, see T. Anwar et al., "Whole Grain and Fiber Intakes and Periodontis in Men," *American Journal of Clinical Nutrition* 83, no. 6 (2006): 1395–400.

6. "Foods That Fight Cancer: Whole Grains," American Institute for Cancer Research.

7. Sarah Knapton, "Daily Bowl of Quinoa Could Save Your Life, Says Harvard University," *Telegraph*, March 24, 2015.

8. Nancy Shute, "Gluten Goodbye: One-Third of Americans Say They Are Trying to Shun It," *NPR*, March 9, 2013.

9. Julie Upton, "Think You're Sensitive to Gluten? Think Again," *US News and World Report*, June 11, 2015.

10. A. Capannolo et al., "Non-Celiac Gluten Sensitivity Among Patients Perceiving Gluten-Related Symptoms," *Digestion* 92, no. 1 (2015): 8–13.

11. K. C. Maki et al., "Digestive and Physiologic Effects of a Wheat Bran Extract, Arabino-Xylan–Oligosaccharide, in Breakfast Cereal," *Nutrition* 28, no. 11-12 (2012): 1115–21.

12. N. Horiguchi, H. Horiguchi, and Y. Suzuki, "Effect of Wheat Gluten Hydrolysate on the Immune System in Healthy Human Subjects," *Bioscience, Biotechnology, and Biochemistry* 69, no. 12 (2005): 2445–49.

13. D. L. Jenkins et al., "Effect of Wheat Bran on Serum Lipids: Influence of Particle Size and Wheat Protein," *Journal of the American College of Nutrition* 18, no. 2 (1999): 159–65.
14. Ryan Andrews, "Phytates and Phytic Acid," Precision Nutrition.

CHAPTER 16

1. Peter Graham and Carroll Vance, "Legumes: Importance and Constraints to Greater Use," *Plant Physiology* 131, no. 3 (2003): 872–77.
2. University Health Center, "A High Fiber Diet," University of Maryland.
3. D. Aune et al., "Legume Intake and the Risk of Cancer: A Multisite Case-Control Study in Uruguay," *Cancer Causes Control* 20, no. 9 (2009): 1605–15.
4. James Gallagher, "Processed Meats Do Cause Cancer," *BBC News*, October 26, 2015.
5. "Foods That Fight Cancer: Dry Beans and Peas (Legumes)," American Institute for Cancer Research.
6. I. Darmadi-Blackberry, "Legumes: The Most Important Dietary Predictor of Survival in Older People of Different Ethnicities," *Asia Pacific Journal of Clinical Nutrition* 13, no. 2 (2004): 217–20.
7. Ryan Andrews, "Phytates and Phytic Acid," Precision Nutrition.
8. Steven Gundry, "15 Ways to Reduce Lectins in Your Diet," GundryMD, May 23, 2017.
9. Dan Buettner, "The Island Where People Forget to Die," *New York Times Magazine*, October 24, 2012.
10. James Hambin, "The Next Gluten," *Atlantic*, April 24, 2017.
11. Joe Leech, "Dietary Lectins: Everything You Need to Know," Healthline Authority Nutrition, April 1, 2015.
12. N. D. Noah, A. E. Bender, G. B. Reaidi, and R. J. Gilbert, "Food Poisoning from Raw Red Kidney Beans," *British Medical Journal* 281, no. 6234 (1980): 236–37.
13. Okinawa Centenarian Study, okicent.org/study.html.
14. H. Wiseman, J. D. O'Reilly, H. Adlercreutz, et al. "Isoflavone Phytoestrogens Consumed in Soy Decrease F2-Isoprostane Concentrations and Increase Resistance of Low-Density Lipoprotein to Oxidation in Humans," *American Journal of Clinical Nutrition* 72 (2000): 395–400.
15. Y. Seiichiro et al., "Soy, Isoflavones, and Breast Cancer Risk in Japan," *Journal of the National Cancer Institute* 95, no. 12 (2003): 906–13.
16. Allison Aubrey, "For Breast Cancer Survivors, Eating Soy Tied to a Longevity Boost," *NPR*, March 7, 2017.
17. Sally Fallon and Mary Enig, "Tragedy and Hype: Third International Soy Symposium," Weston Price Foundation, March 6, 2000.
18. L. Rizzi, I. Rosset, M. Roriz-Cruz, "Global Epidemiology of Dementia: Alzheimer's and Vascular Types," *BioMed Research International* 2014.
19. "What Adventists Mean to You," World Life Expectancy.
20. S. E. File et al., "Eating Soya Improves Human Memory," *Psychopharmacology (Berlin)* 157, no. 4 (2001): 430–36.
21. Josh Wingrove, "Tofu, other soy products linked to memory loss", *Globe and Mail*, July 7, 2008, updated May 2, 2018.
22. Wake Forest University Baptist Medical Center. "Soy Phytoestrogens May Block Estrogen Effects," *ScienceDaily*, January 16, 2006.

23. J. C. Vanegas et al., "Soy Food Intake and Treatment Outcomes of Women Undergoing Assisted Reproductive Technology," *Fertility and Sterility* 103, no. 3 (2015): 749–55.

24. L. Mínguez-Alarcón et al., "Male Soy Food Intake Was Not Associated with In Vitro Fertilization Outcomes Among Couples Attending a Fertility Center," *Andrology* 3, no. 4 (2015): 702–8.

25. J. M. Hamilton-Reeves et al., "Clinical Studies Show No Effects of Soy Protein or Isoflavones on Reproductive Hormones in Men: Results of a Meta-Analysis," *Fertility and Sterility* 94, no. 3 (2010): 997–1007.

26. M. Messina, G. Redmond, "Effects of Soy Protein and Soybean Isoflavones on Thyroid Function in Healthy Adults and Hypothyroid Patients: A Review of the Relevant Literature," *Thyroid* 16, no. 3 (2006): 249–58.

27. World Wildlife Fund, "Soy Facts."

28. Marygrace Taylor, "Is Soy Good or Bad for You? We Have the Science-Backed Answer," *Rodale's Organic Life*, May 17, 2017.

CHAPTER 17

1. International Agency for Research on Cancer, "IARC Monographs Evaluate Consumption of Red Meat and Processed Meat," World Health Organization, October 26, 2015.

2. Casey Dunlop, "Processed Meat and Cancer—What You Need to Know," Cancer Research UK, October 26, 2015.

3. "Higher Risk of Heart Disease, Diabetes from Eating Meat," web video, Harvard School of Public Health, 2010.

4. Sarah Boseley, "Processed Meats Rank Alongside Smoking as Cancer Causes—WHO," *Guardian*, October 26, 2015.

5. Harrison Wein, "Risk in Red Meat?," National Institutes of Health, March 26, 2012.

6. Alex Robinson, "The Ultimate Red Meat: Venison vs. Beef," *Outdoor Life*, May 1, 2013.

7. C. Daley et al., "A Review of Fatty Acid Profiles and Antioxidant Content in Grass-Fed and Grain-Fed Beef, *Nutrition Journal* 9 (2010): 10.

8. R. Sinha et al., "2-Amino-1-Methyl-6-Phenylimidazo[4,5-b]Pyridine, a Carcinogen in High-Temperature-Cooked Meat, and Breast Cancer Risk," *Journal of the National Cancer Institute* 92, no. 16 (2000): 1352–54.

9. C. P. Chiu, D. Y. Yang, B. H. Chen, "Formation of Heterocyclic Amines in Cooked Chicken Legs," *Journal of Food Protection* 61, no. 6 (1998): 712–19.

10. Jill Ettinger, "Chickens Fed Arsenic, Food and Water Contaminated," Organic Authority, March 9, 2011.

11. "The High Cost of Cheap Chicken," *Consumer Reports*.

12. "Milestone: 50 Percent of Fish Are Now Farmed," Live Science, September 8, 2009.

13. M. Chen et al., "Dairy Fat and Risk of Cardiovascular Disease in 3 Cohorts of US Adults," *American Journal of Clinical Nutrition* 104, no. 5 (2016): 1209–17.

14. B. Melnik, J. Swen, and G. Schmitz, "Over-Stimulation of Insulin/IGF-1 Signaling by Western Diet May Promote Diseases of Civilization: Lessons Learnt from Laron Syndrome," *Nutrition & Metabolism (London)* 8 (2011): 41.

15. M. Huncharek, J. Muscat, and B. Kupelnick, "Dairy Products, Dietary Calcium and Vitamin D Intake as Risk Factors for Prostate Cancer: A Meta-analysis of 26,769 Cases from 45 Observational Studies," *Nutrition and Cancer* 60, no. 4 (2008): 421–41.

16. D. M. Swallow, "Genetics of Lactase Persistence and Lactose Intolerance," *Annual Review of Genetics* 37, no. 1 (2003): 197–219.

17. B. Pribila et al., "Improved Lactose Digestion and Intolerance Among African-American Adolescent Girls Fed a Dairy-Rich Diet," *Journal of the American Dietetic Association* 100, no. 5 (2000): 524–28.

18. S. Mishkin, "Dairy Sensitivity, Lactose Malabsorption, and Elimination Diets in Inflammatory Bowel Disease," *American Journal of Clinical Nutrition* 65, no. 2 (1997): 564–67.

19. D. F. Hebeisen et al., "Increased Concentrations of Omega-3 Fatty Acids in Milk and Platelet Rich Plasma of Grass-Fed Cows," *International Journal for Vitamin and Nutrition Research* 63, no. 3 (1993): 229–33.

20. L. J. Schurgers et al., "Nutritional Intake of Vitamins K1 (Phylloquinone) and K2 (Menaquinone) in the Netherlands," *Journal of Nutritional & Environmental Medicine* 9, no. 2 (1999): 115–22.

21. S. Rautianen et al., "Dairy Consumption in Association with Weight Change and Risk of Becoming Overweight or Obese in Middle-Aged and Older Women: A Prospective Cohort Study," *American Journal of Clinical Nutrition* 103, no. 4 (2016): 979–88.

22. K. Aleisha Fetters, "5 Reasons to Start Eating Full-Fat Dairy, According to Science," *US News and World Report*, October 28, 2016.

23. "Top Trends in Prepared Foods 2017: Exploring Trends in Meat, Fish and Seafood; Pasta, Noodles and Rice; Prepared Meals; Savory Deli Food; Soup; and Meat Substitutes," Global Data, June 2017.

24. "Adventist Health Studies: Finding for AHS-2," Loma Linda University School of Public Health.

PART THREE: Gather

1. Markham Heid, "Feeling Lonely Is as Unhealthy as Smoking 15 Cigarettes a Day," *Prevention*, May 13, 2014.

2. For heart disease, see P. M. Eng, E. B. Rimm, G. Fitzmaurice, and I. Kawachi, "Social Ties and Change in Social Ties in Relation to Subsequent Total and Cause-Specific Mortality and Coronary Heart Disease Incidence in Men," *American Journal of Epidemiology* 155, no. 8 (2002): 700–9. For breast cancer, see "Kaiser Permanente Study Shows Women with More Social Connections Have Higher Breast Cancer Survival Rates," Kaiser Permanente, December 11, 2016.

CHAPTER 19

1. N. Christakis and J. Fowler, "The Spread of Obesity in a Large Social Network over 32 Years," *New England Journal of Medicine* 357 (2007): 370–79.

CHAPTER 20

1. Mary Brophy Marcus, "Feeling Lonely? So Are a Lot of Other People, Survey Finds," *CBS News*, October 12, 2016.

CHAPTER 21

1. Kimberly Warner, PhD, et al, "Oceana Reveals Mislabeling of America's Favorite Fish: Salmon," October 2015.

2. Hart Research Associates, "Key Findings from a Survey of Women Fast Food Workers," memorandum, October 5, 2016.

3. E. Helander et al., "Weight Gain over the Holidays in Three Countries," *New England Journal of Medicine* 375 (2016): 1200–2.

CHAPTER 22

1. "Stress and the Sensitive Gut," Harvard Health Publishing, August 2010.

2. Elizabeth Heubeck, "Boost Your Health with a Dose of Gratitude," WebMD, January 11, 2006.

3. Amy Morin, "7 Scientifically Proven Benefits of Gratitude That Will Motivate You to Give Thanks Year-Round," *Forbes*, November 24, 2014.

4. R. A. Emmons and M. E. McCullough, "Counting Blessings Versus Burdens: An Experimental Investigation of Gratitude and Subjective Well-Being in Daily Life," *Journal of Personality and Social Psychology* 84, no. 2 (2003): 377–89.

5. Mikaela Conley, "Thankfulness Linked to Positive Changes in Brain and Body," *ABC News*, November 23, 2011.

6. Rick Hamlin, "What Saying Grace Says About You," *Huffington Post*, March 3, 2011.

7. Lauren F. Winner, "Saying Grace: An Ode to an Old-Fashioned Ritual," *O, The Oprah Magazine*, August 2004.

CHAPTER 23

1. Marisa Tsai, "Eight Countries Taking Action Against Harmful Food Marketing," Foodtank, 2016.

2. Sam Rourke, "Failing to Make the Grade: How the School Lunch System Is Falling Short of Its Purpose," *Artifacts*, September 2012.

3. Rachael Rettner, "Family Meals Help Kids Eat More Fruit & Veggies," LiveScience, December 19, 2012.

4. Laurie Tarkin, "Benefits of the Dinner Table Ritual," *New York Times*, May 3, 2005.

CHAPTER 24

1. Holly Bailey, "Martin Luther King's Unfinished Legacy Is Visible in Desperately Poor Selma," *Yahoo News*, April 2, 2018.

2. "Child Poverty," National Center for Children in Poverty, January 2018.

3. Hannah Richardson, "Child Poverty: Pale and Hungry Pupils 'Fill Pockets with School Food,'" *BBC News*, April 2, 2018.

4. H. C. Storey et al., "A Randomized Controlled Trial of the Effect of School Food and Dining Room Modifications on Classroom Behaviour in Secondary School Children," *European Journal of Clinical Nutrition* 65, no. 1 (2011): 32–38.

5. Shula Edelkind, ed., *The Feingold Bluebook* (Feingold Association of the United States, 2003).

6. Ibid.

7. Ibid.

8. Ed Bruske, "New Study Says School Food May Make Kids Fatter," *Grist*, March 15, 2010.

9. Food and Nutrition Service, *White Paper: USDA Foods in the National School Lunch Program* (USDA, February 2016).

10. "Shifts Needed to Align with Healthy Eating Patterns," chapter 2 in *Dietary Guidelines 2015–2020*, Health.gov.
11. "School Lunch Standards in Europe," European Food Information Council, May 9, 2012.
12. Jenny Anderson, "A Typical Week of School Lunch for Kids in Paris vs. New York," *Quartz*, October 9, 2015.
13. Pauliina Siniauer, "The EU Is Starting a Massive Program to Improve School Lunch Across Europe," *Saveur*, June 26, 2017.
14. "New Data Find Climate-Friendly, Healthy Meals Within Reach for Public Schools," Friends of the Earth, February 15, 2017.
15. Soumya Karlamangla, "L.A. County Launches Campaign Against Childhood Obesity," *Los Angeles Times*, October 11, 2015.
16. S. Whaley et al., *Achieving Healthy Weight Early in Life* (Connecting the Dots, 2014).
17. Lisa Lagasse MHS and Roni Neff, PhD, "Balanced Menus: A Pilot Evaluation of Implementation in Four San Francisco Bay Area Hospitals," Johns Hopkins School of Public Health, April 12, 2010.
18. Katherine Martinko, "What Happens When a School District Reduces Meat and Dairy Consumption?," Treehugger, February 27, 2017.
19. "Historic Meat Reduction Project Launched in Bahia, Brazil," Humane Society International, March 21, 2018.

CHAPTER 25

1. Allison Kopicki, "Strong Support for Labeling Genetically Modified Foods," *New York Times*, July 27, 2013.
2. Dan Flynn, "Early Editorials Against GMO Labeling Initiative in Washington State," Food Safety News, September 6, 2013.
3. AgriSystems International, "Whole Foods Market Announces Mandatory Labeling of GMO Foods," *AgriSystems Newsletter*, May 10, 2013.
4. "Five Major Food Companies Announce GMO Labeling. What Should We Expect at the Grocery Store?," GMO Inside, March 28, 2016.
5. "Verification FAQs," Non-GMO Project.
6. Dean Chase, "The Death of the 'Big Food' Era Is Imminent After the Industry's Biggest Lobbying Group Crumbles," *Quartz*, March 5, 2018.
7. John Fagan, "GMO Myths and Truths Report," Earth Open Source, May 19, 2014.
8. Michael Hansen, "Reasons for Labeling of Genetically Engineered Foods," *Consumer Reports*, March 19, 2012.
9. Anne Steele, "Bayer's Deal For Monsanto," *Wall Street Journal*, September 14, 2016.
10. Douglas Main, "Glyphosate Now the Most-Used Agricultural Chemical Ever," *Newsweek*, May 11, 2018.
11. Doug Gurian-Sherman, "The Battle Over the Most Used Herbicide Heats Up as Nearly 100 Scientists Weigh In," Civil Eats, March 10, 2016.
12. C. Benbrook, "Trends in Glyphosate Herbicide Use in the United States and Globally," *Environmental Sciences Europe* 28, no. 3 (2016).
13. International Agency for Research on Cancer, "IARC Monographs Volume 112: Evaluation of Five Organophosphate Insecticides and Herbicides," World Health Organization, March 20, 2015.

14. Cheryl Hogue, "California to List Glyphosate as a Carcinogen," *Chemical and Engineering News*, July 3, 2017.

15. J. D. Heyes, "Monsanto Roundup Harms Human Endocrine System at Levels Allowed in Drinking Water, Study Shows," Global Research, April 5, 2015.

16. T. Vered and G. Gad, "New Insights into the Shikimate and Aromatic Amino Acids Biosynthesis Pathways in Plants," *Molecular Plant* 3, no. 6 (2010): 956–72; "Glyphosate Formulations and Their Use for the Inhibition of 5-Enolpyruvylshikimate-3-Phosphate Synthase," Google Patents, August 30, 2002; "2017 Could Be a Terrible Tipping Point for Antibiotic Resistance," Food Revolution Network, January 12, 2017.

CHAPTER 26

1. Roger Cohen, "The Organic Fable," *New York Times*, September 6, 2012.

2. "Farm Worker Health Concerns," National Farm Worker Ministry, April 21, 2009.

3. Lorraine Chow, "California Widow Sues Monsanto Alleging Roundup Caused Her Husband's Cancer," BuzzFlash, March 11, 2016.

4. John Reganold, "Can We Feed 10 Billion People on Organic Farming Alone?," *Guardian*, August 14, 2016.

5. E. Cassidy et al., "Redefining Agricultural Yields: From Tonnes to People Nourished per Hectare," *Environmental Research Letter* 8 (2013): 034015.

6. Mark Gold, *The Global Benefits of Eating Less Meat* (New Delhi: Navodanya in collaboration with Compassion in World Farming Trust, 2004).

7. United Nations Conference on Trade and Development, *Wake Up Before It Is Too Late* (Geneva: United Nations, 2013).

8. Maria Trimarchi, "What Is Organic Certification?," HowStuffWorks, January 16, 2008.

9. For lymphoma, see, D. Luo et al., "Exposure to Organochlorine Pesticides and Non-Hodgkin Lymphoma: A Meta-analysis of Observational Studies," *Scientific Reports* 6 (2016): 25768. For brain cancer, see "Heavy Pesticide Exposure Linked to Brain Cancer," *Reuters*, June 12, 2007. For breast cancer, see Lindsay Konkel, "DDT Linked to Fourfold Increase in Breast Cancer Risk," *National Geographic*, June 16, 2005. For ovarian, prostate, stomach, and testicular cancers, see Lorelei Walker and Nancy Hepp, "Cancer Research and Resources," Collaborative on Health and the Environment, September 2016. For liver cancer, see Sara Miller, "Exposure to Pesticides May Increase Risk of Liver Cancer," LiveScience, April 11, 2017.

10. University of Montreal, "Pesticide Exposure May Contribute to ADHD, Study Finds," *ScienceDaily*, May 17, 2010.

11. E. Roberts et al., "Maternal Residence near Agricultural Pesticide Applications and Autism Spectrum Disorders Among Children in the California Central Valley," *Environmental Health Perspectives* 115, no. 10 (2007): 1482–89.

12. L. Oates et al., "Reduction in Urinary Organophosphate Pesticide Metabolites in Adults After a Week-Long Organic Diet," *Environmental Research* 132 (2014): 105–11.

13. "EWG's Shopper's Guide to Pesticides in Produce," Environmental Working Group, 2018.

14. Walter Krol, "Removal of Trace Pesticide Residues from Produce," June 28, 2012, Connecticut Agricultural Experiment Station.

15. Janet Pelley, "Baking Soda Washes Pesticides from Apples," *Chemical and Engineering News*, November 3, 2017.

CHAPTER 27

1. Tim DeChant, "The Great (Big) American Lawn," Per Square Mile, April 8, 2011.
2. Beth Huxta, "The Dark Side of Lawns," Rodale Organic Life, November 26, 2010.
3. "Edible Gardens Versus Lawns," Urban Plantations, July 2015.

CHAPTER 28

1. International Energy Agency, *Energy Technology Perspectives 2008: Scenarios and Strategies Until 2050* (Paris: OECD/IEA, 2008).
2. E. Stehfest et al., "Climate Benefits of Changing Diet," *Climatic Change* 95, no. 1-2 (2009): 83–102.
3. "Spending on Health: A Global Overview," World Health Organization, April 17, 2012.
4. "On Average, How Many Pounds of Corn Make One Pound of Beef?," Cooperative Extension System, October 7, 2008.
5. Jess McNally, "Can Vegetarianism Save the World?," *Stanford Magazine*, January 2010.
6. John Lawrence and Shane Ellis, "Monthly Returns from Cattle Feeding," *Iowa State University Extension and Outreach*, September 2008.
7. Rosie Nold, "How Much Meat Can You Expect from a Fed Steer?," *iGrow*, January 2, 2013.
8. P. Thornton et al., "Livestock and Climate Change," *Livestock Exchange*, International Livestock Research Institute issue brief, November 2011.
9. Cornell University, "U.S. Could Feed 800 Million People with Grain that Livestock Eat, Cornell Ecologist Advises Animal Scientists," *Cornell Chronicle*, August 7, 1997.
10. For methane, see "The Climate Impacts of Methane Emissions," Environmental Defense Fund, April 2012. For nitrous oxide, see "Nitrous Oxide," Scottish Environment Protection Agency.
11. "Main Sources of Nitrous Oxide Emissions," What's Your Impact.
12. Food and Agriculture Organization of the United Nations, "Livestock a Major Threat to Environment," FAO Newsroom, November 2006.
13. P. Scarborough et al., "Dietary Greenhouse Gas Emissions of Meat-Eaters, Fish-Eaters, Vegetarians and Vegans in the UK," *Climatic Change* 125, no. 2 (2014): 179.
14. Laura Parker, "What You Need to Know About the World's Water Wars," *National Geographic*, July 14, 2016.
15. Nathan Halverson, "9 Sobering Facts About California's Groundwater Problem," *Reveal*, June 25, 2015.
16. Eric Holthaus, "The Thirsty West: 10 Percent of California's Water Goes to Almond Farming," *Slate*, May 14, 2014.
17. Dennis Silverman, *Beef in California Agriculture*, UCI Sites, Office of Information Technology, University of California, Irvine.
18. "USGS Estimates Vast Amounts of Water Used in California," *Desert Sun*, August 21, 2014.
19. Michael Jacobson and the Center for Science in the Public Interest, *Six Arguments for a Greener Diet* (Washington, DC: Center for Science in the Public Interest, 2006), 90.
20. "Thirsty Food," *National Geographic*.
21. "Soil Quality," Grace Communications Foundation.
22. Preston Sullivan, "Soil Management," National Sustainable Agriculture Information Service, May 2004.

23. Chris Arsenault, "Only 60 Years of Farming Left If Soil Degradation Continues," *Scientific American*.

24. "9 Interesting Facts About the Sahara Desert," Conservation Institute, June 12, 2013.

25. "7 Important Facts About the Sahara Desert," *Asia-Pacific Economics Blog*, March 26, 2015.

26. Ronnie Cummins and Regeneration International.

27. "Higher Quality Food Through Regenerated Soils & Reduced Inputs," Soils for Life, September 2012.

CHAPTER 29

1. "Barren, Cramped Battery Cages," Humane Society of the United States.

2. "Debeaking Birds Has Got to Stop," *Poultry Press* 17, no. 3 (2007).

3. Yuzhi Li, "Research Reaffirms the Necessity of Tail Docking for Pigs," National Hog Farmer, December 30, 2016.

4. "Crammed into Gestation Crates," Humane Society of the United States.

5. "Animal Rights Group Releases Video from Veal Farm," *Columbus Dispatch*, August 30, 2010.

6. Tom Regan, *Empty Cages: Facing the Challenge of Animal Rights* (Lanham: Rowan & Littlefield, 2005), 90.

7. R. F. Wideman et al., "Pulmonary Arterial Hypertension (Ascites Syndrome) in Broilers: A Review," *Poultry Science* 92 (2013): 64–83.

8. Katherine Hessler and Tanith Balaban, "Agricultural Animals and the Law," *GPSOLO*, 26, no. 5 (July/August 2009).

9. American Society for the Prevention of Cruelty to Animals, "ASPCA Research Shows Americans Overwhelmingly Support Investigations to Expose Animal Abuse on Industrial Farms," press release, February 17, 2012.

10. Cody Carlson, "The Ag Gag Laws: Hiding Factory Farm Abuses from Public Scrutiny," *Atlantic*, March 20, 2012.

11. Rachel Tepper, "George Steinmetz, National Geographic Photographer, Arrested Taking Photos of Kansas Feedlot," *Huffington Post*, July 11, 2013.

12. U.S. Department of Agriculture, "USDA Announces Additional Food Safety Requirements, New Inspection System for Poultry Products," Release No. 0163.14, July 31, 2014.

13. "Whistleblower Profile: Jim Schrier," Food Integrity Campaign.

14. "Help a Meat Inspector Punished for Reporting Inhumane Conditions!," Change.org, December 3, 2013.

15. Victoria Kim, "Chino Slaughterhouse to Pay $300,000 in Settlement," *Los Angeles Times*, November 16, 2012; Cindy Galli and Brian Ross, "Plant Closed by USDA Supplied Beef for In-N-Out Burger," *ABC News*, August 21, 2012.

16. For the U.S., see Bryan Walsh. "New Report Says FDA Allowed 'High Risk' Antibiotics to Be Used on Farm Animals," *Time*, January 28, 2014. For Europe, see "Massive Overuse of Farm Antibiotics Continues in Europe," Compassion in World Farming, October 17, 2016.

17. Environmental Working Group, "Superbugs Invade American Supermarkets," press release, 2013.

18. "UK Supermarkets 'Contributing to Antibiotics Crisis,'" *The Week*, November 14, 2017.

19. "Antibiotic-Resistant Infections Cost the U.S. Healthcare System in Excess of $20 Billion Annually," CISION PR Newswire, October 12, 2009.

20. For antiobiotic resistance statistics, see Centers for Disease Control, "Antibiotic Resistance Threats in the United States," 2013. For terrorism statistics, see "Number of Casualties Due to Terrorism Worldwide Between 2006 and 2016," Statista, July 2017.

21. Candy Sagon, "Antibiotic-Free Meat: What the Label Isn't Telling You," *AARP Healthy Living Blog*, July 12, 2012.

CHAPTER 30

1. For world data, see "World Hunger Falls to Under 800 Million, Eradication Is Next Goal," Food and Agricultural Organization of the United Nations, May 27, 2015. For American data, see "Poverty and Hunger Fact Sheet," Feeding America, September 2017. For Canadian data, see "Household Food Insecurity in Canada," PROOF Food Insecurity Policy Research, February 22, 2018. For European data, see R. Loopstra et al., "Rising Food Insecurity in Europe," *Lancet* 385, no. 9982 (2015): 2041.

2. L. Pan et al., "Food Insecurity Is Associated with Obesity Among US Adults in 12 States," *Journal of the Academy of Nutrition and Dietetics* 112, no. 9 (2012): 1403–9.

3. F. Heidery et al., "Poverty as a Risk Factor in Human Cancers," *Iranian Journal of Public Health* 42, no. 3 (2013): 341–43.

4. "UNNATURAL CAUSES: Is Inequality Making Us Sick?," Episode One, "In Sickness and In Wealth," California Newsreel with Vital Pictures, Inc., 2008.

5. Eric Painin, "How Billions in Tax Dollars Subsidize the Junk Food Industry," *Fiscal Times*, July 25, 2012.

6. Ibid.

7. David Dayen, "The Farm Bill Still Gives Wads of Cash to Agribusiness. It's Just Sneakier About It," *New Republic*, February 4, 2014.

8. Painin, "Tax Dollars Subsidize the Junk Food Industry."

9. Joe Leech, "High Fructose Corn Syrup: Just Like Sugar, or Worse?," Healthline Authority Nutrition, January 8, 2015.

10. K. Siegal et al., "Association of Higher Consumption of Foods Derived from Subsidized Commodities with Adverse Cardiometabolic Risk Among US Adults," *JAMA Internal Medicine* 176, no. 8 (2016): 1124–32.

11. Stefan Tangermann, "Farming Support: The Truth Behind the Numbers," *OECD Observer*, May 2004.

12. Daniel Sumner, "Agricultural Subsidy Programs," Concise Encyclopedia of Economics, 2008.

13. Chris Arsenault, "Family Farms Produce 80 Percent of World's Food, Speculators Seek Land," *Reuters*, October 16, 2014.

14. A. N. Rao, ed. *Food, Agriculture and Education: Science and Technology Education and Future Human Needs* (Oxford: Pergamon Press, 2013), 222.

15. "Women Do 80% of Farm Work, Own Only 13% Land: Oxfam," *Hindu Business Line*, October 2016.

16. "Africa: Women Are Behind 80 Percent of Continent's Food Production," AllAfrica, October 31, 2009.

17. "The Female Face of Farming," Food and Agriculture Organization of the United Nations.

18. "Investing in Small-Scale Farmers Can Help Lift Over 1 Billion People out of Poverty— UN Report," *United Nations News*, June 4, 2013.

19. Sarah Sugar, "Oases in the Urban 'Food Desert'?," *Yale Environment Review*, March 26, 2015.

20. "America's First Sustainable Urban Agrihood," Michigan Urban Farming Initiative, November 2016.

21. Amanda Hurley, "Detroit Is Designing a City with Space for Everyone, Including Goats," Next City, June 6, 2016.

22. Jessica Leigh Hester, "Growing Pains for Detroit's Urban Farms," *CityLab*, August 30, 2016.

Index

JOIN THE FOOD REVOLUTION

If you've been touched by the message of this book, please join us in standing for healthy, ethical, sustainable food for all. You'll gain access to potent resources, a robust global community, and cutting-edge insights to support and deepen your Food Revolution journey.

Find out more at 31dayfoodrevolution.com/join.

ABOUT THE AUTHOR

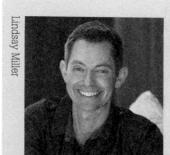

Lindsay Miller

Ocean Robbins is cofounder and CEO of Food Revolution Network—a global community of more than 500,000 members dedicated to healthy, ethical, sustainable food for everyone who eats.

Ocean has hosted and organized online summits and classes that have reached more than a million participants from 190 nations. He's served as an adjunct professor in Chapman University's Peace Studies department and is founder of Youth for Environmental Sanity (YES!), a global nonprofit organization that he launched at age 16 and directed for 20 years.

Ocean has led live in-person events and public presentations for hundreds of thousands of people from more than 65 nations. He is a recipient of many awards, including the National Voting Rights Museum and Institute's Freedom's Flame Award, the Harmon Wilkinson Award for distinguished contribution to the humanities and social sciences, and the national Jefferson Award for Outstanding Public Service. He lives with his wife and identical twin sons in California.

www.31dayfoodrevolution.com

HAY HOUSE
Look within

Join the conversation about latest products,
events, exclusive offers and more.

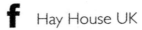   Hay House UK

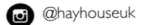   @HayHouseUK

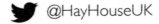   @hayhouseuk

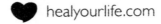   healyourlife.com

We'd love to hear from you!